The
Cigarette
Papers

The Cigarette Papers

Stanton A. Glantz
John Slade
Lisa A. Bero
Peter Hanauer
Deborah E. Barnes

Foreword by C. Everett Koop,
former Surgeon General

UNIVERSITY OF CALIFORNIA PRESS
Berkeley • Los Angeles • London

The electronic version of *The Cigarette Papers* and 8,000 pages of source documents are available on the World Wide Web at the University of California, San Francisco, Digital Library: http://www.library.ucsf.edu/tobacco

Some material in chapters 1, 3, 7, 8, and 10 formed the basis for a series of articles published in *JAMA* (vol. 274) in 1995: S. A. Glantz et al., Looking through a Keyhole at the Tobacco Industry: The Brown and Williamson Documents (pp. 219–224); J. Slade et al., Nicotine and Addiction: The Brown and Williamson Documents (pp. 225–233); P. Hanauer et al., Lawyer Control of Internal Scientific Research to Avoid Products Liability Lawsuits: The Brown and Williamson Documents (pp. 234–240); L. Bero et al., Lawyer Control of the Tobacco Industry's External Research Program: The Brown and Williamson Documents (pp. 241–247); D. E. Barnes et al., Environmental Tobacco Smoke: The Brown and Williamson Documents (pp. 248–253). Figure 11.2 is from S. A. Glantz, Actual Causes of Death in the United States (letter), *JAMA* 1994 (vol. 271, p. 660). This material is copyrighted in the year of publication by the American Medical Association and used with permission of the AMA.

University of California Press
Berkeley and Los Angeles, California

University of California Press, Ltd.
London, England

Library of Congress Cataloging-in-Publication Data

The cigarette papers / Stanton A. Glantz . . . [et al.].
    p. cm.
    Includes bibliographical references and index.
    ISBN 0-520-20572-3 (alk. paper)
    1. Tobacco industry—United States.   2. Tobacco—Health aspects.
   3. Smoking—Health aspects.   I. Glantz, Stanton A.
HD9135.C5   1996
362.29'6—dc20   95-44169
                                      CIP

Printed in the United States of America
9 8 7 6 5 4 3 2 1

Contents

Illustrations

FIGURES

Foreword

It was my privilege to serve as surgeon general of the United States Public Health Service from 1981 to 1989. The issue of smoking was on my desk when I arrived; it was on my desk when I left. As I learned more and more about smoking during my tenure as surgeon general, I was increasingly disturbed by the way the tobacco industry treated the American and world public. The analysis of the previously secret papers from a major tobacco company presented in this book demonstrates that the tobacco industry was even more cynical than even I had previously dared believe.

The surgeon general is perhaps best known for the Surgeon General's reports on smoking and health. During my tenure, eight reports on smoking and health were submitted to Congress and the American public, including the 1988 report, *Nicotine Addiction,* which concluded that nicotine is an addictive drug similar to heroin and cocaine. At the time—as it does today—the tobacco industry vigorously attacked the report (and me) for going beyond the scientific evidence. But now this book confirms that scientists and executives from Brown and Williamson and British American Tobacco routinely appreciated the addictive nature of nicotine a quarter century earlier, in the early 1960s.

All the Surgeon General's reports are modeled on the original 1964 report, *Smoking and Health: A Report to the Surgeon General,* which was made by an advisory committee appointed by the surgeon general to investigate whether or not smoking causes disease. This initial report was mild in its condemnation of smoking, finding primarily that smoking causes lung cancer in men. It did not identify tobacco as an addictive substance—just habituating. These conclusions were much weaker than those the tobacco industry's own scientists were making at the time. They considered nicotine an addictive drug. This information—as well as a wealth of other important information the tobacco industry possessed—was simply not made available to the Surgeon General's Advisory Committee and the public.

One can speculate, with enormous regret, how different that 1964 Surgeon General's report would have been had the tobacco companies shared their research with the Surgeon General's Advisory Committee. What would have been the history of the tobacco issue in the United States—and the world—if that report had had the benefit of all of the information available on tobacco and held privy to the inner circles of the cigarette manufacturing companies? The contrast of public and private statements from the tobacco industry reveals their deceit.

During my years as surgeon general and since, I have often wondered how many people died as a result of the fact that the medical and public health professions were misled by the tobacco industry. Now we can see in retrospect, as the documents discussed in this book reveal, that the tobacco industry was demoralized and in disarray in the mid-1960s, but the public voluntary health agencies and others did not take the kind of decisive action against the industry that some inside the industry expected and feared.

In the course of my own annual press conferences on the release of the Surgeon General's reports to Congress, I frequently spoke of the sleazy behavior of the tobacco industry in its attempts to discredit legitimate science as part of its overall effort to create controversy and doubt. Well-funded tobacco interests attacked (and continue to attack) not only the surgeon general, but also the Environmental Protection Agency, the Food and Drug Administration, the Occupational Safety and Health Administration, and individual scientists who are working to end the scourge of tobacco. This book reveals these campaigns from the inside.

But, although the tobacco companies possess enormous clout with Congress and almost inexhaustible funds for advertising, promotion, and propaganda, the public knows about the deleterious effects of smoking, and most smokers would like to quit—a difficult task because they are addicted. Even smokers do not believe what they hear from the tobacco industry. Smokers and nonsmokers alike should feel misled by the tobacco companies and their deceptive practices.

This book is a vital weapon in the battle against tobacco. I do not believe that anyone who reads it can remain passive in the struggle against tobacco. We all need to raise our voices to clear the air for a healthier America.

C. Everett Koop, M.D., Sc.D.
Surgeon General USPHS 1981–1989

Preface

Tobacco is the leading preventable cause of death: cigarettes and other tobacco products kill 420,000 American smokers and 53,000 non-smokers every year. This toll exceeds the deaths resulting from alcohol abuse, AIDS, traffic accidents, homicides, and suicides *combined*. Nevertheless, the tobacco industry continues to promote and sell its products, unhampered by any meaningful government regulation except for mostly local restrictions designed to protect nonsmokers from the toxins in secondhand tobacco smoke. In fact, the tobacco industry is unique among American and worldwide industries in its ability to forestall effective government regulation and to hold effective public health action at bay while marketing its lethal products. The industry manages this, despite the overwhelming scientific evidence that tobacco products kill, through a combination of skilled legal, political, and public relations strategies designed to confuse the public and to allow it to avoid having to take responsibility for the death and disease it inflicts.

Many public health workers and tobacco control professionals—including the authors of this book—have long suspected that the tobacco industry has known that smoking is dangerous and addictive. But proof to substantiate this suspicion has not been available to the medical and scientific communities, much less to the public. This situation changed dramatically in mid-1994, when an unsolicited box containing several thousand pages of documents from the Brown and Williamson Tobacco Corporation (B&W) arrived at Professor Stanton Glantz's office at the University of California, San Francisco. Like the Pentagon Papers, which revealed private doubts about the Vietnam War inside the government a generation ago, these documents, combined with other material obtained from Brown and Williamson by the House of Representatives Subcommittee on Health and the Environment, and some private papers from a former research director at B&W's parent, British American Tobacco (BAT), provide a candid, private view of the tobacco industry's thoughts and actions over the past thirty years. This view differs dramatically from the public image presented by the industry during that time.

Early in this period B&W and BAT frankly recognized that nicotine is an addictive drug and that people smoke to maintain a target level of nicotine in their bodies. The companies also recognized that smoking causes a variety of diseases, and they actively worked to identify and remove the specific toxins in tobacco smoke that cause these diseases. This scientific work was undertaken many years before the mainstream scientific community had a similar understanding of these issues. Nevertheless, in the mid-1960s, when the US Surgeon General's Advisory Committee was preparing the first Surgeon General's report on smoking, B&W and BAT withheld this important information, even though the Surgeon General's Advisory Committee had requested that the tobacco industry voluntarily provide the relevant results of its research for the committee's deliberations. Later, when it became clear that a "safe" cigarette could not be developed, tobacco industry lawyers took increasing control of scientific research as they tried to insulate the companies against products liability lawsuits. In the process, concerns about legal matters and the public's perceptions of the dangers of smoking and the tobacco industry increasingly took precedence over public health.

This book represents our complete analysis of the Brown and Williamson documents. On July 19, 1995, we published a series of five articles, based on these materials, in the *Journal of the American Medical Association*. The decision to publish these papers represented a courageous stance on the part of the editors of *JAMA* and the leadership of the American Medical Association. We are grateful to the editors of *JAMA,* in particular Drummond Rennie, for providing the first forum for our work.

We are likewise grateful to the National Cancer Institute (Grant CA-61021) and the University of California Tobacco Related Diseases Research Program (Grants 2KT-0072 and 4RT-0035) for supporting this work. We also thank Phil Lollar of UCSF and Robin Barthalow and Tim Nolan of Lieff, Cabraser and Heimann, who provided assistance in indexing the documents. Adriana Marchione of UCSF was invaluable in final manuscript preparation, particularly in helping us track down all those irritating last-minute details. We thank Karen Butter, Nancy Zinn, Valerie Wheat, and Florie Berger of the UCSF Library and Center for Knowledge Management for being good-natured when B&W tried to have the documents removed from the UCSF archive, particularly when B&W had private investigators stake out the library. Henry and Edith Everett provided funds to help the library put the documents on the Internet, and Jane Dystel tried to find a publisher. Naomi Schneider served as our sponsoring editor at UC Press, Dorothy Conway did a superlative job of editing the final manuscript, and Bill Hoffman provided a thoughtful legal review. Joseph Cowan and Cynthia Lynch of the UCSF legal office provided valuable advice on how to navigate the legal shoals that surround these documents, and Christopher Patti of the UC Office of the General Counsel did a fine job of protecting our academic and intellectual freedom to pursue this project, in the face of B&W's efforts to keep the documents from public scrutiny.

Finally, in an era in which public institutions are increasingly held in disdain, we would like to thank the University of California for providing an environment committed to academic freedom and the public interest. It would have been simpler—and cheaper—for the university simply to walk away from this project. After all, the history of the tobacco issue is one in which many large institutions have followed the path of least resistance and failed to confront the issues raised in these documents. No administrator or other official ever told us to stop. Quite the contrary, we were encouraged and protected in our work. This behavior is what makes the University of California a great public institution.

Most of all, we owe thanks to Frieda Glantz, who tolerated the authors' tiptoeing through her room at all hours to get to the computer in the study. No teenager should have to make such a sacrifice.

These documents provide an opportunity to see firsthand how the brown plague of tobacco has been allowed to flourish and to spread. Although the papers are sometimes technical, we hope that readers will find them as eye-opening as we have. Perhaps this understanding will finally lead the public and public policy makers to deal with the tobacco industry in a manner appropriate to the amount of death and suffering it knowingly creates.

San Francisco
October 1995

CHAPTER 1

Looking through a Keyhole at the Tobacco Industry

[The documents] may be evidence supporting a "whistle-blower's" claim that the tobacco company concealed from its customers and the American public the truth regarding the health hazards of tobacco products.

> *Federal Judge Harold Greene*
> *[Maddox v Williams 855 Fed. Supp.*
> *406, at 414, 415 (D.D.C. 1994)]*

INTRODUCTION

Tobacco has been controversial at least since its introduction into Europe shortly after Columbus reported that North American natives used its dried leaves for pleasure (1, 2). The first medical report of tobacco's ill effects dates to 1665, when Samuel Pepys witnessed a Royal Society experiment in which a cat quickly expired when fed "a drop of distilled oil of tobacco." In 1791 the London physician John Hill reported cases in which use of snuff caused nasal cancers. Not until the late 1940s, however, did the modern scientific case that tobacco causes disease begin to accumulate rapidly. Epidemiological and experimental evidence that smoking causes cancer led to the "cancer scares" in the 1950s and, ultimately, to the 1964 Surgeon General's report on smoking and health, which concluded that smoking causes lung cancer (3). By responding to these challenges from the scientific community with aggressive legal, public relations, and political strategies, the tobacco industry has been largely successful in protecting its profits in spite of overwhelming scientific and medical evidence that tobacco products kill and disable hundreds of thousands of smokers and nonsmokers every year (1, 4).

What did the tobacco industry actually know about the addictive nature of nicotine and the dangers of smoking? How did the industry develop its successful legal, public relations, and political programs? Until now, the public's understanding of these questions has been based largely on observation of the industry's behavior and suppositions by a few journalists and public health professionals. This situation changed abruptly in mid-1994, when several thousand pages of internal documents from the Brown and Williamson Tobacco Corporation (B&W) and its parent, BAT Industries (formerly British American Tobacco) of the United Kingdom, became public. These documents reveal that the tobacco industry's public position on smoking and health has diverged dramatically not only from the generally accepted position of the scientific community but also from the results of its own internal research (see table 1.1, p. 15). While even these documents do not provide a complete picture, they offer a candid look at the tobacco industry's internal workings during the smoking and health "controversy" during the last half of the twentieth century.

BAT is the second-largest private cigarette manufacturer in the world. In 1992 the company sold 578 billion cigarettes (5), 10.7 percent of the total world output and more than were consumed in the entire US market that year (6). Its wholly owned US subsidiary, B&W, is now the third-largest cigarette maker in this country. Its US sales increased from about 10 percent of the market during the 1960s to about 18 percent in the 1970s, then fell back to about 10 percent in the 1980s (7). In 1994 it had an 18 percent share of the $48 billion US market, including the domestic cigarette business of American Brands, which B&W purchased in 1995 (8). B&W's domestic brands (before buying American Brands) include Kool, Viceroy, Raleigh, Barclay, Belair, Capri, Fact, and Richland, as well as GPC generic cigarettes.

The tobacco industry has used three primary arguments to prevent government regulation of its products and to defend itself in products liability lawsuits. First, tobacco companies have consistently claimed that there is no conclusive proof that smoking causes diseases such as cancer and heart disease. Second, tobacco companies have claimed that smoking is not addictive and that anyone who smokes makes a free choice to do so. And, finally, tobacco companies have claimed that they are committed to determining the scientific truth about the health effects of tobacco, both by conducting internal research and by funding external research.

These arguments have been essential to the industry's success in claiming that its products should not be subject to further government regulation and that it should not be held legally responsible for the health effects of its products. By refusing to admit that tobacco is addictive and that it causes disease, the tobacco industry has been able (so far) to resist efforts to regulate its products. In addition, the industry has been able to argue that cigarette smoking is a matter of "individual choice," thereby essentially blaming its customers for the diseases they contract by using tobacco products. Finally, the industry's stated willingness to support health-related research has added credibility to its claim that the health effects of smoking have not been scientifically proven, thus helping to allay public fears about its products.

This book analyzes internal documents from the files of Brown and Williamson—documents that were delivered to us, as well as other related documents that have been released to the public during the past year. The documents consist primarily of internal memoranda, letters, and research reports related to B&W and BAT. Many of them are marked "confidential" or "attorney work product," suggesting that the authors never expected them to be released outside the corporation, not even for legal proceedings. These documents demonstrate that the tobacco industry in general, and Brown and Williamson in particular, has engaged in deception of the public for at least thirty years. They show that other cigarette manufacturers participated in some of these activities. The documents are listed at the back of the book under the heading "List of Available Documents" and are cited in the text in curly braces (e.g., {1234.56}). Copies of the actual documents are deposited in the Archives and Special Collections Department of the Library at the University of California, San Francisco, where they are available to the public. They are also available over the Internet at World Wide Web address http://www.library.ucsf.edu/tobacco. The library also has a CD-ROM version of the Documents for sale.

In the documents nicotine is routinely seen as addicting and is always treated as the pharmacologically active agent in tobacco. There is no question that B&W and BAT regarded nicotine's pharmacological (drug) effects as key to the intended smoking experience. The documents also demonstrate that the tobacco industry's professed public-spirited approach to pursuing the truth about smoking and health has been a sham. Its purported willingness to engage in and disseminate health-related research was, in reality, always subservient to commercial and litigation considerations. Initially, the companies' researchers tried to discover the toxic elements in cigarette smoke so that a "safe" cigarette, which would deliver nicotine without also delivering the toxic substances, could be developed. When that objective proved to be unattainable, largely because of the number of toxins involved, decisions about health-related research passed almost exclusively to lawyers. The documents show that lawyers from B&W and other tobacco companies played a central role in research decisions, both within B&W and BAT and also in industry-sponsored research organizations.

The principal aim of this lawyer-controlled research effort was not to improve existing scientific or public understanding of the effects of smoking on health but, rather, to minimize the industry's exposure to litigation liability and additional government regulation. Where the goals of determining and disseminating the truth conflicted with the goal of minimizing B&W's liability, the latter consistently won out. In particular, even after B&W's research had shown that cigarettes cause disease and are addictive, under its lawyers' direction B&W sought to avoid generating any new results reconfirming that smoking causes disease or that nicotine is addictive. B&W sought to avoid affiliation with, or even knowledge of, such research results, for fear they could be used to show that B&W believed that smoking causes disease or that nicotine is addictive. B&W also sought to prevent the dissemination or disclosure of such results, either in court or in any public forum—apparently to the point of removing some relevant documents from its files and shipping them offshore.

Many of the documents are correspondence among company lawyers. In addition to providing insight into B&W and BAT's legal thinking, the lawyers effectively serve as candid witnesses for what the company actually believed at any particular time about disease causation and addiction. The lawyers appear to have accepted the causation and addiction hypotheses about smoking. The 1970s–1980s documents from lawyers specifying what could and could not be claimed in company public relations and advertising show that some lawyers regarded those hypotheses as so well established that they could not be denied directly without risking liability.

The documents show that by the 1960s the tobacco industry in general, and B&W and BAT in particular, had proven in its own laboratories that cigarette tar causes cancer in animals. In addition, by the early 1960s BAT's scientists (and B&W's lawyers) were acting on the assumption that nicotine is addictive. BAT responded by secretly attempting to create a "safe" cigarette that would minimize dangerous elements in the smoke while still delivering nicotine. Publicly, however, it maintained that cigarettes are neither harmful nor addictive. The tobacco industry's primary goal has been to continue as a large commercial enterprise by protecting itself from litigation and government regulation. To this day, despite overwhelming scientific evidence and official government reports, the tobacco industry contends that tobacco products are not addictive and do not cause any disease whatsoever.

B&W'S AND BAT'S CORPORATE STRUCTURE

Brown and Williamson and its parent company, BAT Industries, have a close corporate relationship that has evolved over the years. The Brown and Williamson Tobacco Company was formed in 1906. It was purchased in 1927 by the British American Tobacco Company (BATCo), and its name was changed to the Brown and Williamson Tobacco Corporation {1006.01}. In 1976 BATCo merged with Tobacco Securities Trust to form BAT Industries.

BAT Industries is the parent company of many cigarette manufacturers throughout the world, including Brown and Williamson (US), BAT Cigarettenfabriken (Germany), Souza Cruz (Brazil), and British American Tobacco (which produces cigarettes in more than forty-five countries for domestic and export markets in Europe, Australia, Latin America, Asia, and Africa). In addition, BAT Industries is associated with Imasco in Canada, which is the parent company for Imperial Tobacco. BAT is also the parent company of several insurance and financial services, including Farmers Group (US), Eagle Star (UK), and Allied Dunbar (UK) (9).

Given B&W's status as a subsidiary of BAT, it was natural that the two companies would share information, not only about product development and sales and marketing strategies but also about their scientific research on the health dangers of cigarettes. As we discuss in chapter 2, B&W and the other domestic tobacco companies jointly formed an organization to study smoking and health issues in the mid-1950s, and British tobacco companies formed a similar group in England. In addition, as we discuss in chapter 3, BAT established research facilities (both internally and through contract laboratories) in Europe (England, Germany, and Switzerland) to study the health effects of smoking. The documents are replete with examples of information from all these research efforts, which was shared between B&W and BAT.

This sharing of information, although obviously of mutual benefit, also caused problems. As the evidence of the health dangers of smoking accumulated, B&W realized that it might become a defendant in products liability lawsuits by plaintiffs who claimed that their illnesses had been caused by cigarettes. Tobacco industry lawyers began to realize that the scientific research results that the companies were sharing could be extremely damaging if they became accessible to plaintiffs through discovery procedures. Tobacco companies in the United States were particularly concerned about the potential for lawsuits because products liability laws had been significantly strengthened during the 1960s. B&W therefore began to explore ways to avoid receiving unwanted information (i.e., information useful to a plaintiff) or to protect such information from discovery. In the United Kingdom, on the other hand, products liability laws have not historically been as strong as in the United States. BAT has therefore been more concerned about being dragged into a US lawsuit, because of its status as B&W's parent company, than about products liability suits in the United Kingdom (see chapter 7). A further problem for both companies was the possibility that statements attributable to subsidiary companies, including nontobacco companies, might be harmful to them in products liability litigation.

HISTORY OF THE B&W DOCUMENTS

On May 12, 1994, an unsolicited box of what appeared to be tobacco company documents was delivered to Professor Stanton Glantz at the University of California, San Francisco (UCSF). The documents in the box dated from the early 1950s to the early 1980s. They consisted primarily of confidential internal memoranda related to B&W and BAT. Many of the documents contained internal discussions of the tobacco industry's public relations and legal strategies over the years, and they were often labeled "confidential" or "privileged." The return address on the box was simply "Mr. Butts."

A few days earlier, US news media had started running stories based on what they said were internal documents from Brown and Williamson. In addition, internal documents related to Brown and Williamson were the subject of hearings held on June 23, 1994, before the US House of Representatives Subcommittee on Health and the Environment. The chairman and CEO of B&W, Thomas Sandefur, testified at these hearings and provided additional B&W documents to the subcommittee. In this book we analyze the documents delivered to Professor Glantz as well as the documents provided to the subcommittee, which were later released to the public, documents on nicotine research that B&W released to the press in May 1994 following a story in the *New York Times* (10), and documents obtained from the estate of a former BAT chief scientist.

Brown and Williamson has claimed that some of the documents were stolen from the law firm of Wyatt, Tarrant and Combs in Louisville, Kentucky, by a former paralegal, Dr. Merrell Williams (11, 12). B&W had hired the Wyatt firm to sort and analyze millions of pages of B&W's internal communications, and Williams was one of the paralegals working on the project. This project involved reviewing about 8,600,000 pages of documents, 70,000 pages of which had been identified as "critical" {1002.01} (figure 1.1). Our analysis is based on roughly 10,000 pages, which represent only about 0.1 percent of the documents that were being reviewed.

Williams was hired by the Wyatt firm in 1988 but was laid off in 1992. The following year, Williams, a smoker, underwent major heart surgery. On July 9, 1993, he informed the Wyatt firm through an attorney that he had possession of some of the documents he had been hired to analyze. He returned the documents with a letter stating that his heart condition had been caused by the stress of reviewing the documents as well

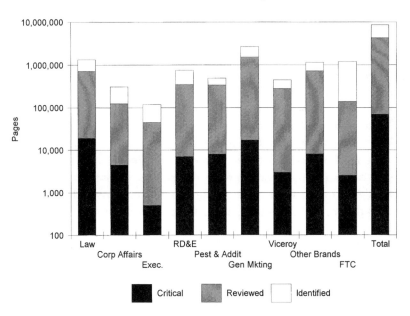

B & W Document Control Project

Figure 1.1. The B&W document control project involved screening millions of pages of documents {1002.01}. Our analysis is based on about 0.1 percent of the screened documents.

as a lifetime of smoking Brown and Williamson brands of cigarettes, and he threatened to sue unless the Wyatt firm settled his claim (13). The Wyatt firm responded by filing a civil suit in the Circuit Court for Jefferson County, Kentucky, accusing Williams of stealing the documents. On January 7, 1994, Judge Thomas Wine issued an order prohibiting Williams from discussing or disseminating any of the information contained in the documents [*Maddox v Williams*, Jefferson Cir. Ct., Case No. 93CI04806]. (On April 3, 1995, Judge Wine modified the order so that Williams could speak with his lawyer about the case. The modification was necessary, according to Judge Wine, because the documents in question were apparently part of the public domain in California, the Congress, and numerous news media, and because B&W had moved for contempt sanctions against Williams.)

On May 17, 1994, the Superior Court for the District of Columbia, at the request of B&W, issued subpoenas against several news agencies that had published or aired articles on some Brown and Williamson documents. The agencies receiving subpoenas were ABC, CBS, National Public Radio, the *New York Times*, the *Washington Post,* the *Louisville Courier-Journal, USA Today,* and the *National Law Review.* Subpoenas were also issued against Congressmen Henry Waxman (D-CA) and Ron Wyden (D-OR), who were members of the House Subcommittee on Health and the Environment. The purpose of the subpoenas, according to B&W, was to obtain copies of the documents so that B&W could determine whether they had been obtained in violation of the Kentucky court order against Merrell Williams.

The news organizations refused to turn over the documents in their possession on the grounds that they did not want to reveal the identity of a confidential source. The matter relating to the subpoenas issued against Congressmen Waxman and Wyden was removed to the US District Court for the District of Columbia on May 19, 1994. In a decision dated June 6, 1994, Judge Harold H. Greene quashed the subpoenas. Because the congressmen were using the documents in connection with a congressional investigation of B&W, the judge concluded, they were protected from the subpoenas under the Speech or Debate Clause of the US Constitution (Article I, Section 6) [*Maddox v Williams*, 855 F. Supp. 406 (D.D.C. 1994)]. That clause, which was designed to preserve legislative independence, provides that senators and representatives may not be questioned in any other place regarding speech or debate in either house of Congress. Despite this provision of the US Constitution, the subpoenas issued against Waxman and Wyden had directed them to submit in person to depositions in the law offices of Brown and Williamson's attorneys and to provide documents or copies to B&W from among the documents in the possession of Congress. According to Judge Greene, "It would be difficult to find orders that more directly impede the official responsibilities of the Congress and are thus in direct violation of the Speech or Debate Clause" [at 410, 411].

Following this decision, subpoenas issued by B&W were also quashed in three separate state court proceedings. On July 22, 1994 [in *Maddox v Williams*, No. 94-202], the Circuit Court for Arlington County, Virginia, quashed subpoenas issued to *USA Today* and one of its reporters. In November 1994 a Massachusetts court, citing "the public interest in the free flow of information," refused to enforce a subpoena issued by B&W against Professor Richard Daynard of Northeastern University School of Law [*Robert J. Maddox v Merrell Williams*, Civil Action No. 94-3389D]. Finally, on April 3, 1995, the Jefferson Circuit Court in Kentucky quashed subpoenas issued to the *Louisville Courier-Journal* and *USA Today*, stating that

> despite B&W's contentions to the contrary, the production of the documents is to identify the source. While the attorney-client privilege may well be a bedrock of our judicial system, freedom of the press and its ability to protect sources of information is a pillar of our Federal Constitution [*Maddox v Williams*, Case No. 93C104806].

In addition to the quashing of the subpoenas, other courts in other contexts have blocked B&W's attempts to suppress the documents. Thus, in April 1995 in an action by the state of Florida against several tobacco companies, the plaintiff introduced a set of B&W documents and the court denied defendants' motion to have the documents sealed, reasoning that

> most, if not all, of the over 800 "stolen" documents filed with the Court as part of Plaintiffs' Request for Admissions were part of the public domain prior to being filed in this Court. These documents have been the subject of newspaper articles, television programs and Congressional hearings. . . . To now seal the court files to protect the confidentiality of these documents would be futile [*State of Florida v American Tobacco Co.* (Cir. Ct. of 15th Judicial District for Palm Beach County, Florida, No. CL95-1466AO)].

During the summer of 1994 Professor Glantz placed the documents in the Archives and Special Collections Department of the UCSF Library, where they were made available to the public. On January 6, 1995, attorneys for a nonsmoker who had developed lung cancer and was suing Philip Morris Tobacco Company for damages attempted to convince a

Mississippi judge to accept these documents into evidence [*Butler v Philip Morris*, Civil Action No. 94-5-53, Cir. Ct., Jones County, Mississippi]. Twenty-five days later, on February 3, 1995, Brown and Williamson demanded that the University of California return the documents on the grounds that they were stolen. B&W also sent private investigators to the library to stake out the archives and to photograph people reading the documents. On February 14, 1995, B&W sued the University of California, demanding return of the documents and access to the library circulation records to learn who had read the documents [*Brown & Williamson Tobacco Corp. v Regents of the University of California* (Super. Ct. for County of San Francisco, No. 967298)].

At a hearing on May 25, 1995, San Francisco Superior Court Judge Stuart Pollak denied B&W's attempt to "recover" the documents from the UCSF Library (11, 14). In reaching his decision, the judge noted the First Amendment concerns raised by B&W's request that the university be prevented from retaining or using the documents:

> But the nature of what is being requested would in fact impinge upon public discussion, public study of this information, which has a bearing on all kinds of issues of public health, public law, documents which may be taken to suggest the advisability of legislation in all kinds of areas.
>
> So, there is . . . a very strong public interest in permitting this particular information, judging from what has been shown in the papers, as to what it concerns, permitting this information to remain available for use by the university or by others who may obtain it from the university [transcript of hearing, at 58, 59].

Again, as the Florida court had done, the San Francisco court noted that much, if not all, of the information in the documents had already been made available to the news media. "The genie is out of the bottle. These documents are out" [at 61].

The San Francisco court stayed its ruling for twenty days to give B&W time to appeal, thus leaving in effect a temporary restraining order against the university, which prevented it from allowing public access to the documents. B&W appealed to California's Court of Appeal and requested that the temporary restraining order be kept in force; the Court of Appeal denied this request without comment on June 22, 1995, as did the California Supreme Court on June 29, 1995. Thus, all the B&W documents used in the preparation of this book have been declared to be in the public domain, either by Congress or by the courts, and, in the case of some of the documents, by two or more authorities. At 12:01 A.M. PST on July 1, 1995, the University of California San Francisco Library and Center for Knowledge Management posted the documents on the Internet (http://www.library.ucsf.edu/tobacco).

Meanwhile, the authors of this book were working on their analysis of the documents and submitted a series of five related articles (which represent about 15 percent of the material in this book) to the *Journal of the American Medical Association* (*JAMA*). After an extensive peer review, the editors of *JAMA* decided to devote most of the July 19, 1995, issue to these papers (15–19), together with an article detailing Brown and Williamson's reaction to the papers (11). In addition, *JAMA* took the unprecedented step of publishing an editorial, signed by the editors of *JAMA* and all the members of the Board of Trustees of the American Medical Association, demanding strong action to control the tobacco industry (20).

Publication of these papers attracted international attention, including that of President Bill Clinton, who read the papers and used them as part of his decision-making process to ask the federal Food and Drug Administration (FDA) to propose regulations of nicotine as an addictive drug and cigarettes and smokeless tobacco products as drug delivery devices (21). The fact that nicotine was in the product to affect the function of the body and that cigarettes could be engineered to control the dose of nicotine delivered got to the core of the issue of FDA jurisdiction to regulate cigarettes.

LIMITATIONS OF THE EVIDENCE

As noted above, the documents provide our first look—through a keyhole—at the inner workings of the tobacco industry during the crucial period in which the scientific case that smoking was addicting smokers and killing them solidified. Our view, however, is a limited one. One of its limitations has to do with the possibility of selection bias; that is, the documents may have been picked by a whistle-blower with an eye toward smoking guns. Another limitation, which shows up particularly in the legal and public relations aspects, is that we cannot always determine from the discussion in the documents whether particular ideas were actually carried out. In some cases the public record clearly shows that the contemplated actions were taken. In others—particularly when the industry's more sub rosa activities are being discussed—it is not obvious where the line between contemplated and actual action lies. As part of our analysis, we have tried to indicate which of these situations existed.

In particular, the attorneys often discuss proposed courses of action, but the documents do not always clearly indicate which course of action the company ultimately chose. Lawyers by nature are asked to evaluate the legal risks of proposed courses of action, but their advice is not always followed. Nonetheless, we were struck by the active role the lawyers played, not just as advisers but also as managers; they often decided which research would be done or not done, who would be funded, and what public relations and political actions would be pursued. Generally speaking, the documents authored by attorneys did not outline possible courses of action or recommend which course to follow; instead, they strongly advocated that certain policies or actions be taken, some of which appear to raise serious ethical questions.

Another possible limitation is that the documents came from a single tobacco company and primarily reflect only the plans and actions of that company. Nevertheless, the documents include correspondence between B&W and other tobacco companies and trade organizations, as well as discussions of the actions of other companies and the industry in general. Many of the documents relate to industry-wide cooperation and reflect the views of participants, including lawyers, representing other companies and trade groups. In addition, other evidence—such as that presented in the *Haines* case, discussed in chapter 7—paints a similar picture of the actions of other tobacco companies. In any event, in our analysis of the documents, we have attempted to keep clear the distinction between the actions of B&W alone and the actions of the tobacco industry generally.

Despite these limitations, we are confident about the conclusions we draw from the documents. When lawyers are shown steering away from projects on the addictiveness or health effects of tobacco, we believe we can reasonably conclude that B&W and BAT knew that tobacco is addictive and causes disease; if it had been genuinely unconvinced of the dangers of smoking, then it would have had no concern that new research would provide ammunition for the enemy. The analogy would be to a criminal defense lawyer who doesn't ask the defendant whether he actually committed the crime because he does not want to be hampered in making his defense by embarrassing knowledge of the defendant's guilt. It will be easier to claim that the defendant is innocent, or even to put the defendant on the stand to testify to his innocence, if the lawyer does not ask the hard questions. The lawyers and scientists who wrote many of the documents were unusually candid in their remarks—possibly because they believed that the documents would be protected by the work product rule or attorney-client privilege, and therefore would never become public.

CONCLUSION

Although, as noted, this book analyzes only a tiny fraction of the documents that B&W had selected for review, the material in that small sample contains overwhelming evidence of the irresponsible and deceptive manner in which B&W has conducted its tobacco business. As will be seen in the following chapters, for more than thirty years B&W has been well aware of the addictive nature of cigarettes, and in the course of those years it has also learned of numerous health dangers of smoking. Yet, throughout this period, it chose to protect its business interests instead of the public health by consistently denying any such knowledge and by hiding adverse scientific evidence from the government and the public, using a wide assortment of scientific, legal, and political techniques.

The documents also demonstrate that B&W's conduct was representative of the tobacco industry generally. B&W acted in concert with the other domestic tobacco companies on numerous projects, the most important of which were specifically designed to prevent, or at least delay, public knowledge of the health dangers of smoking and to protect the tobacco companies from liability if that knowledge became public.

In his opinion quashing B&W subpoenas against Congressmen Waxman and Wyden, Judge Greene stated that it would be inappropriate to withhold the information in the documents from public scrutiny:

> [The documents] may be evidence supporting a "whistle-blower's" claim that the tobacco company concealed from its customers and the American public the truth regarding the health hazards of tobacco products, and that he was merely bringing them to the attention of those who could deal with this menace. With the situation in that posture, to accept blindly the B&W "stolen goods" argument would be to set a precedent at odds with the law, with equity, and with the public interest.
>
> If the B&W strategy were accepted, those seeking to bury their unlawful or potentially unlawful acts from consumers, from other members of the public, and from law enforcement or regulatory authorities could achieve that objective by a simple yet ingenious strategy: all that would need to be done would be to delay or confuse any charges of health hazard, fraud, corruption, overcharge, nuclear or chemical contamination, bribery, or other misdeeds, by focussing instead on inconvenient documentary evidence and labelling it

as the product of theft, violation of proprietary information, interference with contracts, and the like. The result would be that even the most severe public health and safety dangers would be subordinated in litigation and in the public mind to the malefactor's tort or contract claims, real or fictitious.

The law does not support such a strategy or inversion of values. There is a constitutional right to inform the government of violations of federal laws— a right which under [United States Constitution] Article VI supersedes local tort or contract rights and protects the "informer" from retaliation [*Maddox v Williams*, 855 F. Supp. 406, at 414, 415 (D.D.C. 1994)].

In this spirit, we will describe in detail the contents of the Brown and Williamson documents and the story that they tell. There is little doubt that, had the information contained in the documents come to light at an earlier time, the history of tobacco control in the United States would have been vastly different.

TABLE I.I   PUBLIC VERSUS PRIVATE STATEMENTS
MADE BY THE TOBACCO INDUSTRY

Nicotine and Addiction

Summary	By the early 1960s BAT and B&W had developed a sophisticated understanding of nicotine pharmacology and knew that nicotine was pharmacologically addictive. Publicly, however, the tobacco industry has maintained and continues to maintain that nicotine is not addictive. The scientific community was much slower to appreciate nicotine addiction: the Surgeon General did not conclude that nicotine was addictive until 1988 (22).
Surgeon General's Reports	*1964:* "The tobacco habit should be characterized as an habituation rather than an addiction" (3).
	1979: "[It] is no exaggeration to say that smoking is the prototypical substance-abuse dependency and that improved knowledge of this process holds great promise for prevention of risk" (23).
	1988: "After carefully examining the available evidence, this Report concludes that:
	• Cigarettes and other forms of tobacco are addicting.
	• Nicotine is the drug in tobacco that causes addiction.
	• The pharmacologic and behavioral processes that determine tobacco addiction are similar to those that determine addiction to drugs such as heroin and cocaine" (22, pp. 1–2).
B&W/BAT Research Results	"There is increasing evidence that nicotine is the key factor in controlling, through the central nervous system, a number of beneficial effects of tobacco smoke, including its action in the presence of stress situations. In addition, the alkaloid [nicotine] appears to be intimately connected with the phenomena of tobacco habituation (tolerance) and/or addiction." From *The Fate of Nicotine in the Body,* a report describing results of contract research conducted for BAT by Battelle Memorial Institute in Geneva, Switzerland, 1963 {1200.20}.
	"Chronic intake of nicotine tends to restore the normal physiological functioning of the endocrine system, so that ever-increasing dose levels of nicotine are necessary to maintain the desired action. . . . This unconscious desire explains the addiction of the individual to nicotine." From "A Tentative Hypothesis on Nicotine Addiction," an essay written by scientists at Battelle and distributed to senior executives at BAT and B&W, 1963 {1200.01, p. 1}.
B&W/BAT Private Statements	"Moreover, nicotine is addictive. We are, then, in the business of selling nicotine, an addictive drug effective in the release of stress mechanisms." Addison Yeaman, vice president and general counsel, B&W, 1963 {1802.05, p. 4}.
Tobacco Industry's Public Statements	"I do not believe that nicotine is addictive . . . nicotine is a very important constituent in the cigarette smoke for taste." Thomas Sandefur, chairman and CEO, B&W, testifying before the Health and Environment Subcommittee, Energy and Commerce Committee, House of Representatives, June 23, 1994 (24).

TABLE 1.1   (*continued*)

Low-Tar, Low-Nicotine Cigarettes and Smoker Compensation

Summary	Smokers compensate for the lack of nicotine in low-tar, low-nicotine cigarettes by puffing more frequently, by increasing the depth or duration of smoke inhalation, by smoking more cigarettes per day, and by smoking cigarettes to a shorter butt length. This means that smokers of low-tar, low-nicotine cigarettes are exposed to more "tar" and other harmful chemicals than would be indicated by an analysis of the cigarette smoke. This phenomenon, known as smoker compensation, was acknowledged internally in the tobacco industry by the early 1970s but was not appreciated in the scientific community until the 1980s.
Surgeon General's Reports	*1966:* "The preponderance of scientific evidence strongly suggests that the lower the 'tar' and nicotine content of cigarette smoke, the less harmful would be the effect" (25).
	1979: "[The public] should be warned that, in shifting to a less hazardous cigarette, they may in fact increase their hazard if they begin smoking more cigarettes or inhaling more deeply" (23).
	1981: "Smokers may increase the number of cigarettes they smoke and inhale more deeply when they switch to lower yield cigarettes. Compensatory behavior may negate any advantage of the lower yield product or even increase the health risk" (25).
B&W/BAT Research Results	"[W]hatever the characteristics of cigarettes as determined by smoking machines, the smoker adjusts his pattern to deliver his own nicotine requirements." Minutes from BAT's research conference held in Duck Key, Florida, 1974, taken by SJG [S. J. Green of BAT R&D] {1125.01, p. 2}.
	"Compensation study conducted by Imperial Tobacco Co., a BATCo affiliate, [shows that a smoker] adjusts his smoking habits when smoking cigarettes with low nicotine and TPM [total particulate matter] to duplicate his normal cigarette nicotine intake." From document titled "Chronology of Brown & Williamson Smoking and Health Research," regarding research conducted in 1975. Chronology dated 1988 {1006.01, p. 27}.
B&W/BAT Internal Statements	"In most cases, however, the smoker of a filter cigarette was getting as much or more nicotine and tar as he would have gotten from a regular cigarette." Ernest Pepples, vice president and general counsel, B&W, 1976 {2205.01, p. 2}.
Tobacco Industry's Public Statements	"All the fuss about smoking got me to thinking I'd either quit or smoke True. I smoke True." Advertisement for Lorillard's True cigarettes in *Ms.* magazine, October 1975.
	"I like to smoke, and what I like is a cigarette that isn't timid on taste. But I'm not living in some ivory tower. I hear the things being said against high-tar smoking as well as the next guy. And so I started looking. For a low-tar smoke that had some honest-to-goodness taste. Advertisement for Vantage cigarettes in *Time* magazine, November 9, 1977, pp. 86–87.

TABLE 1.1 *(continued)*

Role of the Tobacco Industry's Research Committee/Council for Tobacco Research

Summary	The Tobacco Industry Research Committee (TIRC), later renamed the Council for Tobacco Research–U.S.A., Inc. (CTR), was created by US tobacco companies in 1954. The tobacco industry has publicly claimed that TIRC/CTR is an independent organization that funds unbiased research into the health effects of smoking. Internally, however, tobacco industry representatives have stated that TIRC/CTR was created for public relations purposes, and that it later fulfilled political and legal roles.
B&W/BAT Private Statements	"Originally, CTR was organized as a public relations effort. . . . The research of CTR also discharged a legal responsibility. . . . Finally the industry research effort has included special projects designed to find scientists and medical doctors who might serve as industry witnesses in lawsuits or in a legislative forum." Ernest Pepples, vice president and general counsel, B&W, 1978 {2010.02, p. 2}.
Tobacco Industry's Public Statements	"From the outset, the Tobacco Industry Research Committee has made clear that the object of its research program is to encourage scientific study for facts about tobacco use and health. Its position is that research will help provide the knowledge about lung cancer and heart disease for a full evaluation of all factors being studied in connection with these diseases." Public relations document, circa 1963 {1903.03, p. 1}.
	"The Council for Tobacco Research–U.S.A., Inc., is the sponsoring agency of a program of research into questions of tobacco use and health. . . . The Council awards research grants to independent scientists who are assured complete scientific freedom in conducting their studies. Grantees alone are responsible for reporting or publishing their findings in the accepted scientific manner—through medical and scientific journals and societies" (26).

TABLE I.I   *(continued)*

Smoking and Disease, 1960's

Summary	By the early 1960s the scientific community had determined that smoking is causally related to lung cancer and probably related to heart disease. Results from tobacco industry laboratories supported these conclusions, but the tobacco industry publicly denied that the links had been proven.
Surgeon General's Reports	*1964:* "Cigarette smoking is causally related to lung cancer in men; the magnitude of the effect of cigarette smoking far outweighs all other factors. The data for women, though less extensive, point in the same direction" (3).
	"Cigarette smoking is the most important of the causes of chronic bronchitis in the United States, and increases the risk of dying from chronic bronchitis" (3).
	"Male cigarette smokers have a higher death rate from coronary artery disease than non-smoking males, but it is not clear that the association has causal significance" (3).
	"Cigarette smoking is a significant factor in the causation of cancer of the larynx [and] an association exists between cigarette smoking and cancer of the urinary bladder in men" (3).
B&W/BAT Research Results	"Scientists with whom I talked [at BAT's laboratories in Great Britian] were unanimous in their opinion that smoke is weakly carcinogenic under certain conditions and that efforts should be made to reduce this activity." Dr. R. B. Griffith, head of R&D, B&W, 1965 {1105.01, p. 2}.
B&W/BAT Private Statements	"At the best, the probabilities are that some combination of constituents of smoke will be found conducive to the onset of cancer or to create an environment in which cancer is more likely to occur." Addison Yeaman, vice president and general counsel, B&W, 1963 {1802.05, p. 1}.
Tobacco Industry's Public Statements	"The smoking of tobacco continues to be one of the subjects requiring study in the lung cancer problem, as do many other agents and influences in modern living. Science does not yet know enough about any suspected factors to judge whether they may operate alone, whether they may operate in conjunction with others, or whether they may affect or be affected by factors of whose existence science is not yet aware." Public relations document, circa 1967 {1903.03, p. 3}.

TABLE 1.1 *(continued)*

Smoking and Disease, 1970s

Summary	Throughout the 1970s B&W and BAT (and probably the other tobacco companies as well) privately engaged in a massive research campaign to identify and remove any toxic compounds identified in tobacco smoke. Privately, B&W and BAT scientists concluded there was no scientific controversy about the dangers of smoking. Their goal was to create a "safe" cigarette. However, their research showed that it would be very difficult to remove all the different toxic compounds in tobacco smoke. Publicly, the industry continued to deny that smoking had been proven harmful to health.
Surgeon General's Reports	*1972:* "Tobacco use is associated with increased risk of coronary heart disease; cerebrovascular disease (stroke); aortic aneurysm; peripheral vascular disease; chronic obstructive bronchopulmonary disease (COPD); cancers of the lung, lip, larynx, oral cavity, esophagus, urinary bladder, and pancreas; and gastrointestinal disorders such as peptic ulcer disease. In addition, maternal smoking during pregnancy retards fetal growth" (27).
B&W/BAT Research Results	"Carbon monoxide [CO] will become increasingly regarded as a serious health hazard for smokers. The methods of control available are ventilation, diffusion and the choice of smoking materials. But the inverse relationship of polycyclic aromatics and carbon monoxide is still observed, e.g. lithium hydroxide reduces CO substantially but is coupled with an increase in tumorigenic activity." Minutes from BAT research conference held in Duck Key, Florida, 1974, taken by S. J. Green of BAT R&D {1125.01, p. 3}.
B&W/BAT Private Statements	"There has been no change in the scientific basis for the case against smoking. Additional evidence of smoke-dose related incidence of some diseases associated with smoking has been published. But generally this has long ceased to be an area for scientific controversy." Minutes from BAT research conference held in Sydney, Australia, 1978, taken by S. J. Green of BAT R&D {1174.01, p. 1}.
Tobacco Industry's Public Statements	"Taking all the above into consideration, we believe there is sound evidence to conclude that the statement 'cigarettes cause cancer' is not a statement of fact but merely an hypothesis" [emphasis in original]. B&W public relations document, 1971 {2110.06, p. 10}.

TABLE 1.1   (*continued*)

Smoking and Disease, 1980s

Summary	B&W and BAT continued their efforts to develop a "safer" cigarette during the 1980s. The focus of their research was on minimizing the "biological activity," or carcinogenic potential, of their products. Unfortunately, that proved more difficult than expected. In addition, as the scientific community noted, even if less carcinogenic cigarettes could be designed, these cigarettes would still cause some cancer, as well as heart disease and other noncancer diseases.
Surgeon General's Reports	*1981:* "Smoking cigarettes with lower yields of 'tar' and nicotine reduces the risk of lung cancer and, to some extent, improves the smoker's chance for longer life, provided there is no compensatory increase in the amount smoked. However, the benefits are minimal in comparison with giving up cigarettes entirely" (25).
	1989: "Smoking is responsible for more than one of every six deaths in the United States. Smoking remains the single most important preventable cause of death in our society" (28).
B&W/BAT Research Results	"Cigarette <u>brands</u> can be readily distinguished [in terms of mutagenicity as judged by an Ames test]. This is in contrast with the earlier mouse skin painting results. An unfortunate side-effect is that the sensitivity increases the probability of an Ames League Table [which would rank different brands of cigarettes according to mutagenicity using the Ames test] appearing. A further unfortunate examination is that, to date, it is not uncommon for BAT brands to have a higher result [i.e., greater mutagenicity] than those from the opposition." Minutes from BAT biological conference held in Southampton, England, 1984, author unknown {1181.06, p. 1}.
B&W/BAT Private Statements	"Despite intense research over the past 25 years, the biological activity of smoke remains a major challenge. In particular, it is not known in quantitative terms whether the smoke from modern low and ultra-low delivery products has a lower specific biological activity than that from previous high delivery products. Nor is it clearly established . . . what are the main factors that influence biological [carcinogenic] activity." Minutes from BAT research conference held in Montebello, Canada, 1982, prepared by L. C. F. Blackman of BAT R&D {1179.01, p. 4}.
Tobacco Industry's Public Statements	"Cigarette smoking has not been scientifically established to be a cause of chronic diseases, such as cancer, cardiovascular disease, or emphysema. Nor has it been shown to affect pregnancy outcome adversely." Sheldon Sommers, M.D., scientific director of the CTR in congressional testimony, March 1983 (29).

TABLE 1.1   *(continued)*

Mouse Skin–Painting Experiments

Summary	Both the tobacco industry and the general scientific community have relied on mouse skin–painting experiments to evaluate the carcinogenicity of elements in tobacco smoke. Publicly, however, the tobacco industry has criticized the validity of these tests.
Surgeon General's Reports	*1964:* "[I]nduction of cancer by a compound in one species does not prove that the test compound would be carcinogenic in another species under similar circumstances. Therefore, tests for carcinogenicity in animals can provide only supporting evidence for the carcinogenicity of a given compound or material in man. Nevertheless, any agent that can produce cancer in an animal is suspected of being carcinogenic in man also" (3).
	"Almost every species that has been adequately tested has proved to be susceptible to the effect of certain polycyclic aromatic hydrocarbons identified in cigarette smoke and designated as carcinogenic on the basis of tests in rodents. Therefore, one can reasonably postulate that the same polycyclic hydrocarbons may also be carcinogenic in one or more tissues of man with which they come in contact" (3).
B&W/BAT Research Results	"Studies in instant [fresh] condensate are showing a biological activity towards mouse-skin of the same order as that of stale condensate, suggesting that the biological activity is not time-dependent. The clear possibility of producing cigarettes with reduced mouse-skin biological activity therefore becomes of greater importance and a research solution to the whole problem is more likely." Minutes from BAT research conference held in Hilton Head Island, South Carolina, 1968, prepared by S. J. Green of BAT R&D {1112.01, p. 1}.
	"The meeting agreed that it would be worthwhile to make a cigarette with lower biological activity on mouse skin painting, provided this did not adversely affect the position with respect to irritation and other factors. It was recognized that this implied certain assumptions about the relevance of mouse skin painting." Minutes from BAT research conference held in Montreal, Canada, 1967, author unknown {1165.02, p. 3}.
B&W/BAT Private Statements	"Historically, bioassay experiments were undertaken by the Industry with the object of clarifying the role of smoke constituents in pulmonary carcinogenesis. The most widely used of these methods [was] mouse-skin painting. . . . (a) In the foreseeable future, say five years, mouse-skin painting would remain as the ultimate court of appeal on carcinogenic effects." Minutes from BAT research conference held in Kronberg, Germany, 1969, prepared by S. J. Green of BAT R&D {1169.01, pp. 2–4}.
Tobacco Industry's Public Statements	"Much of the experimental work involves mouse-painting or animal smoke inhalation experiments. . . . [T]hese condensates are artificially produced under laboratory conditions and, as such, have little, if any, relation to cigarette smoke as it reaches the smoker. Further, the results obtained on the skin of mice should not be extrapolated to the lung tissue of the mouse, or to any other animal species. Certainly such skin results should not be extrapolated to the human lung." B&W public relations document, 1971 [emphasis in original] {2110.06, pp. 6–7}.

TABLE I.I   (*continued*)

Environmental Tobacco Smoke (ETS)

Summary   During the 1970s and 1980s scientific evidence began to suggest that exposure to environmental tobacco smoke could cause adverse health effects, such as lung cancer and cardiovascular disease, in nonsmokers. B&W and BAT responded by privately attempting to create a product that produced less hazardous sidestream smoke. Publicly, however, the industry has denied that passive smoking has been proven harmful to health.

Surgeon   *1972:* "1. An atmosphere contaminated with tobacco smoke can
General's   contribute to the discomfort of many individuals.
Reports   2. The level of carbon monoxide attained in experiments using
                            rooms filled with tobacco smoke had been shown to be equal,
                            and at times to exceed, the legal limits for maximum air
                            pollution permitted for ambient air quality. . . .
                        3. Other components of tobacco smoke, such as particulate
                            matter and the oxides of nitrogen, have been shown in various
                            concentrations to affect adversely animal pulmonary and
                            cardiac structure and function. The extent of the contribution
                            of these substances to illness in humans exposed to the
                            concentrations present in an atmosphere contaminated with
                            tobacco smoke is not presently known" (27).

1982: Epidemiologic studies on ETS and lung cancer "raise the concern
that involuntary smoking may pose a carcinogenic risk to the
nonsmoker" (30).

1986: "This review leads to three major conclusions:
     1. Involuntary smoking is a cause of disease, including lung
         cancer, in healthy nonsmokers.
     2. The children of parents who smoke compared with the children of
         nonsmoking parents have an increased frequency of respiratory
         infections, increased respiratory symptoms, and slightly smaller
         rates of increase in lung function as the lung matures.
     3. The simple separation of smokers and nonsmokers within
         the same air space may reduce, but does not eliminate, the
         exposure of nonsmokers to environmental tobacco smoke" (31).

B&W/BAT   "SIDESTREAM RESEARCH AND DEVELOPMENT.
Research   Strategic objectives remain as follows:
Results   1. Develop cigarettes with reduced sidestream yields and/or reduced
                odour and irritation.
            2. Conduct research to anticipate and refute claims about the health
                effects of passive smoking."
            Summary of BAT Group Research and Development Centre Activities on
            Sidestream, Psychology, circa 1984 {1181.12, p. 1}.

B&W/BAT   "We must get hard data both to help counter anti-smoking attacks, and
Private   to support the design of future products. . . . We should keep within BAT:
Statements   i)   animal results on sidestream activity
            ii)   thoughts on the biological activity [carcinogenicity] of sidestream
                  [smoke]
            iii) research findings on the consumer annoyance aspects of
                  environmental [tobacco] smoke—since these have potential
                  commercial value."
            Minutes from BAT research conference held in Montebello, Canada,
            1982, prepared by L. C. F. Blackman of BAT R&D {1179.01, p. 7}.

TABLE 1.1 *(continued)*

Environmental Tobacco Smoke (ETS)

Tobacco Industry's Public Statements	"[E]vidence relating ETS to health effects is scanty, contradictory and often fundamentally flawed. . . . [M]ore and better research needs to be done" (32, p. 1).
	"[E]xposure to environmental tobacco smoke has not been shown to cause lung cancer in nonsmokers. . . . [S]uch exposure has not been shown to impair the respiratory or cardiovascular health of nonsmoking adults or children, or to exacerbate preexisting disease in these groups, or to cause 'allergic' symptoms on a physiological basis" (32, p. 51).

SOURCE: S. A. Glantz, D. E. Barnes, L. Bero, P. Hanauer, and J. Slade, Looking through a keyhole at the tobacco industry: The Brown and Williamson documents, *JAMA* 1995;274:219–224.

REFERENCES

1. Wagner S. *Cigarette Country: Tobacco in American History and Politics.* New York: Praeger, 1971.
2. Glantz S. *Tobacco: Biology and Politics.* Waco, TX: HealthEdCo, 1992.
3. USDHEW. *Smoking and Health. Report of the Advisory Committee to the Surgeon General of the Public Health Service.* Washington, DC: US Department of Health, Education and Welfare, 1964. Public Health Service Publication No. 1103.
4. Taylor P. *The Smoke Ring: Tobacco, Money, and Multi-national Politics.* New York: Pantheon Books, 1984.
5. Maxwell JJ. *The Maxwell Consumer Report: Top World Cigarette Market Leaders.* Richmond, VA: Wheat, First Securities, 1993.
6. Maxwell JJ. *Historical Sales Trends in the Cigarette Industry.* Richmond, VA: Wheat, First Securities, 1993.
7. Maxwell JC Jr. *Historical Sales Trends in the Cigarette Industry: A Statistical Summary Covering 64 Years.* Richmond, VA: Wheat, First Securities, 1989.
8. Weisz P. Smokes "R" Us: Cigarette retailers are coming category among category killers. *Brandweek* 1995 March 6:20–24.
9. B.A.T. Industries. *Annual Review and Summary Financial Statement* London: B.A.T. Industries, 1993.
10. Hilts PJ. Tobacco company was silent on hazards. *New York Times* 1994 May 7:A1.
11. Graham T. The Brown and Williamson documents: The company's response. *JAMA* 1995;274:254–255.
12. Orey M. A mole's tale. *The American Lawyer* 1995 July/August:86–92.
13. Shapiro E. The insider who copied tobacco firm's secrets. *Wall Street Journal* 1994 June 20:B1.
14. Siegel M. University counsel battles Brown and Williamson over tobacco documents. *The American Lawyer* 1995 July/August:48.
15. Glantz SA, Barnes DE, Bero L, Hanauer P, Slade J. Looking through a keyhole at the tobacco industry: The Brown and Williamson documents. *JAMA* 1995;274:219–224.
16. Slade J, Bero L, Hanauer P, Barnes DE, Glantz SA. Nicotine and addiction: The Brown and Williamson documents. *JAMA* 1995;274:225–233.
17. Hanauer P, Slade J, Barnes DE, Bero L, Glantz SA. Lawyer control of internal scientific research to avoid products liability lawsuits: The Brown and Williamson documents. *JAMA* 1995;274:234–240.

18. Bero L, Barnes DE, Hanauer P, Slade J, Glantz SA. Lawyer control of the tobacco industry's external research program: The Brown and Williamson documents. *JAMA* 1995;274:241–247.
19. Barnes DE, Hanauer P, Slade J, Bero LA, Glantz SA. Environmental tobacco smoke: The Brown and Williamson documents. *JAMA* 1995;274:248–253.
20. Todd JS, Rennie D, McAfee RE, et al. The Brown and Williamson documents: Where do we go from here? (editorial). *JAMA* 1995;274:256–259.
21. Cohn B, Turque B. Firing up the politics of teen smoking; Clinton: Why he decided to target tobacco. *Newsweek* 1995 August 21:25–26.
22. USDHHS. *The Health Consequences of Smoking: Nicotine Addiction. A Report of the Surgeon General.* US Department of Health and Human Services, Public Health Service, Centers for Disease Control, Center for Health Promotion and Education, Office on Smoking and Health, 1988. DHHS Publication No. (CDC) 88-8406.
23. USDHEW. *Smoking and Health. A Report of the Surgeon General.* US Department of Health, Education and Welfare, Public Health Service, Office of the Assistant Secretary for Health, Office on Smoking and Health, 1979. DHEW Publication No. (PHS) 79-50066.
24. Sandefur TJ. *Testimony before the House Subcommittee on Health and the Environment.* Committee on Energy and Commerce, US House of Representatives, June 23, 1994.
25. USDHHS. *The Health Consequences of Smoking: The Changing Cigarette. A Report of the Surgeon General.* US Department of Health and Human Services, Public Health Service, Office of the Assistant Secretary of Health, Office on Smoking and Health, 1981. DHHS Publication No. (PHS) 81-50156.
26. Council for Tobacco Research. *Organization and Policy Statement.* New York, NY: Council for Tobacco Research, 1985.
27. USDHEW. *The Health Consequences of Smoking. A Report of the Surgeon General.* US Department of Health, Education and Welfare, Public Health Service, Health Services and Mental Health Administration, 1972. DHEW Publication No. (HSM) 72-7516.
28. USDHHS. *Reducing the Health Consequences of Smoking: 25 Years of Progress.* US Department of Health and Human Services, Public Health Service, Centers for Disease Control, Center for Chronic Disease Prevention and Health Promotion, Office on Smoking and Health, 1989. DHHS Publication No. (CDC) 89-8411.
29. Wolinsky H. When researchers accept funding from the tobacco industry, do ethics go up in smoke? *NY State J Med* 1985;85(7):451–455.
30. USDHHS. *The Health Consequences of Smoking: Cancer. A Report of the Surgeon General.* US Department of Health and Human Services, Public Health Service, Office on Smoking and Health, 1982. DHHS Publication No. (PHS) 82-50179.
31. USDHHS. *The Health Consequences of Involuntary Smoking. A Report of the Surgeon General.* US Department of Health and Human Services, Public Health Service, Centers for Disease Control, 1986. DHHS Publication No. (CDC) 87-8398.
32. Tobacco Institute. *Tobacco Smoke and the Nonsmoker: Scientific Integrity at the Crossroads.* Washington, DC: Tobacco Institute, 1986.

CHAPTER 2

Smoking and Disease: The Tobacco Industry's Earliest Responses

The significant expenditures on the question of smoking and health have allowed the industry to take a respectable stand along the following lines—"After millions of dollars and over twenty years of research, the question about smoking and health is still open."

Ernest Pepples, B&W vice president and general counsel, 1976 {2205.01, p. 2}

INTRODUCTION

During the early 1950s scientists began to publish scientific studies suggesting that cigarette smoking causes lung cancer and other diseases. One of the most influential of the early studies, published by Drs. Ernst L. Wynder and Evarts A. Graham in 1950 (1), showed that smokers had a greater risk of lung cancer than nonsmokers did. Later, Wynder and Graham showed that mice who had cigarette "tar" painted on their backs were more likely to develop malignant tumors than control mice that were not painted with tobacco tar (2). These results were interpreted as important evidence that smoking could cause cancer in humans, and they were widely reported in newspapers and magazines such as the *New York Times* (May 27, 1950), *Reader's Digest* (December 1952), and *Life* (December 21, 1953). The tobacco industry's earliest response to this growing body of scientific evidence was to promote new types of cigarettes, such as cigarettes with filters and "low-tar" cigarettes. The industry implied in its advertisements that these new cigarettes were healthier than the old ones. However, the documents show that the new brands had been created for marketing and public relations purposes, to lull the public into a false sense of security regarding the health effects of smoking.

Part of the industry's response to the evidence linking smoking and disease was the formation of the Tobacco Industry Research Committee (TIRC), later renamed the Council for Tobacco Research (CTR). The industry claimed that TIRC was an independent organization that would determine the truth about the health effects of smoking by funding independent scientific research. The documents show, however, that TIRC was originally created for public relations purposes, to convince the public that there was a "controversy" as to whether smoking is dangerous. As chapter 8 describes, CTR funded "special projects" whose research results could be used by industry lawyers to defend tobacco companies in court and to influence public opinion and public policy.

The release of two major government reports on the health dangers of smoking—the 1962 report of the Royal College of Physicians in the United Kingdom (3) and the 1964 report of the Surgeon General in the United States (4)—apparently sparked a debate in the industry over how to respond to the growing body of evidence that its products kill. The documents suggest that in the United States B&W and, probably, the other tobacco companies were deeply concerned about the potential for regulation and litigation and reacted to the reports primarily by trying to protect themselves from litigation while maintaining their sales and profits. In the United Kingdom, on the other hand, BAT seemed genuinely concerned about the health problems and embarked on an elaborate effort to develop a "safe" cigarette. Chapter 4, however, shows that this effort ultimately failed.

FILTER CIGARETTES AND THE "TAR DERBY"

Tobacco companies responded to the growing public concern over the health effects of smoking by heavily promoting new types of cigarettes, such as cigarettes with filters in the 1950s and "low-tar" cigarettes beginning in the mid-1960s. The documents show that these new brands were not clearly "healthier" than the old brands. Instead, the new brands were designed for marketing purposes, so that tobacco companies could claim in their advertisements that their brand had "lower tar" than the others, even though low-tar cigarettes did not necessarily reduce the health risks of smoking. (BAT scientists made a distinction between "health-oriented" cigarettes, which incorporated technological advances that had been tested and were known to reduce hazards, and "health-image" cigarettes, which were designed to give smokers the illusion of smoking a safer product. This distinction was later formalized at the BAT Hilton Head research conference in 1968; see chapter 4.)

The tobacco industry's strategy of developing filter and low-tar cigarettes is the subject of a memorandum titled "Industry Response to the Cigarette/ Health Controversy" {2205.01}. This memo, written in 1976 by Ernest Pepples, B&W's vice president and general counsel, provides an overview of the industry's public relations strategies. (This memo, which describes the industry's response to the "smoking and health controversy," is discussed in more detail in chapter 7. We limit our discussion here to the portion that refers to the industry's development of filter cigarettes.)

In his memo Pepples points out that the tobacco industry's first response to the growing public concern over the health effects of smoking was to "produce more filter brands and brands with lower tar delivery" {2205.01}. As a result of this strategy, he notes, the market share of filter cigarettes had grown rapidly during the 1950s and 1960s, giving rise to an atmosphere of fierce competition that became known as the "tar derby," because tobacco companies were competing to deliver the lowest tar possible. Perhaps most important, toward the end of his discussion Pepples concedes that the filters did not actually make the cigarettes healthier, but only gave smokers the illusion of smoking a healthier product.

> The industry has moved strongly toward filter cigarettes, which have increased from .6% in 1950 to 87% in 1975. KENT cigarettes were introduced in 1952 with an unusually heavy promotion campaign discussing the micronite filter. Other companies moved strongly into the rapidly growing filter market. In 1951, nine out of twenty brands on the market accounted for as much as 1% of market share. By 1964, 17 of 41 brands had more than 1% share of market. [This proliferation of brands reflects the impact the introduction of filter cigarettes had on consumption patterns.]
>
> This became known as the "tar derby" of the late 1950's. It was characterized by sharply intensified advertising competition. By 1963 well over half of the total unit output was composed of brands which were unknown before 1950.
>
> The new filter brands vying for a piece of the growing filter market made extraordinary claims. There was an urgent effort to highlight and differentiate one brand from the others already on the market. It was important to have the most filter traps. Some claimed to possess the least tars. *In most cases, however, the smoker of a filter cigarette was getting as much or more nicotine and tar as he would have gotten from a regular cigarette.* He had abandoned the regular cigarette, however, on the ground of reduced risk to health [emphasis added]. {2205.01, p. 2}

Pepples adds that government regulation had actually helped the industry put a stop to the "tar derby" by allowing tobacco companies to end their expensive television advertising campaigns.

> This sort of advertising led to the first attempts by the Federal Trade Commission to regulate the industry. A further consequence of the "tar derby"

was the rapid increase in advertising expenditures during this period. Advertising expenditures in selected media jumped from over $55 million in 1952 to approximately $150 million in 1959. The "tar derby" was ended by a voluntary agreement between the FTC and the cigarette companies in 1960. The competition in advertising continued to be fierce, however, with expenditures doubling again by 1970 to a figure of approximately $314 million.

In announcing the agreement, Earl W. Kintner, then FTC Chairman, stated that in "the absence of a satisfactory uniform test and proof of advantage to the smoker, there will be no more tar and nicotine claims in advertising." Kintner said the tar and nicotine blackout was "a landmark example of industry-government cooperation in solving a pressing problem." *The Consumers Union, however, felt that the end of the "tar derby" was to the industry's advantage and to the public's disadvantage. It said that the cigarette industry had succeeded in extricating itself from [an] embarrassing position* [emphasis added; pages 3–5 of this nine-page document are missing from our files]. {2205.01, p. 2}

This memo suggests that the tobacco industry promoted filter and low-tar cigarettes primarily for public relations purposes. (Filter cigarettes had been marketed since the 1930s.) Tobacco companies realized that their customers were concerned about the reports that cigarette smoking might be dangerous, and they therefore introduced new products designed to calm those fears.

EARLY ADVERTISING CLAIMS

Ironically, even before scientific evidence began to suggest that smoking causes lung cancer and other diseases, tobacco companies in the United States were promoting cigarettes with advertisements suggesting that some brands were "healthier" or "less irritating" than others. The documents contain several examples of early advertising claims made by B&W and other tobacco companies {1700.04; 1703.01; 1703.02; 1704.01}.

One document simply lists the advertising slogans for various brands of cigarettes from the 1920s through the 1950s, including Kool, Camel, Lucky Strike, Old Gold, and Viceroy, among others {1700.04}. For example, an advertising slogan for Lucky Strike in 1928 was:

It's toasted. <u>No Throat Irritation—No Cough</u> [emphasis in original]. {1700.04, p. 11}

And in 1929 Lucky Strike advertisements claimed that

20,679 physicians have confirmed the fact that <u>Lucky Strike</u> is less irritating to the throat than other cigarettes. {1700.04, p. 11}

Similarly, advertisements for Kool cigarettes in the 1930s and 1940s suggested that Kools would not irritate the throat. They contained slogans such as

> For your throat's sake Switch from 'Hots' to <u>Kools</u>. {1700.04, p. 1}

By the 1950s, when the public was becoming more apprehensive about the health dangers of smoking that were being described in the press, the tobacco industry heavily promoted filter cigarettes and made claims about less tar. In B&W's advertising of Viceroy cigarettes, for example, the "Health-Guard" filter introduced in 1952 was touted:

> New HEALTH-GUARD Filter Makes VICEROY Better For Your Health Than Any Other Leading Cigarette! {1703.01, p. 2}

This statement was supported in the advertisements with "facts" designed to downplay the ad claims of other companies. For example, in 1952, at a time when Lorillard was extolling the low nicotine delivery of Kent, B&W trumpeted:

> Although most filters help to remove tobacco tars, laboratory analysis <u>proved</u> that smoke from other leading filter-tip cigarettes contain [*sic*] up to 110.5% <u>more nicotine</u> than VICEROY [emphasis in original]. {1703.01, p. 2}

Reduced nicotine was a key claim made for several other brands at the time. Before filters, Camel, Chesterfield, and Old Gold all made low-nicotine claims. Kent's health claims were also based on nicotine data, but this claim was not explicit in the advertising at the time (5, 6).

In 1955 B&W drew additional contrasts between Viceroy's Health-Guard filter, which was made from cellulose acetate, and the crocidolite asbestos (Micronite) filter of Kent. Ads in college newspapers posed this question:

> Why do more college men and women smoke VICEROYS than any other filter cigarette? . . .
> Because only VICEROY gives you 20,000 filter traps in every filter tip, made from a pure natural substance—cellulose—found in delicious fruits and other edibles! . . .
> Besides being non-mineral and non-toxic, this cellulose acetate filter never shreds or crumbles. {1703.01, p. 9}

A 1955 magazine ad proclaimed:

> NO OTHER FILTER LIKE VICEROY! NO COTTON! NO PAPER! NO ASBESTOS! NO CHARCOAL! NO FOREIGN SUBSTANCES OF ANY KING! [*sic*]. {1703.01, p. 10}

Nonetheless, after an article published in *Reader's Digest* in 1957 (7) cited Kent as the least toxic filter cigarette, a finding based on a comparison of tar deliveries, Viceroy's sales dropped sharply {1703.02, p. 11}.

These examples of the tobacco industry's advertising claims, along with the "tar derby" memo from Pepples, indicate that the industry began promoting filter and reduced-tar cigarettes during the 1950s primarily to calm public fears about the health effects of smoking. Although the advertisements of the era suggested that the new cigarettes were "healthier," there was no real evidence that this was so. When the evidence finally began to come in (beginning only twenty years later, in 1977), the verdict was that lowering tar with filters had only a very modest effect in lowering the enormous risk of lung cancer caused by cigarettes and no effect in protecting the consumer from the more common threat, fatal heart disease (8, 9).

Today the tobacco industry claims that it markets filter and "low-tar" cigarettes because of public demand, and not because it believes that these products are "safer." For instance, R. J. Reynolds—in its monograph about Premier, a novel nicotine delivery system—refers to the development of filter and "low-tar" cigarettes as manufacturer responses to consumer demand (10). However, the industry itself, through its advertising campaigns, has helped create the illusion that these products are safer.

B&W'S INTERNAL RESEARCH PROGRAM

Before the 1950s the tobacco companies, or at least Brown and Williamson, apparently had conducted very little research on the health effects of smoking, even though they discussed the purported health benefits long before that in their advertisements. Beginning in the early 1950s, however, the industry began to conduct more scientific research to determine the health effects of its products.

The history of B&W's research program is described in a document that chronologically lists all the smoking and health research conducted by B&W from 1906 to 1986 {1006.01}. The entry for 1946 states:

> Prior to 1946, the only research done at Brown & Williamson was performed in a laboratory established under the control of the Manufacturing Department. In 1946, the Technical Research Department was formed with Dr. R. C. Ernst as the Director of Research on a consulting basis. . . . The majority of research conducted at this time was still in the form of technical support. {1006.01, p. 1}

This entry suggests that, until 1946, B&W had only studied technical issues related to cigarette marketing and development. By 1948, however, B&W had begun developing a cellulose acetate filter. In 1950 the company began work to "eliminate the harsh, irritating smoke in a cigarette that comes from the paper wrapper" {1006.01, p. 2}.

The entry for 1952 suggests that B&W was becoming more concerned about the health effects of its products with each passing year. It also indicates that B&W was particularly concerned about the tar and nicotine content of its cigarettes.

> The Tennessee Eastman cellulose acetate filter known as the "Health Guard Tip" is reported to be in production. Cigarettes with this filter produce 42–46% less tar and 19–35% less nicotine than the non-filtered competitors. A review of the scientific literature on arsenic and cancer and the presence of arsenic in smoke and insecticides is conducted. Cancer is "investigated from a literature standpoint" in light of "frightening testimony" from epidemiology studies. A carcinogenic hydrocarbon, benzo(a)pyrene, is partially isolated from tobacco leaf and smoke. {1006.01, p. 2}

By 1952 early epidemiological studies in the United States and the United Kingdom were showing substantial risks for lung cancer related to cigarette smoking. At the time, arsenic and benzo(a)pyrene (or benzpyrene) were the only two known carcinogenic materials suspected of being in tobacco smoke (11). As of 1952, only a single, unconfirmed report, published in 1939, had indicated that benzo(a)pyrene could be found in tobacco smoke. The next published report of similar findings appeared in 1954 (11). Therefore, the unpublished work B&W scientists were doing in 1952, achieving a "partial isolation" of benzo(a)pyrene from tobacco leaf and tobacco smoke, was at the leading edge of the field at the time.

By 1953 B&W had begun a more intensive effort to study tobacco and its effects. Dr. I. W. Tucker was appointed as the first full-time director of B&W's Technical Research Department. In his departmental report at the end of 1953, according to the B&W chronology {1006.01, p. 2}, Dr. Tucker said that the smoking and health situation "will be an important factor in establishing the direction which our research department will take." A few months later, at an industry conference in Bristol, England, Dr. Tucker stated that "tobacco companies' research departments must now conduct work on smoke constituents not only for technological improvements but also for better understanding of their products as a result of the smoking and health controversy" {1006.01, p. 3}.

Unfortunately for the tobacco industry, the results of these early studies were discouraging. As we discuss in the following chapters, by the 1960s BAT scientists had concluded that nicotine is addictive and company-sponsored laboratory tests showed that components of tobacco smoke cause cancer in animals. The company responded to these findings at first by attempting to create a "safe" cigarette, although it publicly maintained that cigarettes had not been proven dangerous to health. When the scientists had concluded that they would not be able to create a "safe" cigarette, the company retreated behind a stone wall of denial, where it remains to this day.

THE COUNCIL FOR TOBACCO RESEARCH

The same memo {2205.01} that discussed the "tar derby" also discussed another public relations strategy adopted by the tobacco industry during the 1950s—the sponsorship of supposedly independent scientific research. (The memo, written in 1976 by Ernest Pepples, describes the industry's response to the "cigarette/health controversy" over time. As stated above, other aspects of this memo are discussed in detail in chapter 7.) This strategy allowed the tobacco industry to claim that there was a "controversy" over the effects of smoking and that more research was needed to resolve the debate.

Pepples notes that, besides producing filter and low-tar cigarettes, the industry reacted to the evidence linking its products to various diseases by supporting scientific research. The purpose of this research was "to refute unfavorable findings or at a minimum to keep the scientific question open" {2205.01, p. 1}. In addition, Pepples states:

> *The significant expenditures on the question of smoking and health have allowed the industry to take a respectable stand along the following lines— "After millions of dollars and over twenty years of research, the question about smoking and health is still open"* [emphasis added]. {2205.01, p. 1–2}

The Tobacco Industry Research Committee (TIRC), formed jointly by US tobacco companies in 1954, was the primary institution that helped the industry promote this message. (TIRC was renamed the Council for Tobacco Research–U.S.A. [CTR] in 1964. We will therefore refer to this organization as TIRC when discussing periods from 1954 to 1964 and as CTR when discussing periods after 1964.) By 1985 CTR's annual budget reached $11,278,000.

The industry stated publicly that it was forming TIRC in response to scientific reports suggesting a link between smoking and lung cancer, and that the purpose of TIRC was to fund independent scientific research to determine whether these reports were true. However, the documents show that TIRC was actually formed for public relations purposes, to convince the public that the hazards of smoking had not been definitively proven.

The formation of TIRC is described in detail in a series of internal memos from the public relations firm of Hill and Knowlton, Inc. (H&K), which was hired by the tobacco companies in 1953 to help them devise a public relations campaign (12). The H&K memos state that late in 1953 the president of American Tobacco, Paul M. Hahn, sent telegrams to the presidents of the other major tobacco companies, inviting them to meet in New York to develop a campaign to counter the negative publicity surrounding cigarettes. The meeting was convened on December 15, 1953, at the Plaza Hotel in New York City and was attended by the presidents of American Tobacco Company, Benson & Hedges, Brown and Williamson, P. Lorillard, Philip Morris, R. J. Reynolds, and U.S. Tobacco, as well as the chief executives of Hill and Knowlton. The president of Liggett & Myers was invited to the meeting but did not attend (12). (Liggett & Myers did join TIRC on March 5, 1964, but resigned four years later, on January 8, 1968 {1920.01, p. 23}.)

Following the meeting, H&K submitted a proposal regarding the tobacco industry's public relations campaign (12). H&K recommended that the tobacco companies jointly form a research committee that would sponsor independent scientific research on the health effects of smoking. In addition, an announcement describing the formation of the research committee should be distributed widely as news and placed as an advertisement in newspapers and magazines nationwide. The tobacco industry followed Hill and Knowlton's advice. On January 4, 1954, the industry announced formation of the Tobacco Industry Research Committee (TIRC) in an advertisement titled "A Frank Statement to Cigarette Smokers" (figure 2.1). This advertisement appeared in 448 newspapers in 258 cities, reaching an estimated circulation of 43,245,000 (12). The advertisement states,

> Recent reports on experiments with mice [conducted by Wynder, Graham, and Croninger (2), who found that painting mice with tobacco tar caused cancer] have given wide publicity to a theory that cigarette smoking is in some way linked with lung cancer in human beings. . . . Many people have asked

A Frank Statement

to Cigarette Smokers

RECENT REPORTS on experiments with mice have given wide publicity to a theory that cigarette smoking is in some way linked with lung cancer in human beings.

Although conducted by doctors of professional standing, these experiments are not regarded as conclusive in the field of cancer research. However, we do not believe that any serious medical research, even though its results are inconclusive should be disregarded or lightly dismissed.

At the same time, we feel it is in the public interest to call attention to the fact that eminent doctors and research scientists have publicly questioned the claimed significance of these experiments.

Distinguished authorities point out:

1. That medical research of recent years indicates many possible causes of lung cancer.

2. That there is no agreement among the authorities regarding what the cause is.

3. That there is no proof that cigarette smoking is one of the causes.

4. That statistics purporting to link cigarette smoking with the disease could apply with equal force to any one of many other aspects of modern life. Indeed the validity of the statistics themselves is questioned by numerous scientists.

We accept an interest in people's health as a basic responsibility, paramount to every other consideration in our business.

We believe the products we make are not injurious to health.

We always have and always will cooperate closely with those whose task it is to safeguard the public health.

For more than 300 years tobacco has given solace, relaxation, and enjoyment to mankind. At one time or another during those years critics have held it responsible for practically every disease of the human body. One by one these charges have been abandoned for lack of evidence.

Regardless of the record of the past, the fact that cigarette smoking today should even be suspected as a cause of a serious disease is a matter of deep concern to us.

Many people have asked us what we are doing to meet the public's concern aroused by the recent reports. Here is the answer:

1. We are pledging aid and assistance to the research effort into all phases of tobacco use and health. This joint financial aid will of course be in addition to what is already being contributed by individual companies.

2. For this purpose we are establishing a joint industry group consisting initially of the undersigned. This group will be known as TOBACCO INDUSTRY RESEARCH COMMITTEE.

3. In charge of the research activities of the Committee will be a scientist of unimpeachable integrity and national repute. In addition there will be an Advisory Board of scientists disinterested in the cigarette industry. A group of distinguished men from medicine, science, and education will be invited to serve on this Board. These scientists will advise the Committee on its research activities.

This statement is being issued because we believe the people are entitled to know where we stand on this matter and what we intend to do about it.

TOBACCO INDUSTRY RESEARCH COMMITTEE

5400 EMPIRE STATE BUILDING, NEW YORK 1, N. Y.

SPONSORS:

THE AMERICAN TOBACCO COMPANY, INC.
Paul M. Hahn, President

BENSON & HEDGES
Joseph F. Cullman, Jr., President

BRIGHT BELT WAREHOUSE ASSOCIATION
F. S. Royster, President

BROWN & WILLIAMSON TOBACCO CORPORATION
Timothy V. Hartnett, President

BURLEY AUCTION WAREHOUSE ASSOCIATION
Albert Clay, President

BURLEY TOBACCO GROWERS COOPERATIVE ASSOCIATION
John W. Jones, President

LARUS & BROTHER COMPANY, INC.
W. T. Reed, Jr., President

LORILLARD COMPANY
Herbert A. Kent, Chairman

MARYLAND TOBACCO GROWERS ASSOCIATION
Samuel C. Linton, General Manager

PHILLIP MORRIS & CO., LTD., INC.
O. Parker McComas, President

R. J. REYNOLDS TOBACCO COMPANY
E. A. Darr, President

STEPHANO BROTHERS, INC.
C. S. Stephano, D'Sc., Director of Research

TOBACCO ASSOCIATES, INC.
(An organization of flue-cured tobacco growers)
J. B. Hutson, President

UNITED STATES TOBACCO COMPANY
J. W. Peterson, President

Figure 2.1. The tobacco industry ran this advertisement in January 1954 announcing the creation of the Tobacco Industry Research Committee in response to growing public concern that smoking causes cancer.

us what we are doing to meet the public's concern aroused by the recent reports. Here is the answer:

1.   We are pledging aid and assistance to the research effort into all
phases of tobacco use and health. . . .

2.   For this purpose we are establishing a joint industry group consisting initially of the undersigned. This group will be known as TOBACCO IN-
DUSTRY RESEARCH COMMITTEE.

3.   In charge of the research activities of the Committee will be a scientist of unimpeachable integrity and national repute. In addition there
will be an Advisory Board of scientists disinterested in the cigarette
industry. . . .

This statement is being issued because we believe the people are entitled to
know where we stand on this matter and what we intend to do about it.
{1901.01}

The "Frank Statement" advertisement also clearly expresses the tobacco industry's concern for the health of its customers:

*We accept an interest in people's health as a basic responsibility, paramount
to every other consideration in our business* [emphasis added]. {1901.01}

The documents demonstrate that in subsequent years the tobacco industry did not meet the goal it established for itself in 1954.

TIRC'S ORGANIZATION AND POLICY

A document on TIRC's general organization and policy {1903.03} states
that TIRC is independent of the industry and that its purpose is to fund
research into the health effects of tobacco. Although this document was
prepared for internal use by B&W staff, it contains the same statements
about the role of TIRC that were made publicly at the time—possibly because it was written by a member of B&W's public relations department.

The Tobacco Industry Research Committee is the sponsoring agency of a research program into questions of tobacco use and health. It was organized in
early 1954 by representatives of tobacco manufacturers, growers and ware-
housemen.

Shortly after organization, the T.I.R.C. invited doctors and scientists who
were well known for their work in cancer and other diseases to serve on a
Scientific Advisory Board to administer a grants-in-aid program. This Board
currently consists of nine scientists who maintain their respective institutional
affiliations.

Grants by the Board through 1962 have been made to nearly 140 scientists in over 90 hospitals, universities, and research institutions from funds
that now total $6,250,000 appropriated by the T.I.R.C. {1903.03, p. 1}

The document then discusses the role of TIRC's Scientific Advisory Board (SAB), which was always described as being an independent group of scientists that had complete control over awarding funding.

> *The Scientific Advisory Board has full responsibility for research policy and programming.* As a Board it does not directly engage in research for the T.I.R.C. and the T.I.R.C. itself does not operate any research facility.
>
> *Grants-in-aid for research are made by the Board to independent scientists who are assured complete scientific freedom in conducting their research.* They alone are responsible for reporting or publishing their findings in the accepted scientific manner—through medical and scientific journals and societies. From the outset, the Tobacco Industry Research Committee has made clear that the object of its research program is to encourage scientific study for facts about tobacco use and health. Its position is that research will help provide the knowledge about lung cancer and heart disease for a full evaluation of all factors being studied in connection with these diseases [emphasis added]. {1903.03, p. 1}

Table 2.1 lists the members of TIRC's and CTR's advisory boards from 1964 through 1994. In general, the members of the SAB were well-respected academic researchers whose presence lent credibility to CTR. TIRC and CTR also had a scientific director who was responsible for outlining a research program and allocating research funds to best advance this program {1920.01, p. 34}. However, as described in chapter 8, the SAB and the scientific director did not always make the final decisions about which projects could be funded by CTR. Tobacco industry lawyers were responsible for many of the funding decisions. Nevertheless, in all the public statements that the industry has released over the years, it has staunchly maintained that TIRC, and later CTR, was an independent organization devoted to determining the health effects of tobacco. As we show later in this section and in chapter 8, however, the industry privately admitted that the main purpose of TIRC was public relations: to keep the "controversy" over smoking and health alive.

The document on TIRC's organization and policy also describes its position on the health effects of tobacco—namely, that the links between smoking and disease had not been proven and that more research was needed to determine the role of tobacco in various diseases.

> During the past year, the Tobacco Industry Research Committee has continued and extended its support of research.
>
> While these research studies have increased our factual knowledge, they have at the same time continued to make clear and to emphasize the great and critical gaps in that knowledge. . . .

TABLE 2.1   MEMBERS OF TIRC/CTR
SCIENTIFIC ADVISORY BOARD

Name	Affiliation	Dates of Service
Howard B. Andervont, ScD	Scientific Editor, Journal of the National Cancer Institute.	4/20/64 to 12/31/66; 1970 to 12/31/74
Richard J. Bing, MD	Professor of Medicine, Washington University; Director, Washington University Medical Service, V.A. Hospital; Professor and Chairman, Dept. of Medicine, Wayne State University College of Medicine; Director of Cardiology and Intramural Medicine, Huntington Memorial Hospital; Professor of Medicine, University of Southern California School of Medicine; Director of Experimental Cardiology and Scientific Development, Huntington Medical Research Institute; Visiting Associate, California Institute of Technology.	6/6/58 to present[1]
Roswell K. Boutwell, PhD	Professor of Oncology, McArdle Laboratory for Cancer Research, University of Wisconsin.	7/28/80 to 5/31/84
Drummond H. Bowden, MD	Professor and Head, Department of Pathology, University of Manitoba Health Sciences Center.	4/24/81 to present[1]
Michael J. Brennan, MD	President and Medical Director, Michigan Cancer Foundation.	3/23/81 to present[1]
McKeen Cattell, PhD, MD	Professor of Pharmacology, Cornell University Medical College.	3/30/54 to 4/13/73
Julius H. Comroe, Jr., MD	Director, Cardiovascular Research Institute, University of California Medical Center; Chairman and Professor, University of Pennsylvania Graduate School of Medicine.	8/12/54 to 3/16/60
John E. Craighead, MD	Professor and Chairman, Department of Pathology, and Director of Laboratories, University of Vermont College of Medicine and Medical Center Hospital of Vermont.	11/76 to 10/77
Joseph D. Feldman, MD	Head, Department of Immunopathology, Scripps Clinic and Research Foundation; Member, Research Institute of Scripps Clinic; Editor, Journal of Immunology.	3/74 to present[1]
William U. Gardner, PhD	E. K. Hunt Professor of Anatomy, Yale University School of Medicine.	11/15/71 to 2/26/85
Peter M. Howley, MD	Laboratory of Pathology, National Cancer Institute.	7/7/82 to present[1]
Robert J. Huebner, MD	Chief, Viral Carcinogenesis Branch, National Cancer Institute; Chief, Laboratory of RNA Tumor Viruses, National Cancer Institute; Laboratory of Cellular and Molecular Biology, National Cancer Institute.	4/68 to 12/31/81

TABLE 2.1 *(continued)*

Name	Affiliation	Dates of Service
Leon O. Jacobson, MD	Professor and Chairman, Dept. of Medicine, Dean of the Division of Biological Sciences, Regenstein Professor of Biological Sciences, University of Chicago; Director, Argonne Cancer Research Hospital; Director, The Franklin McLean Memorial Research Institute.	4/5/54 to present[1]
Manfred L. Karnovsky, PhD	Harold T. White Professor of Biological Chemistry, Dept. of Biological Chemistry, Harvard Medical School.	5/3/85 to present[1]
Paul Kotin, MD	Paul Pierce Professor of Pathology, University of Southern California School of Medicine; Chief, Carcinogenesis Studies Branch and Associate Director of Field Studies, National Cancer Institute.	4/12/54 to 11/26/65
Averill A. Liebow, MD	Professor and Chairman, Department of Pathology, University of California School of Medicine, San Diego.	9/10/73 to 2/1/77
Clarence Cook Little, ScD, LLD, LittD	Director, Roscoe B. Jackson Memorial Laboratory.	3/31/54 to 12/23/71
Clayton G. Loosli, PhD, MD	Hastings Professor of Medicine and Pathology, University of Southern California School of Medicine.	10/19/66 to 8/1/73
Henry T. Lynch, MD	Professor and Chairman, Department of Preventive Medicine and Public Health, Creighton University School of Medicine; Professor of Medicine, President, Hereditary Cancer Institute, Creighton University School of Medicine.	11/15/73 to present[1]
Kenneth M. Lynch, MD, ScD, LLD	President, Dean of Faculty, Professor of Pathology, and Chancellor, Medical College of South Carolina.	3/31/54 to 11/29/74 (became board member emeritus in 1973)
Hans Meier, DVM, Dr.Med. Vet, MRSH	Senior Staff Scientist, The Jackson Laboratory.	10/31/71 to 5/14/81
G. Barry Pierce, MD	American Cancer Society Centennial Research Professor, University of Colorado Health Sciences Center.	3/18/82 to present[1]
Stanley P. Reimann, MD, ScD	Scientific Director, Institute for Cancer Research; Director, Lankenau Hospital Research Institute.	3/29/54 to 2/21/68
Gordon H. Sato, PhD	Professor of Biology, University of California, San Diego; Director, W. Alton Jones Cell Science Center.	4/28/80 to present[1]
William F. Rienhoff, Jr., MD	Professor of Surgery, Johns Hopkins University, School of Medicine.	4/2/54 to 9/19/72

TABLE 2.1   *(continued)*

Name	Affiliation	Dates of Service
Sheldon C. Sommers, MD	Professor of Pathology, Columbia University College of Physicians and Surgeons; Director of Laboratories, Lenox Hill Hospital.	7/66 to present[1]
Lee W. Wattenberg, MD	Professor of Pathology, Department of Laboratory Medicine and Pathology, University of Minnesota Medical School.	10/9/75 to 1/9/79
Edwin B. Wilson, PhD, LLD	Professor of Vital Statistics, Harvard University.	7/12/54 to 12/28/64
John P. Wyatt, MD	Professor and Head, Department of Pathology, University of Manitoba Faculty of Medicine; Director, Tobacco and Health Research Institute, University of Kentucky.	10/13/72 to 1/22/80

[1]"Present" is December 1994.
SOURCE: {1920.01, p. 28}.

The smoking of tobacco continues to be one of the subjects requiring study in the lung cancer problem, as do many other agents and influences in modern living. Science does not yet know enough about any suspected factors to judge whether they may operate alone, whether they may operate in conjunction with others, or whether they may affect or be affected by factors of whose existence science is not yet aware. Indeed, it is not known whether these factors actually are "causative" in any real sense.

As the tobacco industry continues its support of the search for truth and knowledge, it must recognize, as is always the case in true scientific research, there can be no promise of a quick answer. The important thing is to keep on adding to knowledge until the accumulative facts provide the basis for a sound conclusion. {1903.03, pp. 1–3}

THE ROLE OF HILL AND KNOWLTON

As described earlier, the Hill and Knowlton public relations firm was integral in the formation of TIRC. In fact, from 1954 to 1958, the tobacco industry's public relations activities were carried out at TIRC with the help of H&K staff (12). In 1958 several states began to propose tobacco regulations, and the industry decided that it needed a more vocal lobbying group than TIRC. The Tobacco Institute was formed in 1958 to take over the industry's lobbying and public relations needs (12). However, Hill and Knowlton continued to provide public relations guidance for both TIRC and the Tobacco Institute. This role of H&K is described in a memo from John V. Blalock (B&W public relations) to J. W. Burgard (B&W marketing){1902.05}. The memo begins:

> This organization [Hill and Knowlton] serves as the Public Relations Counsel to The Tobacco Institute and the Tobacco Industry Research Committee. It is so intimately involved in the affairs of both that a proper separation of functions, as well as a strict definition of operations, is virtually impossible in this brief summary.
>
> However, aside from performing the usual P.R. functions . . . Hill and Knowlton can be described as "straddling both T.I. and T.I.R.C. and acting as a buffer for each." {1902.05, p. 1}

The document then explains what he means by "buffer":

> Hill and Knowlton decides whether questions from outside individuals or organizations are to be directed to The Tobacco Institute or to the T.I.R.C. {1902.05, p. 1}

Blalock also mentions the substantial overlap of staffs between H&K, the Tobacco Institute, and TIRC. Two of H&K's staff members worked full-time on the Tobacco Institute account; in addition, William T. Hoyt of H&K was the executive director of TIRC as well as the executive secretary for TIRC's Scientific Advisory Board. "Without question, he [Hoyt] is the administrative head of T.I.R.C." {1902.05, p. 2}. The close relationship between H&K, the Tobacco Institute, and TIRC supports the hypothesis that all three were acting as arms of the tobacco industry's public relations efforts.

PUBLIC RELATIONS STATEMENTS ABOUT TIRC: CREATING A FALSE CONTROVERSY

The tobacco industry often referred to TIRC in its public relations statements. TIRC was used to reinforce the claim that there was a "controversy" regarding the health effects of smoking and that more research was needed. For example, a document titled "Cigarette Smoking and Health: What Are the Facts?" {1903.02}, written after the Royal College of Physicians report was issued (3), disputes the claim that there is "mounting evidence" against smoking and notes that TIRC is attempting to learn the answers to the smoking and health debate, since "medical science has not found the basic causes of lung cancer." The paper does not mention the increased risk of lung cancer among smokers and emphasizes the fact that most people who smoke do not get lung cancer, as though that somehow implies that smoking is not an important cause

of the disease. It diverts attention from any possible role cigarettes may play in the causation of lung cancer by noting that a wide variety of possible causes of lung disease are under study, including "viruses, previous lung ailments, air pollutants, heredity, stress and strain, and other factors." By pointing to the efforts made by TIRC and its Scientific Advisory Board in developing an understanding of the lung cancer problem, the paper, in effect, keeps alive the "controversy" about the dangers of smoking.

The "What Are the Facts" document begins by listing ten common questions about the dangers of smoking and then answering them with the tobacco industry's standard claim that the dangers had not been proven. For example:

> Is there "mounting evidence" to link cigarette smoking with lung cancer?
> The "evidence" is not medical in the usual sense, because clinical and experimental research does not bear out the anti-cigarette theory. There is no scientific cause-and-effect proof. Only statistical studies provide the "evidence." The curious thing is that most of what has been written against cigarette smoking in recent years is based on a relatively few statistical reports. The "mounting evidence" impression is mainly the result of mounting publicity, rather than scientific findings [emphasis in original]. {1903.02, p. 3}

The statement is grossly misleading. The answer to the question is (and was, of course) "yes," but neither "yes" nor "no" is offered. Instead, the answer seeks to sow doubt and confusion. The reader is led through a maze of different *types* of evidence mixed up with prejudicial but high-sounding language about medicine, science, clinical work, and experimental work, leaving the false impression that the association of cigarettes and lung cancer must be flimsy.

In the spring of 1962, the Royal College of Physicians issued the first major report reviewing the data on cigarettes and disease (3). Since "What Are the Facts" quotes from this report, it was available to the author. The report meticulously reviewed the literature and carefully evaluated all alternative explanations for the increase in lung cancer. Its conclusion, "Cigarette smoking is a cause of lung cancer and bronchitis," was the only reasonable one considering all the data available in 1962, and nothing that has been learned since then about smoking and disease has brought this conclusion into doubt. On the contrary, subsequent data have confirmed it many times over.

The "What Are the Facts" memo explains how the industry is responding to the scientific evidence linking its products to cancer and heart disease. Specifically, it describes the research being funded through TIRC.

The tobacco industry recognizes that it has a special responsibility to help find the true facts about tobacco and health. Since 1954, it has been supporting a program of independent research through the Tobacco Industry Research Committee.

 . . . These grants are made "with no strings attached" to encourage scientific study into the complex question of tobacco use and health. Scientific Director of the T.I.R.C. is Dr. Clarence Cook Little, world-renowned cancer researcher and for 16 years managing director of what is now the American Cancer Society.

The entire grants-in-aid program is administered by a Scientific Advisory Board of nine noted doctors, scientists, and educators. . . . They determine the research policy and award the grants for research. {1903.02, pp. 3–4}

"What Are the Facts?" also claims that much of the TIRC-supported research has raised uncertainty about the health dangers of smoking and suggests that other things are to blame, so as to deflect attention away from tobacco.

[TIRC research] emphasizes that many clinical and experimental factors still need to be identified, investigated, and evaluated regarding the origin of lung cancer and other diseases. Actually, the number of suspects under study in lung cancer has broadened and now includes viruses, previous lung ailments, air pollutants, heredity, stress and strain, and other factors. {1903.02, p. 4}

Another document summarizes the TIRC's "Position of Tobacco and Health Issue":

While these [TIRC-funded] research studies have increased our factual knowledge, they have at the same time continued to make clear and to emphasize the great and critical gaps in that knowledge. They have confirmed the soundness of the position held and expressed by the T.I.R.C.

This position is that there does not exist the essential experimental and clinical knowledge with which science can even define or identify the multiple factors or influences that may contribute to the origin and progress of these diseases.

 . . . As the tobacco industry continues its support of the search for truth and knowledge, it must recognize, as is always the case in true scientific research, *there can be no promise of a quick answer.* The important thing is to keep on adding to knowledge until the accumulative facts provide the basis for a sound conclusion [emphasis added]. {1903.03, pp. 2, 3}

These statements make it clear that the tobacco industry believed that TIRC-supported research was accomplishing one of its goals of perpetuating controversy about the adverse effects of tobacco.

A document entitled "10 Assertions about Smoking and Health vs. the True Facts," dated October 3, 1967, advises tobacco industry employees on how to respond to data on the adverse health effects of tobacco. In a foreword to the document, E. P. Finch, president of B&W, states:

> Keeping accurately informed on the smoking and health controversy is an increasing problem. Many assertions are being made which tend to condemn smoking and the tobacco industry. Headlines carry these assertions as "news." Unfortunately, the other side is sometimes overlooked.
>
> And there is another side to the controversy! The following section states and gives factual replies to 10 of the most common assertions. {1903.01, p. 1}

The responses to the assertions rely heavily on CTR regular and special projects for support, demonstrating how the projects were used to criticize data on the adverse effects of tobacco. To counter the assertion "All doctors are convinced that smoking is dangerous," the document suggests the following response:

> Doctors are by no means unanimous in condemning smoking. . . . For example, some of the country's most eminent men of medicine and science— from such renowned institutions as Bellevue Hospital, Columbia University Medical School, Yale University Medical School, and New York Medical College—have testified before the U.S. Congress that the charges against tobacco remain unproved. {1903.01, p. 4}

A document entitled "Those Who Expressed Doubt before United States Congress of Smoking-Disease Relationship" contains excerpts of official testimony before the Senate Committee on Commerce and the House Committee on Interstate and Foreign Commerce in 1965. It states:

> Over 30 of this country' most eminent men of medicine and science have submitted their views before the United States Congress that the charges against tobacco remain unproved. They gave detailed evidence as to why they are unwilling to accept statistical evidence as scientific proof of a causal relationship between cigarette smoking and human disease. {1903.07, p. 1}

Five of the thirty scientists (Joseph H. Ogura, M.D., professor of otolaryngology at Washington University in St. Louis; Theodor D. Sterling, Ph.D., professor of biostatistics at the University of Cincinnati; Hiram Langston, M.D., chief of surgery at the Chicago State Tuberculosis Sanitorium; R. H. Rigdon, M.D., professor of pathology at the University of Texas, Galveston; and Henry I. Russek, M.D., former director of cardiovascular research at the US Public Health Service Hospital in Staten

Island, New York) later received funding through CTR's Special Projects Division, which was administered by tobacco industry lawyers and was used to produce scientific data that would be useful to the industry (see chapter 8).

THE EVOLVING ROLE OF CTR

Although CTR was originally formed as a public relations instrument, its role and importance to the tobacco industry evolved over the years. This evolution is described in an April 4, 1978, memo from Ernest Pepples to J. E. Edens, chairman and CEO of B&W.

> *Originally, CTR was organized as a public relations effort.* The industry told the world CTR would look at the diseases which were being associated with smoking. There was even a suggestion by our political spokesmen that if a harmful element turned up[,] the industry would try to root it out. *The research of CTR also discharged a legal responsibility.* The manufacturer has a duty to know its product. The Scientific Advisory Board composed of highly reputable independent scientists constitutes a place where the present state of the art is constantly being updated. Theoretically SAB is showing us the way in a highly complex field. *There is another political need for research. Recently it has been suggested that CTR or industry research should enable us to give quick responses to new developments in the propaganda of the avid anti-smoking groups.* For example, CTR or someone should be able to rebut the suggestion that smokers suffer from a peculiar disease, as widely alleged in the press some few months ago. . . . *Finally the industry research effort has included special projects designed to find scientists and medical doctors who might serve as industry witnesses in lawsuits or in a legislative forum.* All of these matters and more should be considered in asking what kind of research the industry should do [emphasis added]. {2010.02, p. 2}

Pepples's description of CTR is remarkable in several respects. First, he confirms that CTR was formed for public relations purposes. In addition, he notes that CTR has served as a political and legal shield for the industry over the years. Finally, he states outright that CTR's "special projects" were designed to develop research data and scientists that could be used to defend the industry in court and legislative efforts (see chapter 8). All these statements contrast sharply with CTR's publicly stated goal of determining the truth regarding the health effects of smoking.

Similar views on the importance of CTR were expressed by Bill Shinn of Shook, Hardy, and Bacon, a law firm that represents tobacco companies. Shinn's comments are summarized by Pepples in a memo to C. I. McCarty, B&W's chairman and chief operating officer {2010.03}. The memo is marked "privileged" and is dated September 29, 1978. In it Pepples notes that, according to Shinn, CTR is valuable to the industry because it provides legal protection as well as political and public relations advantages.

> Bill [Shinn] mentions two aspects of particular value in CTR: (1) the direct legal protection derived by Brown & Williamson and (2) the political and public relations advantage accruing to the industry. {2010.03}

With regard to legal protection, Pepples mentions the *Monroe* case against Kool cigarettes, evidently an unreported case or one that was dismissed or settled. He notes that B&W was asked in this case to describe what it had done to keep abreast of the science concerning its product.

> Our reply tells about the ten imminent [*sic*] scientists who serve on the SAB in an advisory capacity at CTR and it tells about the grants which CTR has made over 10 years. Stated another way, our answer says CTR is our window on the world of smoking and health research. *This avoids the research dilemma presented to a responsible manufacturer of cigarettes, which on the one hand needs to know the state of the art and on the other hand cannot afford the risk of having in-house work turn sour* [emphasis added]. {2010.03}

Pepples then discusses a problem faced by Liggett. Liggett had filed a report written by an outside lab in support of a patent application, and the report had stated that tumorigenicity was reduced when a particular catalyst was added to the tobacco blend. A newspaper in Charlotte, North Carolina, in a front-page story based on the patent application, declared that Liggett had admitted to laboratory proof of a causal relationship between cigarettes and cancer. Pepples states,

> *The point here is the value of having CTR doing work in a nondirected and independent fashion as contrasted with work either in-house or under B&W contract which, if it goes wrong, can become the smoking pistol in a lawsuit* [emphasis added]. {2010.03}

In other words, CTR gave the tobacco industry not only an opportunity to develop the scientific information it needed to protect its interests but also some insulation against liability for results that could prove to be legally embarrassing. When the work supported the industry's position, it could be trumpeted; when it supported the case against smoking—as in Gary Friedman's work on smoking and heart disease (13), discussed in chapter 8—the industry could walk away from it.

The documents show a marked contrast between what the tobacco industry was saying publicly and what it was saying privately about the purpose of TIRC, and later CTR. Publicly, the industry maintained, and continues to maintain, that the primary purpose of TIRC and CTR has been to fund independent research to determine whether smoking is truly hazardous to health. Privately, however, lawyers for B&W stated that CTR's primary purpose was to allow the tobacco industry to argue that there was a "controversy" about tobacco's effects and that more research was needed to resolve the "controversy." Furthermore, CTR provided legal and political protection for the industry. Beginning in 1966, CTR began to fund "special projects," which were awarded not by CTR's Scientific Advisory Board but by tobacco industry lawyers. This special project funding was not disclosed to the public. As we show in chapter 8, CTR's special projects were used to develop scientific evidence that the tobacco industry could use selectively to defend itself in court, for public relations purposes, and to influence public policy. Developing data for defense is not in itself problematic, of course. But questions do arise when the research is done in secret, so that only favorable results need be shown; when the fact of industry support for what does get published is concealed from the public; and when the attorney-client privilege is invoked in spite of claims that all relevant information will be made public.

INDUSTRY REACTION TO THE 1964 SURGEON GENERAL'S REPORT

At the same time that the tobacco industry was publicly claiming that there was no scientific proof that smoking is dangerous to health, official agencies in the United States and the United Kingdom produced two major reports on the health effects of smoking. The first was the 1962 report of the British Royal College of Physicians (RCP).

RCP REPORT, 1962

The RCP established a committee in 1959 to examine the data about smoking and health. The committee reviewed the scientific literature and considered all the various explanations that had been put forth about the rise in lung cancer cases and, in particular, about the more common occurrence of lung cancer among people who smoked. The committee also reviewed data pertaining to other conditions thought related to smoking. The Royal College issued its report on March 7, 1962, at a press conference headed by Sir Robert Platt, president of the college. The major conclusions were these:

The benefits of smoking are almost entirely psychological and social. It may help some people to avoid obesity. There is no reason to suppose that smoking prevents neurosis.

Cigarette smoking is a cause of lung cancer and bronchitis, and probably contributes to the development of coronary heart disease and various other less common diseases. It delays healing of gastric and duodenal ulcers.

The risks of smoking to the individual are calculated from death rates in relation to smoking habits among British doctors. The chance of dying in the next ten years for a man aged 35 who is a heavy cigarette smoker is 1 in 23, whereas the risk for a non-smoker is only 1 in 90. Only 15% (one in six) of men this age who are non-smokers but 33% (one in three) of heavy smokers will die before the age of 65. Not all this difference in expectation of life is attributable to smoking.

The number of deaths caused by diseases associated with smoking is large. (3, p. S7)

Thirty thousand copies of the report had been sold in the United States by May. *Reader's Digest* and *Scientific American,* among other publications, gave prominence to articles based on it (14, 15).

The tobacco industry's official statement in response to the RCP report avoided direct disagreement with it but called it "incomplete." The *British Medical Journal* reported,

> On publication of the Royal College of Physicians' report the Tobacco Manufacturers' Standing Committee stated: 'The R.C.P. Committee was set up to consider the effects on health of both smoking and air pollution. By deferring to a separate report its consideration of air pollution the R.C.P. Committee has recognized the importance and complexity of this factor, but in so doing the Committee has, in T.M.S.C.'s view, produced an incomplete assessment of the problems involved.' The Tobacco Manufacturers' Standing Committee regards the three following approaches in research as 'both practical and essential': (a) 'A study of environment and personal characteristics, as well as past medical histories,' may throw important new light on the incidence of lung cancer and chronic bronchitis. (b) 'Much more research is undoubtedly needed into the constituents and effects of air pollution.' (c) 'Further investigation is needed into the chemistry and biological effects of tobacco smoke.' (16, p. 810)

The Tobacco Manufacturers' Standing Committee (TMSC), formed in 1956 by the British tobacco companies, was modeled on the American TIRC. TMSC, like TIRC, funded independent researchers to study issues related to smoking and health. Unlike TIRC, however, TMSC also conducted in-house research at a jointly sponsored industry laboratory in Harrogate, England, The Harrogate laboratory was opened in 1962. It conducted several large-scale studies on the effects of tobacco smoke inhalation and skin painting in mice (to study cancer) and also did some work on nicotine (see chapters 3 and 4). Shortly after the Harrogate lab was opened, TMSC was renamed the Tobacco Research Council (TRC). The name was later changed again to the Tobacco Advisory Committee (TAC) {1014.01, pp. 11–12}.

US SURGEON GENERAL'S REPORT, 1964

Shortly after release of the RCP report, the US Surgeon General set up the Surgeon General's Advisory Committee on Smoking and Health to produce a similar report on the effects of smoking. The tobacco industry was allowed to veto any proposed member of the advisory committee that it deemed was not impartial on the issue of smoking and health. The committee therefore consisted entirely of scientists who had not yet publicly expressed any opinion about the health effects of smoking and who were willing to look impartially at the evidence. After working for fourteen months, the advisory committee released its report in 1964.

The major conclusions of the 1964 Surgeon General's report, *Smoking and Health* (4), were these:

The Effects of Smoking: Principal Findings

Cigarette smoking is associated with a 70 percent increase in the age-specific death rates of males. The total number of excess deaths causally related to cigarette smoking in the U.S. population cannot be accurately estimated. In view of the continuing and mounting evidence from many sources, it is the judgment of the Committee that cigarette smoking contributes substantially to mortality from certain specific diseases and to the overall death rate.

Lung Cancer

Cigarette smoking is causally related to lung cancer in men; the magnitude of the effect of cigarette smoking far outweighs all other factors. The data for women, though less extensive, point in the same direction.

The risk of developing lung cancer increases with duration of smoking and the number of cigarettes smoked per day, and is diminished by discontinuing smoking. In comparison with non-smokers, average male smokers of cigarettes have approximately a 9- to 10-fold risk of developing lung cancer and heavy smokers at least a 20-fold risk.

The risk of developing cancer of the lung for the combined group of pipe smokers, cigar smokers, and pipe and cigar smokers is greater than for non-smokers, but much less than for cigarette smokers.

Cigarette smoking is much more important than occupational exposures in the causation of lung cancer in the general population.

Chronic Bronchitis and Emphysema

Cigarette smoking is the most important of the causes of chronic bronchitis in the United States, and increases the risk of dying from chronic bronchitis and emphysema. A relationship exists between cigarette smoking and emphysema but it has not been established that the relationship is causal.

Studies demonstrate that fatalities from this illness are infrequent among non-smokers.

For the bulk of the population of the United States, the relative importance of cigarette smoking as a cause of chronic broncho-pulmonary disease is much greater than atmospheric pollution or occupational exposures.

Cardiovascular Diseases

It is established that male cigarette smokers have a higher death rate from coronary artery disease than non-smoking males. Although the causative role of cigarette smoking in deaths from coronary disease is not proven, the Committee considers it more prudent from the public health viewpoint to assume that the established association has causative meaning than to suspend judgment until no uncertainty remains.

Although a causal relationship has not been established, higher mortality of cigarette smokers is associated with many other cardiovascular diseases, including miscellaneous circulatory diseases, other heart diseases, hypertensive heart disease, and general arteriosclerosis.

Other Cancer Sites

Pipe smoking appears to be causally related to lip cancer. Cigarette smoking is a significant factor in the causation of cancer of the larynx. The evidence supports the belief that an association exists between tobacco use and cancer of the esophagus, and between cigarette smoking and cancer of the urinary bladder in men, but the data are not adequate to decide whether these relationships are causal.

Data on an association between smoking and cancer of the stomach are contradictory and incomplete. (4, pp. 31–32)

After discussing the role of nicotine in tobacco use and recognizing that tobacco use is "reinforced and perpetuated by the pharmacological actions of nicotine" (p. 32), the committee offered the following summary conclusion:

On the basis of prolonged study and evaluation of many lines of converging evidence, the Committee makes the following judgment:

Cigarette smoking is a health hazard of sufficient importance in the United States to warrant appropriate remedial action [emphasis in original]. (4, p. 33)

REACTIONS BY BAT AND B&W

As we discuss in chapters 4 and 5, BAT responded to the RCP report with what appears to be a genuine desire to identify and remove any harmful elements in cigarette smoke. There also appears to have been a spirit of cooperation between different cigarette manufacturers in the United Kingdom, and the British companies stated that they would share any information that would help produce a "safe" cigarette.

The response was quite different in the United States. Even before the US Surgeon General's 1964 report was released, B&W's public relations personnel and its lawyers were discussing how the company and the industry should respond. Despite public commitments to participate openly in the debate over the "smoking and health controversy," as pledged in the "Frank Statement" a decade earlier, B&W and BAT withheld important research findings on nicotine addiction from the Surgeon General's Advisory Committee, which had requested that the industry provide its relevant research. As described in the memos that follow and in chapter 3, B&W appears to have been motivated primarily by a desire to protect itself against regulation and litigation while maintaining its bottom line.

A "GRAVE CRISIS": B&W'S PUBLIC RELATIONS

The level of concern that the Surgeon General's report aroused in the industry's public relations departments is indicated in a report from John V. Blalock, director of public relations for B&W, to J. W. Burgard of B&W's Marketing Department {1902.01}. A copy of this report was also delivered to B&W's president, E. P. Finch. The report is dated June 18, 1963, six months before the Surgeon General's report was actually released.

In this report Blalock discusses meetings he held with various representatives from the Tobacco Institute, the Tobacco Industry Research Committee, and the public relations firm of Hill and Knowlton regarding how the industry as a whole should respond to the Surgeon General's report.

> The consensus is that the industry is in a "grave crisis," and the philosophy is "to expect the worst and work for the best." Of course the greatest cause for alarm is the forthcoming Surgeon General's report, which is expected to be detrimental to the industry. The only degree of hope is the possibility that, instead of singling out tobacco per se, the report will take into account a list of other agents (environmental and otherwise) which are suspect. However, this is deemed a rather dim hope, because indications point to a strong indictment of tobacco, with possible "root-shaking" consequences. {1902.01, pp. 1–2}

Blalock speaks of "an unmistakable note of pessimism" throughout these discussions {1902.01, p. 2} because of the threat of "mounting organized opposition" against tobacco. Those who attended these meetings were particularly fearful that extensive press coverage of anti-smoking reports being issued by organizations such as the American Cancer Society and the American Heart Association would convince the public to accept whatever was said in the Surgeon General's report {1902.01, p. 2}.

Blalock also states that he expects the Surgeon General's report to consist of two phases. First, the Surgeon General will probably release his scientific findings based on a review of the data. Blalock recommends that public relations during this phase be handled by TIRC, which could provide tobacco industry–generated data, with guidance from H&K {1902.01, p. 2}. The second phase will consist of a recommendation for legislative or government action, such as labeling, stricter regulation of advertising, or regulation by the Food and Drug Administration. This phase, Blalock advises, should be handled by the Tobacco Institute, also with guidance from H&K {1902.01, p. 2}.

Apparently, however, neither of these organizations felt prepared to handle the situation that was about to confront them.

> [There are] feelings of frustration, inadequacy, and fear that exist among those engaged in representing the tobacco industry on an organized front. However, perhaps this is more healthy than it would seem at first blush. At least these people want to do something in the face of mounting opposition. They want direction—an opportunity to take effective measures in the interest of the industry. {1902.01, p. 3}

Blalock also discusses the reasons for the industry's current state of underpreparedness. He points to a lack of cooperation among the tobacco companies in developing a public relations strategy and notes that the industry's public relations strategy has been affected by legal concerns, and that it would be unwise to assure the public that cigarettes were not dangerous to health.

> Litigations, of course, have vastly affected the Public Relations posture—and understandably so. *Certainly, no one can quarrel with the urgent necessity of complying with the lawyers' position in regard to assumption of risk. It would be foolhardy indeed to take a form of "aggressive" action which implies assurances, denial of harm, and similar claims* [emphasis added]. {1902.01, pp. 3–4}

Blalock concludes his report by reiterating that the industry does not have a plan of action and by recommending that strong leadership will be needed to steer the industry through the crisis.

[T]he great specter of the Surgeon General's Report looms before us, and the inescapable fact remains that the industry, at the moment, does not have a definite plan of action or reaction. There is talk of possibilities—the first step in planning. Yet the disturbing element is that no one seems disposed to suggest measures for meeting these possibilities. Everyone admits to a "wait-and-see" attitude, but this is without individual endorsement. Invariably, the burden of inaction is placed on "a lack of direction" and the need for "policy decisions."

I would suggest that the time is most propitious for leadership in shoring up industry organization and planning. Such leadership should be applied on all levels of participation—Executive, Legal, Trade, and Public Relations. I see Brown & Williamson as having both this opportunity and obligation. {1902.01, p. 4}

The Blalock report indicates that tobacco companies in the United States felt that the release of the 1964 Surgeon General's report on smoking and health would dramatically alter public perception of their product and would probably lead to government regulation of tobacco. The industry's public relations departments were unsure how they should respond to the report and were scrambling to develop a new strategy that would maintain public acceptance of tobacco while minimizing the potential for lawsuits.

"AN AGGRESSIVE POSTURE": B&W'S LEGAL DEPARTMENT

Just as the tobacco industry's public relations personnel were struggling to develop a strategy for responding to the Surgeon General's report, industry lawyers were analyzing its legal implications—specifically, how to ward off potential lawsuits accusing the tobacco companies of failing to warn consumers about the dangers of smoking once the Surgeon General had issued a statement stating that cigarettes were dangerous to health.

One of the documents {1802.05} describes a strategy proposed by Addison Yeaman, who was B&W's vice president and general counsel at the time. Yeaman's main suggestion is that the industry should engage in a massive program of scientific research to identify and remove any carcinogens present in tobacco smoke. Yeaman begins by stating that his comments are based on an assumption that the Surgeon General's report will conclude that there is a link between smoking and cancer. He recommends that the industry respond by financing an elaborate research campaign to make cigarettes less harmful. While making this suggestion, however, he implies that he believes cigarettes are, in fact, harmful to health.

We must, I think, recognize that in defense of the industry and in preservation of its present earnings position, the industry must either a) disprove the theory of causal relationship or b) discover the carcinogen or carcinogens, co-carcinogens, or whatever, and demonstrate our ability to remove or neutralize them. This means that we must embark—in whatever form of organization—on massive and impressively financed research into the etiology of cancer as it relates to the use of tobacco. . . . *Certainly one would hope to prove there is no etiological factor in smoke but the odds are greatly against success in that effort. At the best, the probabilities are that some combination of constituents of smoke will be found conducive to the onset of cancer or to create an environment in which cancer is more likely to occur* [emphasis added]. {1802.05, p. 1}

Yeaman then explains why the Tobacco Industry Research Committee (TIRC), which had ostensibly been created by the industry to fund research into the health effects of smoking, would not be appropriate for the type of research program he is proposing.

[TIRC] *was conceived as a public relations gesture and (however undefiled the Scientific Advisory Board and its grants may be) it has functioned as a public relations operation.* . . . I suggest that for the new research effort we enlist the cooperation of the Surgeon General, the Public Health Service, the American Cancer Society, the American Heart Association, American Medical Association and any and all other responsible health agencies or medical or scientific associations concerned with the question of tobacco and health. The new effort should be conducted by a new organization lavishly financed, autonomous, self-perpetuating, and uncontrolled save that its efforts be confined to the single problem of the relation of tobacco to human health [emphasis added]. {1802.05, p. 2}

At first glance, Yeaman's statements appear to be motivated by a genuine desire to develop a "safe" cigarette. He later makes clear, however, that a motivation behind this proposal is to allow the industry to be more vocal in its attacks on scientific research suggesting a causal link between smoking and disease.

[To engage in the proposed research campaign] would, I suggest, free the industry to take a much more aggressive posture to meet attack. It would in particular free the industry to attack the Surgeon General's Report itself by pointing out its gaps and omissions, its reliance on statistics, its lack of clinical evidence, etc., etc. True we might worsen our situation in litigation, but that I would risk in contemplation of the greater benefits to be derived from going on the offensive. {1802.05, p. 2}

Yeaman is saying that B&W can both do good and do well: develop a safe cigarette to meet critics on positive turf.

This new offensive strike, Yeaman argues, should be carried out by a stronger and more aggressive Tobacco Institute in response to any regulation that might be imposed following release of the Surgeon General's report—for instance, stricter regulation of advertising and requirements for warning labels or content labels.

> To meet these threats, which will arise not merely at the Federal but at the state level as well, the Tobacco Institute is available but it can be effective only if the industry abandons its timorous approach to the Institute as a functioning trade association. {1802.05, p. 3}

Furthermore, Yeaman recommends that the industry voluntarily agree to use warning labels on its products in order to protect itself from future litigation.

> The question immediately arises: how would such aggressive posture affect litigation? With one exception (Green v. American Tobacco Co.) those actions which have gone to judgement were won by the defendants on the defense of assumption of risk. The issuance of the Surgeon General's Report will, in my opinion, insure the success of that defense as to causes of action arising in the future <u>if the industry can steel itself to issuing a warning</u>. *I have no wish to be tarred and feathered, but I would suggest that the industry might serve itself on several fronts if it voluntarily adopted a package legend such as "excessive use of this product may be injurious to health of susceptible persons" and would embody such a legend in pica in its print advertising.* This is so controversial a suggestion—indeed shocking—that I would rather not try to anticipate the arguments against it in this note but reserve my defense [italic emphasis added]. {1802.05, p. 3}

Yeaman continues his memo by reviewing the likely conclusions of the Surgeon General's report and by reflecting further on how the industry should respond.

> But cigarettes—we will assume the Surgeon General's Committee to say—despite the beneficent effect of nicotine, have certain *unattractive side effects:*
> 1) They cause, or predispose to, lung cancer.
> 2) They contribute to certain cardiovascular disorders.
> 3) They may well be truly causative in emphysema, etc., etc.
>
> We challenge those charges and we have assumed our obligation to determine their truth or falsity by creating the new Tobacco Research Foundation [the hypothetical new research agency]. In the meantime (we say) here is our triple, or quadruple or quintuple filter, capable of removing whatever constituent of smoke is currently suspect while delivering full flavor—and incidentally—a nice jolt of nicotine. And if we are the <u>first</u> to be able to make and sustain that claim, what price Kent? [italic emphasis added]. {1802.05, pp. 4–5}

Yeaman concludes by stating that, if B&W were able to develop a "safe" cigarette, it would be morally obliged to make that knowledge available to other companies. However, he adds, the most important thing is that "we get there firstest with the mostest" {1802.05, p. 5}.

The notion that tobacco companies should engage in certain types of research for legal or political reasons is echoed in another document from the same era. This letter, dated January 2, 1964, and addressed to B&W's president, is marked "private and confidential." Unfortunately, the signature at the end is illegible. However, the return address is BAT's Millbank office, and the contents of the letter suggest that it was written by someone fairly high up in BAT's corporate structure, because it recommends that B&W consider conducting biological tests in case the company is called to testify about the health effects of its products.

> We have been coming to the view that Brown & Williamson, and possibly other Companies in the [BAT] Group, should pay more direct attention to biological tests. We have been fortified in this view by the recent visit of Mr. [Ed] Jacob [of the law firm Jacob and Medinger] who referred to the possibility of a Congressional enquiry at which various cigarette companies might be called upon to testify as to the real efficacy of their filters and the methods by which such efficacy has (or has not) been established.
>
> . . .
>
> I suggest that in view of the repeated Industry statements that more research is needed and is being undertaken, and with an eye to a possible Congressional enquiry, you might have more to gain than to lose. {1804.01, p. 1}

These tests would demonstrate that the companies are doing everything they can to provide a "safer" product to their customers.

> Of course this whole question of biological testing is a very difficult one and in the present state of ignorance of the real causes of cancer and other diseases allegedly connected with smoking (a state which may continue for a long time) *any work undertaken must be with a commercial or political motive as well as a scientific motive.* In other words, we should like to be able to say that certain of our cigarettes provide smoke in which certain suspect ingredients have been diminished, and that the smoke from these cigarettes has been scientifically proved to produce less change than other cigarettes on animal tissues. From this would follow the conclusion that in the light of all available knowledge, the Company is doing its best to supply a 'safer' smoke [emphasis added]. {1804.01, pp. 1–2}

Although B&W's lawyers initially supported research efforts to develop a safe cigarette and to study the carcinogenicity of their products in biological tests, they later changed their philosophy and strongly urged the company not to engage in any research that could produce damaging results.

CONCLUSION

During the 1950s research linking cigarette smoking to adverse health effects was reported. The tobacco industry responded to the growing public concern over the health effects of smoking by promoting filter cigarettes and by forming the Tobacco Industry Research Committee. Although the industry claimed publicly that both of these actions were being taken in the interests of the public health, the documents indicate that the true motivation behind them was to convince the public that the health hazards of smoking had not been proven. The release of the 1964 report of the US Surgeon General, *Smoking and Health,* created a crisis within the industry. The general counsel of B&W advised that the company should attempt to develop a "safer" cigarette, in part to protect itself against lawsuits. As discussed in chapters 3 and 4, during the 1960s and 1970s the industry conducted research to understand nicotine and to identify and remove harmful elements from tobacco smoke. Ultimately, however, the industry failed to make a safer cigarette.

REFERENCES

1. Wynder EL, Graham EA. Tobacco smoking as a possible etiologic factor in bronchiogenic carcinoma: A study of six hundred and eighty-four proved cases. *JAMA* 1950;143(4):329–336.
2. Wynder E, Graham E, Croninger A. Experimental production of carcinoma with cigarette tar. *Cancer Res* 1953;13:855–864.
3. Royal College of Physicians. *Smoking and Health. A Report of the Royal College of Physicians on Smoking in Relation to Cancer of the Lung and Other Diseases.* London: Pitman Medical Publishing Co., 1962.
4. USDHEW. *Smoking and Health. Report of the Advisory Committee to the Surgeon General of the Public Health Service.* US Department of Health, Education and Welfare, 1964. Public Health Service Publication No. 1103.
5. Tye J. *Sixty Years of Deception: An Analysis and Compilation of Cigarette Ads in Time Magazine, 1925–1985.* Palo Alto, CA: Health Advocacy Center, 1986.
6. Friedell M. Effect of cigarette smoke on the peripheral vascular system. *JAMA* 1953;152:897–900.
7. Miller LM, Monahan J. The facts behind filter-tip cigarettes. *Reader's Digest* 1957 July:33–39.
8. USDHHS. *The Health Consequences of Smoking: Cancer. A Report of the Surgeon General.* US Department of Health and Human Services, Public Health Service, Office on Smoking and Health, 1982. DHHS Publication No. (PHS) 82-50179.
9. USDHHS. *Reducing the Health Consequences of Smoking: 25 Years of Progress.* US Department of Health and Human Services, Public Health Service, Centers for Dis-

ease Control, Center for Chronic Disease Prevention and Health Promotion, Office
on Smoking and Health, 1989. DHHS Publication No. (CDC) 89-8411.

10. R. J. Reynolds Tobacco Co. *Chemical and Biological Studies on New Cigarette Prototypes That Heat Instead of Burn Tobacco.* Winston-Salem, NC: R. J. Reynolds Tobacco Co., 1988.

11. Wynder E. Neoplastic diseases. In: Wynder EL, ed. *The Biologic Effects of Tobacco* (pp. 102–132). Boston: Little, Brown, 1955.

12. Pollay RW. *A Scientific Smoke Screen: A Documentary History of Smoke Public Relations Efforts for and by the Tobacco Industry Research Council (TIRC), 1954–1958.* Vancouver, Canada: History of Advertising Archives, 1990. Tobacco Industry Promotion Series.

13. Friedman G, Dales L, Ury H. Mortality in middle-aged smokers and nonsmokers. *New Engl J Med* 1979;300:213–217.

14. Hammond E. The effects of smoking. *Scientific American* July 1962;207(1):39–51.

15. Miller L. Lung cancer and cigarettes: Here are the latest findings. *Reader's Digest* 1962 July:45–50.

16. Tobacco Manufacturers' Standing Committee. [Synopsis of] [s]tatement by tobacco manufacturers. *Brit Med J* 1962;1:810.

CHAPTER 3

Addiction and Cigarettes as Nicotine Delivery Devices

> Moreover, nicotine is addictive. We are, then, in the business
> of selling nicotine, an addictive drug effective in the release of
> stress mechanisms.
>
> *Addison Yeaman, B&W general counsel, 1963*
> *{1802.05, p. 4}*

INTRODUCTION

Of the thousands of chemicals in tobacco smoke, nicotine is the most important. Nicotine makes tobacco addictive. The addictiveness of tobacco keeps people smoking long enough and heavily enough for the other chemicals in tobacco to cause heart disease, cancer, and other diseases. The documents reveal that B&W and BAT had a sophisticated and scientifically accurate understanding of nicotine pharmacology, including an explicit recognition of nicotine's addictiveness, more than thirty years ago. By 1963 B&W and BAT scientists and executives were internally acknowledging that nicotine is an addictive drug and that tobacco companies are essentially in the business of "selling nicotine." Nevertheless, the tobacco industry has publicly maintained over the years that nicotine is not addictive, and that the alkaloid merely adds "taste and flavor" to tobacco.

Addiction to a drug, also called dependence on a drug, is a condition in which an individual has lost control over the use of the drug and continues to use it despite adverse consequences. This conception is the basis for the diagnostic criteria for addiction found in the *Diagnostic and Statistical Manual* of the American Psychiatric Association (1). Although it has long been recognized that people cannot readily stop using tobacco products (2), the modern scientific basis for classifying nicotine as addictive was not highlighted until the 1988 Surgeon General's report, *Nicotine Addiction* (3).

There are several reasons why the tobacco industry has maintained so staunchly that nicotine is not addictive. First, the tobacco industry has argued in products liability lawsuits that smoking is a matter of "personal choice," and that tobacco companies should not, therefore, be held responsible for adverse health effects attributed to smoking. If the industry were to admit that nicotine is addictive, it would have a much harder time arguing that people can choose to quit smoking any time they want. In addition, if the industry were to admit that nicotine is addictive, it would open itself up to increased regulation. Under the Food, Drug and Cosmetic Act, an article (other than a food) is a drug or a device subject to regulation by the Food and Drug Administration (FDA) if its manufacturer intends that it affect the structure or function of the body when used. An intent to cause addiction would clearly qualify nicotine in tobacco products as a drug and the products themselves as drugs or devices and therefore subject to FDA regulation, just as the agency regulates nicotine chewing gum and patches. Intent to cause pharmacological effects besides addiction, such as effects on mood or weight control, would also qualify the nicotine in tobacco products as a drug. The FDA examined this question in 1994 (4, 5) and concluded that cigarettes and smokeless tobacco are, in fact, delivery devices for the drug nicotine (6). On August 10, 1995, the agency proposed regulations under the Food, Drug and Cosmetic Act to protect children from nicotine addiction (7).

Nicotine's addictiveness also has implications for policy regarding tobacco advertising and promotion. Virtually all tobacco use begins in childhood and adolescence. Half of those who smoke cigarettes as adults have started by age 14, and most of those who will smoke as adults are already smoking every day by age 17 (8). Among young people (12–17 years old) who smoke at least twenty cigarettes daily, 84 percent reported that they "needed" or were "dependent" on cigarettes (8). Three out of four adult smokers say that they are addicted. By some estimates, as many as 74 to 90 percent are addicted. Seventeen million Americans (more than a third of all smokers) try to quit each year, but fewer than one out of ten succeeds. For every smoker who quits, nine try but fail (4). Since addiction develops insidiously, those affected only gradually come to appreciate that they cannot stop despite their intentions to do so.

Although the tobacco industry accepted the current series of rotating warnings on cigarette packages in 1984—which mention lung cancer, heart disease, prenatal problems, carbon monoxide exposure, and improved health from stopping smoking—it successfully lobbied against having the word "addiction" appear in any warning (Matthew Myers, personal communication, January 30, 1995).

This chapter discusses what the documents reveal about the tobacco industry's knowledge of nicotine—namely, that both B&W and BAT clearly recognized that nicotine is pharmacologically active, that it is addictive, and that cigarettes are essentially nicotine delivery devices.

SOUTHAMPTON RESEARCH CONFERENCE, 1962

BAT held periodic research conferences so that scientists and executives from its subsidiaries around the world could share the results of their research and discuss various issues affecting the industry. The 1962 BAT research conference was held in Southampton, England, and was attended by twenty-nine BAT representatives from five countries. The United States and Canada sent four delegates each. The report from the conference is fifty-five pages long and discusses a wide range of topics related to smoking and health. In this chapter we limit our discussion to the portions of the Southampton conference that are relevant to nicotine. (Chapter 4 examines the smoking and health dimensions of this conference.)

The keynote address for the Southampton meeting was delivered by Sir Charles Ellis, an executive in the Research and Development Establishment at BAT's Millbank headquarters in London. In his keynote address, Sir Charles attempts to explain the conclusions of the British Royal College of Physicians' (RCP) first report on smoking and health, which had been released a few months earlier (9). The RCP report concluded that smoking causes lung cancer and that the British government should take "decisive steps" to control the rising consumption of cigarettes in the United Kingdom. According to Sir Charles, the authors of this report were predisposed to believing that cigarettes are harmful. One reason for this belief:

> . . . *smoking is a habit of addiction* that is pleasurable; many people, therefore, find themselves sub-consciously prepared to believe that it must be wrong [emphasis added]. {1102.01, p. 4}

Later during his address, Sir Charles acknowledges that nicotine is the substance responsible for the addictiveness of smoking. However, he also appears to believe that nicotine has beneficial properties, which studies supported by the Tobacco Manufacturers' Standing Committee (TMSC, see chapter 2) are now investigating.

One result of the recent public discussions on smoking and health must have been to make each of us examine whether smoking is *just a habit of addiction* or has any positive benefits. It is my conviction that nicotine is a very remarkable beneficent drug that both helps the body to resist external stress and also can as a result show a pronounced tranquillising effect. You are all aware of the very great increase in the use of artificial controls, stimulants, tranquillisers, sleeping pills, and it is a fact that under modern conditions of life people find that they cannot depend just on their subconscious reactions to meet the various environmental strains with which they are confronted: they must have drugs available which they can take when they feel the need. *Nicotine is not only a very fine drug, but the technique of administration by smoking has considerable psychological advantages and a built-in control against excessive absorption.* It is almost impossible to take an overdose of nicotine in the way it is only too easy to do with sleeping pills. Perhaps, therefore, in the midst of all this consideration of the possible harmful effects of smoking you will be pleased to hear that T.M.S.C. is supporting work to elucidate the effects of nicotine as a beneficent alkaloid drug.

We have almost completed arrangements to support Dr. M. J. Rand at the London School of Pharmacy to investigate whether cigarette smoke produces effects on the central nervous system characteristic of tranquillising or stimulating drugs and, if so, to see if such activity is due solely to nicotine. The cost is likely to be about £13,000 in three years.

We attach so much importance to this aspect of our research that we are proposing to start active work at Harrogate with our own permanent staff. Arrangements are practically completed with Dr. [A. K.] Armitage to start at Harrogate to work on the pharmacology of smoke, and we are fortunate in having the distinguished Dr. [J. H.] Burn to act as consultant and advise us on the direction of this work [emphasis added]. {1102.01, pp. 15–16}

The Southampton conference report includes a detailed summary of the discussion following Sir Charles's keynote address. While there was a brisk debate over the directions BAT research should take (discussed in chapter 4), there was no apparent disagreement with Sir Charles's characterization of nicotine as addictive, with his comments on its other pharmacological properties, or with his characterization of nicotine as a drug.

BATTELLE'S NICOTINE RESEARCH PROGRAM

Not disclosed in Sir Charles's 1962 speech was contract research on nicotine that BAT was already having done by the Battelle Memorial Institute laboratory in Geneva, Switzerland. The project was headed by Sir Charles, and its ultimate purpose was to develop a novel nicotine delivery device that would avoid the toxicity of conventional cigarettes.

Battelle undertook several projects for BAT on nicotine from the late 1950s through about 1967. Project Mad Hatter was a comprehensive literature review. Project Hippo I involved animal experiments exploring the effects of nicotine on stress, weight gain, water balance, and hormonal regulation. The investigators regarded each of these diverse phenomena as related to the action of nicotine on the hypothalamus, a part of the brain that was then the focus of intense scientific interest because of its apparent control over the pituitary gland, the so-called "master gland" of the body. Project Hippo II extended this work on the hypothalamic effects of nicotine by exploring whether nicotine acts in ways similar to major tranquilizing drugs such as reserpine. A separate series of experiments traced the basic pharmacokinetics (absorption, distribution, and fate) of nicotine. Finally, Project Ariel sought to develop an alternative nicotine delivery system: a device that would provide the consumer with nicotine while delivering negligible amounts of the other toxins found in tobacco smoke.

PROJECT HIPPO I

Project Hippo I was designed to explore nicotine's role in several areas the investigators thought involved hypothalamic functions, including reduction of stress, inhibition of weight gain, maintenance of water balance (hormonally controlled through the hypothalamus), and regulation of gonadotrophic (sex) hormones. The results of Project Hippo I are described in a January 1962 report from Battelle to BAT {1211.01}. The introduction to this forty-eight-page report describes the background and goals of Project Hippo I:

> It is an everyday experience to each smoker that smoking a cigarette helps mastering the numerous stressful stimuli of modern life.
> This effect is possibly one of the most powerful reasons which make one smoke.
> How does nicotine exert this action? The normal defence mechanism against stressful agents is a nearly immediate release of those hormones synthesized by the adrenal cortex which act upon the cell metabolisms: they are called "corticosteroids" and play the cardinal role in the defence of the organism against stress. Their release from the gland is mediated through a very complicated system involving the stimulation of hypothalamus and pituitary function. . . .
> As a working hypothesis we assumed the idea that nicotine could help to master the stressful stimuli by way of enhancing (or facilitating) the normal defence mechanism.
> If this were true, it would be easier to understand another very important effect of smoking: it is well known that stopping to smoke has an immediate

effect on body weight. As body weight is regulated by the hypothalamo-pituitary system, our working hypothesis could be enlarged in order to assume the idea of an interference of nicotine in the hypothalamic regulation of body weight as well as in the defence against stress. {1212.01, pp. 6–7}

By conducting these experiments, Battelle was testing some of the most advanced neuroendocrine theories of the day. The adrenal corticosteroids had been introduced as wonder drugs into clinical medicine about a decade before this, and since the mid-1950s neuroendocrinologists had been gradually coming to understand the central role of the hypothalamus in the regulation of pituitary gland function (10, 11).

The report also discusses experiments that Battelle's scientists conducted on nicotine tolerance in rats. Tolerance to a drug is said to have developed when an animal requires a larger dose to achieve the same effect as that previously produced by a smaller dose. Tolerance is a common feature of addicting drugs. It need not be present for addiction to exist, but it usually is. Addiction, or dependence, is a clinical syndrome that includes loss of control over use of a psychoactive drug, withdrawal symptoms when the drug is no longer taken, and continued use despite problems caused by the drug. The report notes that tolerance could be induced in *all* rats, although some required several months to achieve this state.

The report describes in detail the effects of nicotine on rats in the various experiments. Of interest here is the importance the authors attached to nicotine's ability to influence the response to stress. For these scientists, this response helped explain the tranquilizing effect of nicotine and provided a direct link to the subsequent project, Hippo II.

Project Hippo I also included an elegant series of experiments on weight control in rats using nicotine. Nicotine was shown to inhibit food intake in both tolerant and nontolerant animals. Reserpine did not modify this action of nicotine. Nicotine rapidly stimulated the mobilization of lipid deposits (fat) and the degradation of free fatty acids. Each of these actions was in the direction expected for a drug that would be of benefit in controlling obesity {1211.01, p. 3}. The work Battelle conducted for BAT under Project Hippo I on weight control preceded published accounts of these phenomena by twenty years (3, 12).

PROJECT HIPPO II

Battelle extended its research on the hypothalamic actions of nicotine in Project Hippo II. Battelle's final report on Project Hippo II, in 1963, spells out why the tobacco industry was interested in comparing nicotine and reserpine: it was concerned that the new tranquilizing agents would compete with cigarettes as stress reducers. The results of Battelle's research must have been reassuring to BAT, since the experiments demonstrated that nicotine had far fewer side effects than the tranquilizer reserpine.

> The aim of the whole research "HIPPO" was to understand some of the activities of nicotine—those activities that could explain why cigarette smokers are so fond of their habit. It was also our purpose to compare these effects with those of the new drugs called "tranquillizers", which might supersede tobacco habits in the near future. We studied mainly the drug called reserpine.
>
> Why does one smoke? It is certainly not because of nicotine's cardiovascular activities, which are so well-known to pharmacologists. The reasons for the "pleasure of smoking" must be found partly in the relief of anxiety that cigarette smoking brings so constantly, and in such a very short time.
>
> This sedative—or soothing—effect of cigarette smoking and of nicotine is however very different from the "tranquillizing" effect as it was defined by pharmacologists after the discovery of the Rauwolfia alkaloids. [Rauwolfia is the plant group in which reserpine is found.] Tranquillizers are highly effective in the management of overactive psychotic patients and, as such, are largely used in psychiatry; nicotine is certainly devoid of such effects.
>
> However, as the new drugs are used increasingly by "the members of our so-called normal population who are subjected to intolerable stress" (see our First Report on HIPPO II, p. 3), they might, from this point of view, supersede tobacco habits.
>
> Our investigation definitely shows that both kinds of drugs act quite differently, and that nicotine may be considered (its cardio-vascular effects not being contemplated here) as more "beneficial"—or less noxious—than the new tranquillizers, from some very important points of view.
>
> The so-called "beneficial" effects of nicotine are of two kinds:
>
> 1.   Enhancing effect on the pituitary-adrenal response to stress;
> 2.   Regulation of body weight.
>
> These effects do not seem to be shared by reserpine, which on the contrary shows undesirable side-actions that are not given by nicotine, i.e. a nearly complete blockade of gonadic and thyroid activities, reflecting most probably a general blockade of the hypothalamo-pituitary system, which normally controls all the endocrine activities. {1211.03, pp. 1–2}

Two pages later, the report indicates that one of the hypotheses under study might explain the phenomena of tolerance, withdrawal, and addiction to nicotine.

> A quantitative investigation of the relations with time of nicotine—and of some possible brain mediators—on adreno-corticotrophic activity could give us the key to the explanation of both phenomena of tolerance and of addiction, in showing the symptoms of withdrawal. {1211.03, p. 4}

So, addiction to nicotine is real. The hypotheses guiding Hippo II were summarized in a diagram, which is reproduced as figure 3.1 {1211.03, p. 5}. In this model nicotine acts in the brain and at the level of the hypothalamus to affect appetite, stress reactions mediated through the adrenal gland, and changes in blood pressure and in water balance (antidiuretic effect). The experimental data gathered by the Battelle scientists in Hippo I and Hippo II provided direct empirical support for this model.

"FATE OF NICOTINE" STUDY

In addition to conducting the Hippo projects, Battelle also studied how nicotine is absorbed into, distributed within, and eliminated from the body. This work seems to have been part of the overall development process for Project Ariel, an alternative nicotine delivery system discussed later in this chapter. To properly design this delivery system, BAT needed basic pharmacological data on how nicotine was absorbed, distributed, and eliminated from the body. The results of these pioneering experiments are described in a report titled *The Fate of Nicotine in the Body,* dated May 1963 {1213.01}. The report begins,

> *There is increasing evidence that nicotine is the key factor in controlling, through the central nervous system, a number of beneficial effects of tobacco smoke, including its action in the presence of stress situations. (Larsen, Haag & Silvette (1960)) In addition, the alkaloid [nicotine] appears to be intimately connected with the phenomena of tobacco habituation (tolerance) and/or addiction. (Larsen et al. (1960))* Detailed knowledge of these effects of nicotine in the body of a smoker is therefore of vital importance to the tobacco industry, not only in connection with their present standard products, but also with regard to future potential uses of tobacco alkaloids.
>
> The numerous effects of nicotine in the body may, at first, be conveniently measured by various physiological and pharmacological experiments. However, the elucidation of the mode(s) of action of nicotine will ultimately depend on biochemical analyses dealing with the behavior of the nicotine molecule on, and its interactions with, the surface of physiologically active, macromolecular cell constituents (enzymes, receptors, etc.). The success of such analyses depends, in turn, on a detailed knowledge of the fate of nicotine in the body, i.e. of the various mechanisms which control the type and the rate of (a) absorption, (b) distribution, (c) breakdown or transformation, and (d) elimination [emphasis added]. {1213.01, pp. 1–2}

Battelle's 1963 report describes a comprehensive series of animal and human experiments on the absorption, distribution, metabolism, and elimination of nicotine.

To study the absorption of nicotine, Battelle used nicotine labeled with radioactive carbon (C^{14}) to measure the amount of nicotine absorbed by

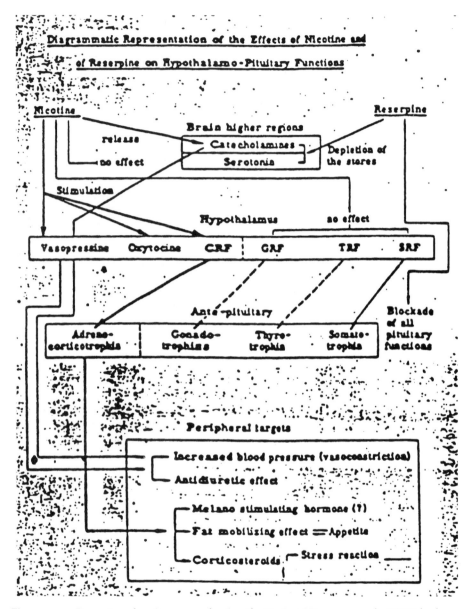

Figure 3.1. By 1962, when it was conducting the Project Hippo research, B&W had a sophisticated understanding of how nicotine acts on the nervous system. Source: {1211.03, p. 5}

different types of smokers. The two subjects described as "non-inhalers" absorbed 22 percent and 42 percent of the nicotine drawn into their mouths, while most of those who inhaled absorbed between 70 and 90 percent of the ingested dose. The two subjects who "eject[ed] the smoke immediately after inhalation" had nicotine absorption rates in the 40 to 50 percent range. Daily consumption of nicotine among all the subjects in this experiment was found to range from 10 to 91 mg {1213.01, p. 8}. These data demonstrate the importance of inhalation for nicotine absorption from cigarette smoke. Inhalation is unrelated to taste or flavor; it is only important for nicotine absorption into the bloodstream (13). Similar work with C^{14}-labeled nicotine was not reported in the general scientific literature until a dozen years later (14).

The Fate of Nicotine in the Body also describes Battelle's animal work on nicotine absorption. Using C^{14}-labeled nicotine in rabbits, the Battelle scientists compared gastric absorption with pulmonary absorption. Gastric absorption was slow, and first pass removal of nicotine by the liver (which transforms nicotine into inactive metabolites) was demonstrated following gastric administration, with consequently low systemic nicotine levels. In contrast, absorption from the lungs was rapid and led to widespread distribution. These results show that nicotine absorbed from the stomach is largely metabolized by the liver before it has a chance to get to the brain. That is why tobacco products have to be puffed, smoked or sucked on, or absorbed directly into the bloodstream (i.e., via a nicotine patch). A nicotine pill would not work because the nicotine would be inactivated before it reached the brain.

Battelle's report also discusses earlier work on nicotine absorption, which had demonstrated that free-base nicotine is absorbed more rapidly than nicotine salts. Nicotine exists in the free-base form at an alkaline pH. In acidic environments nicotine exists as a salt. The more rapid the absorption, the greater the impact nicotine has on the brain. Work such as this on nicotine absorption has nothing to do with taste and flavor.

The *Fate of Nicotine* report concludes with a discussion of the work on nicotine metabolism in the context of tolerance and addiction. Pharmacologists had recognized that tolerance could develop either from breaking down a drug faster with repeated exposure (metabolic tolerance) or from adaptations to the drug at the level of the target tissue (cellular tolerance). They also recognized that there is an important relationship between the development of tolerance and the potential for a drug to cause addiction.

Although tolerance to some drugs may depend on accelerated enzymatic breakdown, prolonged consumption of others, including morphine, appears to induce cellular adaptions. (Axelrod (1956); Shuster (1961); Takemori (1961) (1962)) In any case, the present results offer no conclusive evidence for any particular mechanism involved in tolerance to nicotine, nor do they indicate a lead to the phenomenon of addiction. *We believe that both tolerance and addiction are intimately connected, and that it would be most useful to investigate the two phenomena with regard to cellular adaptation, especially in target organs of the central nervous system* [emphasis added]. {1213.01, p. 27}

Within a few weeks of completion of *The Fate of Nicotine in the Body*, Sir Charles Ellis sent a copy to William S. Cutchins, the president of B&W at the time. In his cover letter, Sir Charles asks that the report be given no wider circulation than the Hippo reports had received.

[The report] is an account of work which has been carried out in association with the other researches which were sent to you recently under the title of HIPPO. I feel sure you will agree that a knowledge of the fate of nicotine in the body is a necessary accompaniment to studying the physiological effects that nicotine can produce. . . .

Would you please treat this as confidential document under the same conditions as I described for the report HIPPO. {1200.16}

The documents do not include any acknowledgment from Cutchins, but the person who would shortly replace him as president, E. P. Finch, received the report along with a summary by the B&W vice president of research, T. M. Wade, Jr. {1200.07, 1200.16}

A TENTATIVE HYPOTHESIS ON NICOTINE ADDICTION

The Battelle scientists who conducted the Hippo projects for BAT also wrote a speculative essay about the mechanism underlying nicotine addiction. The essay, marked "Confidential" and titled "A Tentative Hypothesis on Nicotine Addiction" {1200.01}, sought to explain nicotine tolerance, withdrawal, and addiction in the context of what was then cutting-edge neuroendocrinology.

The hypothalamo-pituitary stimulation of nicotine is the beneficial mechanism which makes people smoke; in other words, nicotine helps people to cope with stress. In the beginning of nicotine consumption, relatively small doses can perform the desired action. *Chronic intake of nicotine tends to restore the normal physiological functioning of the endocrine system, so that ever-increasing dose levels of nicotine are necessary to maintain the desired action. Unlike other dopings, such as morphine, the demand for increasing dose levels is relatively slow for nicotine.*

In a chronic smoker the normal equilibrium in the corticotropin-releasing system can be maintained only by continuous nicotine intake. It seems that those individuals are but slightly different in their aptitude to cope with stress in comparison with a non-smoker. If nicotine intake, however, is prohibited to chronic smokers, the corticotropin-releasing ability of the hypothalamus is greatly reduced, so that these individuals are left with an unbalanced endocrine system. A body left in this unbalanced status craves for renewed drug intake in order to restore the physiological equilibrium. *This unconscious desire explains the addiction of the individual to nicotine* [emphasis added]. {1200.01, pp. 1–2}

The short essay includes a review of the effects of nicotine on appetite and weight control, based on experiments using animals.

It is a well-known fact that fresh smokers show loss of appetite, and therefore loss of weight. Chronic smokers gradually turn to normal food intake. If nicotine is withdrawn from these individuals, the low FFA [free fatty acid] concentration in the blood provokes increased appetite, and therefore increased food intake, or at least a permanent hunger feeling. This feeling can be satisfied either by increased food intake or by renewed smoking.

Laboratory experiments with rats confirm this mechanism: injection of nicotine induces a marked reduction in food intake in the beginning of the treatment. Chronic application of nicotine in the so-called "tolerant rats" shows after a certain time no difference in the growth curves between treated and untreated animals. Interruption of nicotine application provokes a marked increase in food intake of "tolerant rats", which increase, however, turns very rapidly to normal (in our experiments within one week). {1200.01, p. 2}

The essay concludes,

[A] tentative hypothesis for the explanation of nicotine addiction would be that of an unconscious desire to restore the normal physiological equilibrium of the corticotropin-releasing system in a body in which the normal functioning of the system has been weakened by chronic intake of nicotine. {1200.01, p. 3}

In summary, pharmacological research at Battelle sponsored by BAT in the early 1960s was based on a paradigm of addiction. It sought to elucidate "beneficial" effects of nicotine such as "tranquilising" and weight loss effects, and it also explored the extent to which other drugs might compete with cigarettes in the consumer marketplace.

The results of the Hippo projects were distributed to BAT officials around the world, including executives at Brown and Williamson. The speculative paper on nicotine addiction, however, received only limited circulation. In fact, when Sir Charles Ellis sent a copy of the essay to

Brown and Williamson's general counsel, Addison Yeaman, he attached a cover letter advising Yeaman that the essay was "a private working paper" and that it was not being circulated to the other recipients of the Hippo reports {1200.02}.

DEBATE ABOUT SHARING RESEARCH FINDINGS WITH THE US SURGEON GENERAL

The Hippo reports prompted a flurry of correspondence between BAT headquarters and the B&W executive suite in the summer of 1963, particularly over the question of what information, if any, to disclose to the US Surgeon General's Advisory Committee on Smoking and Health, which was to issue its report the following year. Despite the fact that the Battelle research added new insight into the area of nicotine pharmacology, BAT and B&W ultimately decided to withhold the results of the Hippo projects from the Surgeon General's Advisory Committee.

A note dated June 19, 1963, from A. D. McCormick, a senior R&D executive at BAT, to Bill Cutchins, B&W's president, mentions that BAT has decided to send the results of the Battelle work to the Tobacco Research Council (TRC) in the United Kingdom and the Tobacco Industry Research Committee (TIRC) in the United States. (As described in chapter 2, TRC and TIRC were created by the tobacco industry as "independent" organizations that funded scientific research related to the health effects of tobacco.) McCormick then asks about the advisability of submitting the results to the Surgeon General's committee.

> On 4th June [1963] Sir Charles Ellis sent to you copies of reports of research which B.A.T. had sponsored at the Battelle Research Institute in Geneva showing the beneficial effects of nicotine on the smoker. B.A.T. decided to make this research available to the T.R.C. here and it is being evaluated by T.R.C.'s outside medical experts. *Preliminary reports indicate that these experts think the Battelle work to be a sound piece of research. It was always contemplated that if the reports stood up scientifically it might be desirable to get them submitted to the U.S. Surgeon General's Committee.*
>
> Todd of T.R.C., is to-day sending copies to T.I.R.C. with a request that they consider whether it would help the U.S. industry for these reports to be passed on to the Surgeon General's Committee.
>
> I thought you should have this information in case you or any of your colleagues in Louisville [at B&W headquarters] might for any reason think this course of action inadvisable.
>
> Could you please let me know as soon as you get back what your views are [emphasis added]. {1200.10}

A handwritten note on this document indicates that Cutchins asked Addison Yeaman, the general counsel at B&W, to prepare a reply.

In his reply, dated June 28, 1963, Yeaman expresses some regret that the Battelle reports were shared within the industry's jointly funded research groups. Specifically, he mentions the connections between the Battelle work and a project being conducted at B&W by R. B. Griffith, director of R&D, to develop a special filter called the Avalon filter.

> I rather regret that Todd [of TRC] took this action without preliminary consultation here for the reason the Battelle nicotine report ties in so closely to Griffith's work that we would have preferred including both Griffith's work [on the Avalon filter] and the Battelle report in our consideration of submission to the Surgeon General. Moreover, Ed Jacob [a lawyer with Jacob and Medinger] in a talk with me yesterday reported that there was reason to believe that the Surgeon General's report would give particular emphasis to the part played by the aerosols in relation to possible deleterious effects of tobacco smoke. This, again, ties in so closely to Griffith's work, and by extension to Battelle's work, as to lead us to the preliminary opinion that the Battelle work and the Griffith development should—if at all—go into the Surgeon General as part of one package.
>
> Happily Ed Jacob will be with us on Tuesday to give us the benefit of his particular and special knowledge of the Committee, its reports, etc., etc., in deciding what disclosures B&W should make of Griffith's work to the Surgeon General's Committee and, if such disclosure is to be made, whether it should be through TIRC or direct by B&W. The fact that the Battelle report is now in TIRC's hands undoubtedly will have some effect on that decision. {1802.01}

It is not clear from the documents precisely what "special knowledge" Jacob had of the Surgeon General's committee.

McCormick of BAT replied by cable a few days later to say that the independent scientists who had reviewed the Battelle reports had concluded that the results should *not* be submitted to the Surgeon General's committee.

> T.R.C. consultant scientists advise it is too early to submit Battelle reports to Surgeon General's Committee but we think they will agree that continuation by Battelle of this work would be useful. Charles Ellis convinced of beneficial effects of nicotine but agrees further investigation desirable before publication. Please inform T.I.R.C. {1802.02}

B&W's Yeaman cabled back the same day to say that William T. Hoyt, the executive director of TIRC, had not distributed the reports to TIRC's Scientific Advisory Board (figure 3.2):

Prior to receipt your telex July 3 Hoyt of TIRC agreed to withhold disclosure of Battelle report to TIRC members or SAB until further notice from me. *Finch [of B&W] agrees submission Battelle or Griffith developments to Surgeon General undesirable and we agree continuance of Battelle work useful but disturbed at its implication re cardiovascular disorders.*

We believe combination Battelle work and Griffith's developments have implications which increase desirability reevaluation TIRC and reassessment fundamental policy re health. Hope to get off comprehensive note next week [emphasis added]. {1802.03}

McCormick amplified on his cable to Yeaman in a letter written the next day, but before he had received Yeaman's cable.

Charles' [Sir Charles Ellis's] view is that as the situation has now developed it would be wiser for B. & W. not to take the initiative in submitting anything to the Surgeon General's Committee but rather wait and hope that the Committee will ask the individual manufacturers for further details of their research work and then, should this happen, it would give B. & W. the opportunity of submitting the Battelle work and the work on the "Avalon" filter. As further work on both has to be done, the work would be immune from detailed criticism, but its disclosure would demonstrate that B. & W. and its associates had adopted a forward looking positive policy of research. {1803.01}

Yeaman compiled his thoughts on the nicotine research at BAT, Griffith's work on a new filter at B&W, and the Surgeon General's committee in a five-page memorandum dated July 17, 1963 {1802.05}. The memorandum presents an overview of B&W's strategic position on the health question and argues for the aggressive pursuit of selective filtration (the Griffith filter, code named Avalon) and the promotion of the beneficial effects of nicotine as revealed by the Battelle work. In Yeaman's view, the Battelle findings on nicotine could be used to justify smoking because of its positive benefits. If B&W could remove harmful constituents from smoke, it could then—with a clear conscience—promote cigarettes as nicotine delivery devices for people under stress from modern living. The memo opens,

The determination by Battelle of the "tranquilizing" function of nicotine, as received by the human system in the delivered smoke of cigarettes, together with nicotine's possible effect on obesity, delivers to the industry what well may be its first effective instrument of propaganda counter to that of the American Cancer Society, et al, damning cigarettes as having a causal relationship to cancer of the lung. The Battelle work is not in any degree responsive to that indictment nor to the Report expected to be returned by the Surgeon General's Committee on Smoking and Health. I would submit, however, that the Griffith filter offers the bridge over which the industry might

GE 59Á 4½M 2-61

BRO\\ & WILLIAMSON TOBACCO CORI \\TION
OUTGOING CABLE

DATE____July 3, 1963____

TO:____MR. McCORMICK____

CITY:____LONDON____COUNTRY: (____ENGLAND____)

PRIOR TO RECEIPT YOUR TELEX JULY 3 HOYT OF TIRC AGREED TO WITHHOLD DISCLOSURI

BATTELLE REPORT TO TIRC MEMBERS OR SAB UNTIL FURTHER NOTICE FROM ME.   FINCH

AGREES SUBMISSION BATTELLE OR GRIFFITH DEVELOPMENTS TO SURGEON GENERAL

UNDESIRABLE AND WE AGREE CONTINUANCE OF BATTELLE WORK USEFUL BUT DISTURBED

AT ITS IMPLICATIONS RE CARDIOVASCULAR DISORDERS.

WE BELIEVE COMBINATION BATTELLE WORK AND GRIFFITH'S DEVELOPMENTS HAVE

IMPLICATIONS WHICH INCREASE DESIRABILITY REEVALUATION TIRC AND REASSESSMENT

FUNDAMENTAL POLICY RE HEALTH.   HOPE TO GET OFF COMPREHENSIVE NOTE NEXT WEEK.

YEAMAN

Sent by:____mS____

bc: Messrs. Finch, Wade & Griffith
(2 copies to Cable Dept.)

Figure 3.2.   July 3, 1963, cable from Addison Yeaman to Tony McCormick confirming agreement to withhold scientific results on nicotine pharmacology from the Surgeon General's Advisory Committee, which was then preparing the original 1964 Surgeon General's report {1200.12}.

> pass from its present terrain of defense to a field for effective counter attack using the Battelle study as the basic weapon. I will assume for purposes of this note that the "Griffith filter" is one which permits filtration to specification; it filters taste and nicotine (and nicotine in even more effective form) free of constituent #1 to infinity, selectively. I grossly overstate and oversimplify Dr. Griffith's claims deliberately. {1802.05, p. 1}

Yeaman's statement clearly indicates that he regards nicotine as important primarily for its "tranquilizing" effects, not for its taste. In fact, he even mentions taste and nicotine separately, suggesting that they are independent in his mind. This understanding contrasts sharply with the tobacco industry's recent public claims that nicotine only adds taste and flavor.

Yeaman then offers his recommendations for possible responses to the Surgeon General's report. At the end of the paper, he returns to his discussion of nicotine. After quoting extensively from the final summary of the Hippo II report {1211.03}, which describes the beneficial effects of nicotine, he adds,

> *Moreover, nicotine is addictive.*
> *We are, then, in the business of selling nicotine, an addictive drug effec-*
> *tive in the release of stress mechanisms* [emphasis added]. {1802.05, p. 4}

As the documents reveal, B&W management knew about the work BAT had contracted for at Battelle in Geneva. Its decision to withhold important research on nicotine pharmacology from the Surgeon General's Advisory Committee is in stark contrast to the industry's public position of openness advanced in the "Frank Statement" ad and other public statements (see chapter 2).

PROJECT ARIEL

The basic pharmacology work embodied in the Hippo projects and in *The Fate of Nicotine in the Body* was based on the realization that cigarettes are, at root, nicotine delivery systems. They are dirty devices, though. BAT, with help from Battelle, extended the initial work on nicotine pharmacology by developing an alternative delivery system that could administer nicotine to the body free of the toxins from tobacco smoke. The design goal was a safe cigarette (discussed in chapter 4). The device was named Ariel.

Two patents were issued to Battelle on Ariel, but BAT's Sir Charles Ellis is listed in both as the lead inventor (15, 16). The patents were apparently assigned to Battelle to disguise their origin. A 1970 letter from BAT to Addison Yeaman at B&W notes that "the patents were put into Battelle's name rather than B.A.T.'s for security reasons" {1202.01}.

Ariel relied on burning tobacco to heat a centrally arranged tube containing nicotine and an aerosol generator, consisting of a material such as water, which would form an aerosol when heated and then cooled, so that the nicotine could dissolve into the droplets and then be inhaled as part of the aerosol. The consumer would inhale an aerosol enriched in nicotine but relatively deficient in the "tar" elements of cigarette smoke. The device clearly embodies Sir Charles Ellis's vision of the essence of a cigarette—that it is a nicotine delivery device. The fact that BAT funded the work in the first place indicates that this vision was also shared by others at the company at the time.

What did BAT see as Ariel's potential position in the market in the early 1960s? After all, the device was significantly different from a cigarette. It would have been impossible to move all customers over to Ariel right away, so the product needed a beginning niche in the market to become established. To whom, then, would it be targeted initially? While the documents do not directly answer this question, the underlying rationale for the Hippo II project suggests a possible initial positioning: since the cigarette industry was worried about competition from tranquilizing drugs, which would help people deal with stress without the toxicity associated with cigarettes {1211.02}, a way to meet this competition head-on was to develop a substantially less toxic form of a cigarette. Thus, one potential market for Ariel was the group that otherwise might have used tranquilizing drugs to reduce stress.

The patents for Ariel explicitly emphasize the importance of nicotine for the smoking experience and indicate that its action is, at least in part, physiological. (Because nicotine is not a normal part of the body, the actions would have been more accurately described as pharmacological.) The first patent, filed February 4, 1964, begins,

> This invention relates to an improved smoking device whereby an improved smoke stream of a controlled character is delivered to the smoker.
>
> In commercially available conventional smoking devices such as cigarettes, cigars and pipes, tobacco and reconstituted tobacco, or tobacco substitutes, are ignited and the products of combustion, in the form of a smoke stream in filtered or unfiltered form, are delivered to the mouth of the smoker. The smoke stream thus formed of the products of combustion may contain components which do not enhance the quality and characteristics of the smoke.
>
> It is a prime object of the present invention to overcome the difficulties and disadvantages heretofore encountered [presumably, all the toxins generated during the combustion process] and to provide an improved smoking device which delivers an improved smoke stream of a controlled character and which does not contain the products of combustion.
>
>   . . .
>
> The smoking device incorporates a continuous smoke passageway from its outer end to its mouthpiece end and which communicates with the nicotine-releasing composition. The smoke passageway includes an aerosol-nucleating chamber between the nicotine-releasing composition and the mouthpiece. This chamber is arranged so as to cool at an appropriate rate the potentially aerosol-forming materials sufficiently to enable aerosol particles to form, and the nicotine vapor is caused to contact the aerosol particles and condense thereon, whereby the nicotine assumes the transferability of the aerosol particles on which they condense.
>
>   . . .
>
> The nicotine-releasing material employed in this form of device preferably comprises cured, shredded or cut and blended cigarette tobacco or reconstituted tobacco or mixtures thereof. *The nicotine content of the tobacco or*

reconstituted tobacco is preferably enriched by mixing therewith a tobacco
concentrate rich in nicotine so that the available nicotine in the mixture con-
stitutes between approximately 5 and 20% by weight of the tobacco mater-
ial [emphasis added]. (15, column 1, lines 10–63; column 4, lines 2–10)

Conventional cigarettes also transport nicotine in droplets, except that
the droplets are largely composed of the tars produced during the burning of tobacco. In the Ariel cigarettes the droplets were derived from
other "aerosol-forming materials," such as water, making them potentially much less dangerous. Smoke from the burning tobacco around the
core of the Ariel cigarette would be vented to the outside.

The following additional details are from the second patent:

A total and satisfying 'smoke' can be obtained with a high nicotine to tar ratio or, as sometimes expressed, a low ratio of total particulate matter (T.P.M.)
to nicotine. This latter ratio can readily be reduced to one-quarter or less of
the values normally expected of smoke from cigarettes having no special provisions for reducing the ratio. If *desired*, the nicotine content may be made
normal, but with little of the normal particulate and vapor phases.

. . .

Thus, *when the smoking device is smoked the smoker will draw into his*
mouth a small amount of smoke adequate to satisfy the taste of the smoker
along with the nicotine containing aerosol.

. . .

Although the invention thus seeks primarily to furnish a *smoking device*
which will yield nicotine in an acceptable form, both psychologically and
physiologically, but without the necessity for taking into the system so much
of the products of combustion as is usual when smoking a conventional cigarette, it may also be used mainly or partially as a means for achieving greater
freedom for influencing the taste of the smoke, for introducing flavors and so
forth [emphasis added]. (16, column 2, lines 30–38, 52–55, and 66; column
3, line 3)

This patent demonstrates the pharmacological role nicotine plays in cigarettes. It shows that the essence of a conventional cigarette, stripped of
its undesirable elements, is "a smoking device which will yield nicotine
in an acceptable form, both psychologically and physiologically" (or,
more accurately, "pharmacologically," since nicotine is not part of normal human physiology). The patent mentions the provision of tastes and
flavors through this invention, but this benefit is clearly regarded as secondary and as a separate matter, distinct from nicotine delivery.

The Ariel patents preceded patents from R. J. Reynolds and Philip
Morris for analogous alternative nicotine delivery devices by twenty
years or more (17). The best known of these devices, Premier from R. J.

Reynolds, featured an insulated charcoal fuel element at the lit end of a cigarette-like device. The burning charcoal heated alumina beads coated with nicotine and glycerin, which, in turn, produced a nicotine-laden aerosol (18). Premier was sold in test markets briefly but was withdrawn because of poor consumer acceptance and opposition from the public health community (19). In 1994 RJR announced that it was conducting consumer tests on another charcoal-heated nicotine delivery device, called Eclipse, which produces an aerosol by heating glycerin adsorbed onto reconstituted tobacco. The resulting aerosol picks up nicotine and other soluble constituents from tobacco in the proximal portion of the device. As with Ariel and Premier, this device reportedly delivers nicotine while markedly lowering the delivery of other toxic constituents (20).

Brown and Williamson has continued to conduct research on Ariel-like devices. The Ariel formula of a central core that generates the inhaled aerosol and that is heated by a surrounding fuel is illustrated in two patents assigned to B&W in 1990 and one in 1994 (21–23). While the first of these recent patents envisions tobacco as the fuel, the latter two employ carbon in the style of Premier.

The flurry of patent activity in this area in the 1990s may be related to the expiration of the BAT patents on Ariel in 1983 and 1984 (originally issued in 1966 and 1967), in addition to advances in technical feasibility or market potential for these products. RJR seems to have begun the development of Premier in the early 1980s. This class of device incorporates a heating element, a reservoir for nicotine, and a means for dissolving vaporized nicotine in an aerosol for inhalation by the consumer. A cigarette contains each of these functions, but novel devices such as Ariel and Premier compartmentalize them and so make the normal operation of a cigarette easier to understand.

Ariel grew out of the realization that nicotine delivery is the essence of a cigarette and the belief that a nicotine delivery device relatively free of the major toxins of cigarette smoke could be designed. Although the product was never brought to market, its design and conception demonstrate what BAT and B&W thought was the most important part of their tobacco products: nicotine.

BAT'S INTERNAL RESEARCH ON NICOTINE

In addition to contracting with Battelle, BAT also conducted its own studies on nicotine at its laboratory in Southampton and at other laboratories around the world. Some of these research activities are described in BAT's reports of its annual research conferences involving key scientists from BAT member companies with active R&D laboratories. Other research activities on nicotine are described in two site visit reports and in research reports. These documents indicate that over an extended period of time the company recognized the central importance of nicotine because of its pharmacological properties.

In September 1969 D. J. Wood from R&DE (Research and Development Establishment) at BAT gave a presentation to company executives about the R&D work the company was doing. The notes of his talk summarize the work being done on nicotine:

> The presence of nicotine is the reason why the tobacco plant was singled out from all other plants for consumption in this rather unusual way.
>
> Nicotine has well documented pharmacological action. It is claimed to have a dual effect, acting both as a stimulant and a tranquilliser. It is believed to be responsible for the "satisfaction" of smoking, using this term in the physiological rather than the psychological sense.
>
> Investigations at R.&D.E. are aimed at finding out more about the factors controlling nicotine absorption in the human respiratory system.
>
> Extractable and Non-extractable nicotine (define) [see below].
>
> Possibility of getting satisfaction from fairly low nicotine cigarettes, provided sufficient nicotine is in the extractable form.
>
> Certain medical studies would seek to blame nicotine for cardio-vascular disease, so high levels of total nicotine are not likely to be fashionable in health-conscious countries in the future.
>
> Mention absorption of nicotine via the mouth, e.g. cigar smokers.
> {1184.02, p. 7}

The documents provide numerous details about this systematic program of pharmacological research.

OVERVIEW OF PROGRAM, 1967

Robert J. Johnson, a senior scientist with B&W research and development, summarizes a June 20, 1967, meeting at which BAT's past and present research on nicotine was discussed. Johnson described six separate areas of research on nicotine that members of the BAT R&D group at Southampton had on their agenda:

> Project ARIEL—This is dormant for the moment. The first samples tried gave a tremendous kick, even though the nicotine delivery was quite small. It would appear that the project will be reinitiated within a few months.
>
> Dr. S. R. Evelyn is presently investigating the absorption of extractable and non-extractable nicotine in the mouth, albeit with a mechanical mouth.

Dr. J. D. Backhurst is setting up an analysis for pH of whole smoke on a puff-by-puff basis. This correlates with his previous interest in extractable nicotine[.]

Mr. H. G. Horsewell continues to work with alkaline filter additives which selectively increase nicotine delivery.

Dr. R. E. Thornton will be synthesizing ring-labeled nicotine as his first project in the new radiochemical facilities. This will initially be to determine the percentage of nicotine which is destroyed during smoking.

Dr. D. J. Wood will be assigning the new physiologist to a study into the organoleptic [sensory, especially irritation] effects of nicotine. {1201.01, pp. 10–11}

The research program was concerned with understanding the delivery of nicotine in smoke and its absorption. The organoleptic work described comes closer than anything else in the documents to suggesting an interest in the taste and flavor of nicotine, but it actually seems to be more concerned with understanding the irritating properties of nicotine on mucous membranes. This is an important problem in cigarette design, since alkaline nicotine, which is readily absorbed in the mouth, is also irritating to the throat (13).

Some of the internal research reports for the work in progress mentioned by Dr. Johnson were available to us in summary form. These reports deal mainly with the absorption of nicotine.

A 1966 report describes "Further Work on 'Extractable' Nicotine" {1205.01}. Nicotine that is "extractable" (more soluble in chloroform than water) proved to be a better gauge of perceived "strength" by the smoker than whole nicotine content. Most "extractable" nicotine was recognized to be nicotine base, so the "nonextractable" nicotine was the acidic salt. The report speculates on why "extractable" nicotine has a greater perceived strength:

> The reasons for the relationship between smoker response and "extractable" nicotine content of the smoke remain obscure. Several possible explanations have been considered and, at the present time, it would appear that the increased smoker response is associated with nicotine reaching the brain more quickly. {1205.01, p. 1}

It is now widely recognized that what BAT scientists were calling "extractable nicotine," nicotine base (also called free nicotine or unionized nicotine), is readily absorbed in the mouth and nose, while the ionized form that exists in acidic environments is hardly absorbed at all in the mouth (3). The internal research reports indicate that BAT had a sophisticated understanding of this distinction thirty years ago.

A series of reports from 1968 and 1969 document the interest of the research scientists at BAT in the variables that account for nicotine absorption in the mouth, as from pipe and cigar smoke {1214.01; 1205.05; 1205.06}. Nicotine retention in the mouth was found to be a function of the pH (acidity) of the smoke, while absorption was a function of the pH of saliva. "Extractable nicotine content" was directly related to pH. The design criterion for the membrane used in the artificial mouth was that it permit the passage of unionized (free-base) nicotine but not that of ionized nicotine (salt) {1214.01, p. 12}. An appropriate imitation of the way an actual mouth works, absorbing unionized but not ionized nicotine, was an explicit feature for the model system. This is yet another indication that the scientists at BAT knew the importance of nicotine absorption. The last report in this series notes that, in contrast to pipe and cigar smokers, cigarette smokers usually inhale {1205.06}.

These research reports put flesh on Dr. Johnson's brief summary and demonstrate that in the late 1960s BAT's R&DE had a tremendous interest in achieving a better understanding of how nicotine is best absorbed into the body from pipes, cigars, and cigarettes.

MONTREAL RESEARCH CONFERENCE, 1967

The 1967 R&D conference was held in Montreal over three days in October {1165.01; 1165.02; 1165.03}. The document we have is probably a draft, since the official minutes are quoted in the minutes of the 1970 conference and differ somewhat from these notes (see below). The draft lists the main "assumptions made by R&D scientists," noting that they were listed "without any attempt to justify them or to agree on their correctness at this time." Although the draft is explicit that no attempt had been made to agree on these "main" assumptions, the minutes of the 1970 St. Adele conference reviewed the final 1967 assumptions and listed them without this qualification. The following assumptions had to do with nicotine:

> There is a minimum level of nicotine. *Smoking is an addictive habit attributable to nicotine and the form of nicotine affects the rate of absorption by the smoker.*
>
>   . . .
>
> *If there is no inhaling, there is no lung cancer or respiratory disease.*
> *Smoking has both physiological and psychological effects.*
> There will be some government involvement in the tobacco industry in the future [emphasis added]. {1165.01, p. 2}

A handwritten edit in the document changes the phrase "an addictive habit" to "a habit."

The meeting notes reflect a concern with the inevitability of future government regulation.

> It was agreed that smoking is likely to be associated with health continuously in the future and that it was not a passing phase. *It was likely, moreover, that tobacco would be involved in legislation of a food and drug administration nature in respect both of product and of manufacturer* [emphasis added]. {1165.01, p. 4}

Thus, the nine assembled BAT scientists, including B&W representatives from Louisville, acknowledged that health concerns were never going to disappear. Furthermore, they felt that FDA-style product regulation could be justified by the public health community.

In a discussion of concurrent developments in cigarette filters, the use of "an alkaloid additive" to affect "the ratio of extractable to non-extractable nicotine" was emphasized {1165.02, p. 1}. The filter additive PEI (polyethyleneimine) was mentioned as a way to "be helpful in rendering the nicotine more available to the smoker" {1165.02, p. 4} in a "low TPM, normal nicotine" cigarette. TPM is total particulate matter; it consists mostly of tar. The participants also considered the development of a "low TPM, low nicotine cigarette" but wondered whether consumers would be attracted to such a brand. Someone mentioned that in Germany per capita cigarette consumption had risen as nicotine content had fallen. Participants agreed that more information was needed on the "optimal level" of nicotine for the smoker.

Ariel was discussed, as was "a cigarette aimed to be pleasantly non-inhalable" {1165.02, p. 5}. Moreover, "it was noted in passing that the trend towards making cigarlets [little cigars] milder and therefore more easily inhalable was undesirable on health grounds" {1165.02, p. 5}. These two comments echo sentiments recorded at other research conferences. They emphasize the importance of inhalation to the normal functioning of cigarettes as well as the fundamental problem that it poses in the causation of cancer and respiratory disease.

The importance of nicotine was emphasized in the discussion that closed the second day of the conference.

> A general discussion followed on basic assumptions which guided thinking in the field of smoking and health. While recognizing the importance of psychological factors in smoking and the possibility that some smokers would accept non-nicotine cigarettes, *it was felt that nicotine is important for the majority of smokers and that the form of nicotine can be significant.* It was

also considered that nicotine will be increasingly subject to attack. It was agreed that there will be increasing government involvement in the industry [emphasis added]. {1165.02, p. 6}

In the context of the previous and current laboratory work conducted by BAT, these comments about nicotine can only refer to the importance of nicotine as a drug in tobacco products.

HILTON HEAD RESEARCH CONFERENCE, 1968

Twelve members of R&D groups from various BAT companies participated in a research conference at Hilton Head, South Carolina, on September 24–30, 1968. A terse report of conclusions was prepared by the conference chairman, Dr. S. J. Green, head of BAT's Research and Development Establishment at Southampton. The participants recognized the emerging evidence that nicotine has adverse effects on the cardiovascular system {1112.01, p. 2} and agreed that researchers should look for substances that would have the actions of nicotine in the brain but would not be toxic to the circulation. The intended effects were "brain stimulation and stress-relief":

> *In view of its pre-eminent importance, the pharmacology of nicotine should continue to be kept under review and attention paid to the possible discovery of other substances possessing the desired features of brain stimulation and stress-relief without direct effects on the circulatory system.* The possibility that nicotine and other substances together may exert effects larger than either separately (synergism) should be studied and if necessary the attention of Marketing Departments should be drawn to these possibilities.
>
> It was, however, agreed that nicotine or tobacco extracts should not be put in a part of the cigarette, e.g. the filter, where they could be readily ingested.
>
> In a discussion of devices for the controlled administration of nicotine, the current position of the ARIEL project was reviewed, and it was requested that Southampton should supply some ARIEL devices to the overseas laboratories for examination [emphasis added]. {1112.01, p. 3}

The fact that the inhalation of tobacco smoke was an expected part of smoking a cigarette came through in the discussion of the "non-inhalable" cigarette. Finally, Ariel remained a focus of interest in relation to the "controlled administration of nicotine."

KRONBERG RESEARCH CONFERENCE, 1969

The minutes of the research conference at Kronberg, Germany (June 1969), deal mostly with smoking and health concerns (discussed in detail in chapter 4), but there are several salient comments related to nicotine.

PEI (polyethyleneimine), a filter additive that boosted the delivery of "extractable nicotine" in cigarette smoke, was used in a series of human test panel experiments {1205.03}. Increased levels of "extractable nicotine" increased the "impact of inhaling" while producing a "small increase" in throat and nose irritation. The minutes note that a suggested upper limit for PEI is 3 percent of the filter by weight, because of concern about adverse effects on bioassay results {1169.01, p. 8}. The PEI work is discussed at several different places in the documents.

Nicotine received specific attention when the participants discussed the development of nontobacco materials for smoking.

> There was a general discussion on non-tobacco materials and, largely due to the difficulties foreseen with the addition of nicotine, the Conference did not envisage at present the likely success of a totally non-tobacco cigarette. However, it now seems quite likely that non-tobacco materials will be successfully incorporated into cigarettes as blend constituents, particularly in health oriented products. *A large usage of non-tobacco materials would be likely to increase the demand for high-nicotine tobaccos* [emphasis added]. {1169.01, p. 8}

The development of a completely tobacco-free product was seen as unlikely because nicotine would have to be added. In making this judgment, the participants may have been thinking about a regulatory barrier. If nicotine were added to a tobacco substitute material, a drug regulatory authority such as the FDA might raise questions about whether the nicotine in this instance was a drug.

ST. ADELE RESEARCH CONFERENCE, 1970

At the 1970 research conference, held at St. Adele, Quebec, the consensus statements agreed upon at the Montreal conference three years earlier (see above) were reviewed. The changes in the wording of the consensus statements between these two meetings appear to reflect a growing awareness of the legal implications of scientific statements. On nicotine, the 1970 conference agreed,

> Nicotine is important, and there is probably a minimum level necessary for *consumer acceptance* in any given market. The chemical form of nicotine has been shown to affect the rate of absorption by the smoker [emphasis added]. {1170.01, p. 1}

In contrast, the corresponding statement in the minutes of the 1967 meeting (which, in turn, differs from that quoted from the draft minutes, in the above section headed "Montreal Research Conference, 1967") reads:

> Nicotine is important and there is probably a minimum level of nicotine to which for many people the *habituated effects of smoking* are attributable. The form of nicotine probably affects the rate of absorption by the smoker [emphasis added]. {1170.01, p. 1}

The statement on inhalation was changed markedly. The 1967 draft statement that we have reads:

> If there is no inhaling, there *is* no lung cancer or respiratory disease [emphasis added]. {1165.01, p. 2}.

The 1970 version:

> It was accepted that, without inhalation, *no association* between smoking and respiratory disease could reasonably be alledge [*sic*] [emphasis added]. {1170.01, p. 2}

The corresponding 1967 statement is not quoted in the 1970 minutes, which note somewhat ambiguously, "In 1967 the corresponding statement was not agreed" {1170.01, p. 2}.

Participants agreed that R&D was an essential activity for the company and that one of the general objectives of R&D was to "enhance the technological base of the company, and specifically to *create a framework for product design*" (emphasis added) {1170.01, p. 2}. This objective emphasizes the commercial intent behind much of the work done in R&D, presumably including the work on nicotine and the work on developing technologies to reduce toxicity. This explicit objective may be relevant to the matter of intent and the potential for FDA regulation.

The participants considered what their company's business might look like in a world in which cigarettes were no longer acceptable.

> It was agreed that, if and when total cigarette consumption declined, great opportunities for supplying the demand of other socially acceptable habits could follow. Discussion followed on those opportunities which might arise. Amongst those discussed were a) chewing products, and b) wet snuff. It was felt that this whole area, much of which is already in the tobacco industry, should be examined more thoroughly. Particular attention should be given to buccal administration of nicotine and other physiologically active ingredients. At the same time, it was re-affirmed that we would not contemplate the incorporation of nicotine in edible products. {1170.01, p. 3}

This discussion fits into the wishful thinking evident at other conferences about a noninhalable cigarette. Once again, nicotine is central to this speculation. Pure nicotine was not to be used as an additive in a tobacco product, but a high-nicotine tobacco extract was within the rules.

> The addition of nicotine to SM [substitute smoking materials] was considered, and it was recommended that nicotine per se, should not be used inside any tobacco factory. However, high nicotine content tobacco extract might be added. So long as SM remains a blend constituent, it would not be considered desirable for the supplier to include nicotine in the formulation. Nevertheless, for purposes of laboratory experimentation under suitable controls, nicotine-containing materials offered by suppliers may be used. {1170.01, p. 4}

The development of tobaccos with high nicotine content was expected, but the participants also called for research into the role of other nicotinic alkaloids and encouraged the Canadian subsidiary to explore the development of reconstituted tobacco with high nicotine content {1170.01, p. 5}. They recommended that cigarettes made by competitors be compared on the basis of extractable nicotine per puff, since such comparisons might provide a coherent basis for understanding market segmentation among consumers {1170.01, p. 7}.

Finally,

> It was agreed that insufficient work is being done on those benefits perceived by the consumer, and that psychological and pharmacological studies should be initiated, both at industry and group level, to identify the consumers' needs. {1170.01, p. 9}

This stress on pharmacological research to determine consumer needs illustrates again the underlying intent of BAT and B&W to deliver controlled amounts of pharmacologically active nicotine to their customers.

STUDIES ON CENTRAL NERVOUS SYSTEM EFFECTS OF NICOTINE

The documents include summaries of several research reports that examine the effects of nicotine on the central nervous system (CNS). All but one are internal BAT reports. The exception is a 1971 report from the labs of the Imperial Tobacco Group, Limited, in the United Kingdom.

G. Lawrence Willey and D. Neville Kellett of the Huntingdon Research Centre of the Imperial Tobacco Group reported their preliminary work with nicotine administration to squirrel monkeys in early 1971 {1218.01}. Experiments in this series of studies were to include measurements at the brain surface of acetylcholine, the naturally occurring neurotransmitter that nicotine mimics; effects of nicotine on the electroencephalogram; electrical stimulation studies of the brain; and behavioral effects. In their report the authors explicitly acknowledge that their experiments with monkeys sought to model the human experience.

> Actions of nicotine at peripheral sites in the body have been extensively investigated, but much less is known about its central effects. The aim of the studies to be reported here is to determine whether, in doses comparable to those taken into the blood by smokers, nicotine affects physiological processes and behavioural functions of the central nervous system of the primate. {1218.01, p.1}

Later in the report, the authors again explicitly acknowledge that the experiment was based on the conceptualization of nicotine as a drug.

> We also intend to compare changes produced by nicotine with those elicited by other drugs which are known to affect central nervous system function e.g. caffeine, amphetamine, chlorpromazine [an antipsychotic drug], meprobamate [a sedative]. {1218.01, p. 4}

Two electroencephalograph (EEG) studies of smoking were reported in late 1974 {1205.15; 1221.01}. The first, by R. F. Brotzge and Dr. J. E. Kennedy of B&W, describes an increase in alpha brain wave activity of adults after they smoked a cigarette {1121.01}. The report speculates that the effect "may reflect both psychological and physiological responses." (In this context, as mentioned, the term "physiological" appears to mean "pharmacological.") Evidently, this study was undertaken at B&W to facilitate product development.

> The development of new products and the modification of existing ones requires that we have some knowledge of the smoker toward whom these efforts are directed. The work described in this report is focused on the acute, or immediate physiological response of smokers. {1221.01, p. 1}

By saying that product design can be guided by pharmacological studies such as this, the authors reveal an intention to affect the structure or function of the body. As with other material in this chapter, it contributes to a determination that the FDA has jurisdiction over tobacco products.

The second EEG study was conducted by A. K. Comer and R. E. Thornton at BAT's Southampton laboratory {1205.15}. The study found that smoking increased the activity being measured in some subjects but decreased it in others. In their discussion the authors note that nicotine "has been assumed to be the main pharmacologically active component in smoke." They speculate that the disparate results may be explained by the hypothesis "that smoking may assist some people to optimise the level of activity in the brain."

These three reports illustrate the fact that, twenty years ago, Imperial, B&W, and BAT each thought that it was useful to examine the effects of nicotine on the central nervous system.

SMOKER COMPENSATION STUDIES

Compensation, the tendency of a person to smoke a cigarette having a lower machine-measured nicotine delivery more vigorously than a higher-delivery product, was mentioned for the first time in documents from the mid-1970s. The studies reported at the research conference held at Duck Key, Florida, in 1974 show that the tobacco industry was years ahead of the general scientific community in examining and understanding this phenomenon. The first study of compensation listed in the Surgeon General's 1988 report on nicotine addiction (3) is from 1980 (24). The work was confirmed three years later (25).

Specifically, the report of the conference notes:

> The Kippa study [a study of nicotine delivery at the German BAT laboratory] in Germany suggests that *whatever the characteristics of cigarettes as determined by smoking machines, the smoker adjusts his pattern to deliver his own nicotine requirements (about 0.8 mg per cigarette).*
>
> It is recommended that such studies should be considered for application in other countries where B.A.T. has a substantial interest in understanding more about smoking behaviour either for direct commercial or for health reasons [emphasis added]. {1125.01, p. 2}

Later in the report, an additional experiment to measure compensation in the context of cigarette ventilation is recommended: putting small holes in the filter or paper so that air is drawn into the smoke stream, thereby diluting it and reducing smoke delivery.

> The effect of ventilation on smoking behaviour should be explored in a McKennell-type test. {1125.01, p. 3}

By the 1970s dilution of mainstream cigarette smoke with room air had become a major technique for reducing machine-measured tar and nicotine deliveries. Termed "ventilation," dilution was accomplished with a variety of techniques, including the use of porous cigarette paper and the drilling of holes around the filter tip. We do not know what a "McKennell-type test" is.

An apparent replication of the German work was completed the following year in Canada. The "Chronology of B&W's Smoking and Health Research" includes the following item for 1975:

> Compensation study conducted by Imperial Tobacco Co., a BATCo affiliate, [shows that a smoker] *adjusts his smoking habits when smoking cigarettes with low nicotine and TPM* [total particulate matter] *to duplicate his normal cigarette nicotine intake* (Imperial Tobacco Project T-8077) [emphasis added]. {1006.01, p. 27}

Overall cigarette consumption data in the United Kingdom between 1965 and 1973 demonstrated a compensation effect {1190.09}. In 1975 G. F. Todd of the Tobacco Research Council analyzed per capita cigarette consumption for men and women for each year over this nine-year period, during which tar yields were steadily declining. Per capita cigarette consumption rose for both men and women through the period, indicating that smokers were smoking more in partial compensation.

Additional work on compensation was conducted by an outside contractor but reported through the R&D lab at Southampton by J. R. Courtney and A. K. Comer {1208.02}. Completed in 1978, the study analyzed the butts of cigarettes smoked by humans and compared the smoke constituents with those found in machine-smoked cigarettes. The technique permitted an estimation of actual delivery of smoke to the consumer. The study found compensation effects.

By 1980 B&W was beginning to recognize the legal and political dimensions of smoker compensation. In response to a questionnaire circulated by Dr. Alan Heard of BAT R&D about the proposed agenda for the upcoming research conference at Sea Island, Georgia {1132.01}, Dr. R. A. Sanford, vice president of R&D at B&W, indicated that B&W had "definite interest" in the proposed discussion of "compensation/smoker behaviour," but he also noted that this area of research was "dangerous" and questioned, "Is this in our best interests?" {1132.01, p. 3}. Research on smoker compensation was showing that consumers smoked cigarettes in ways that defeated the low-tar designs of the products. This finding undermined the implied benefit of low-tar smoke as less hazardous than normal cigarettes. In any event, the minutes of the conference did not include a discussion of compensation {1177.01}.

The 1983 research conference in Rio de Janeiro covered a variety of topics related to nicotine {1180.07}, including smoker compensation. The minutes of the conference note,

Compensation is now attracting the interest of Government and medical authorities in many parts of the world. This is based on the increasing number of new studies and, in part, by the evidence submitted by the industry to the FTC [Federal Trade Commission] in the Barclay investigation—much of which has already been communicated to Government authorities in Australia, Belgium, Finland, Holland, Switzerland and the UK.

There is now an urgent need to assess whether there are ways in which the industry can either counter the situation or alternatively turn it into a commercial advantage.

A direct consequence of this growing interest in compensation is the possibility that the FTC, and other authorities, may call for a change in the standard smoking machine test procedure for all products. If this were simply to be a modification to the existing standard procedure (increased puff volume, duration or interval) the effect would be to increase delivery levels but it would probably have little effect on League Table rankings [relative tar and nicotine yields]. A more extreme possibility is that an entirely new test procedure could be developed, eg a biological index. . . .

Either move would weaken the concept of low tar and would both confuse and concern the smoker. Operating Companies around the Group should, therefore, do everything possible to defend and maintain the present standard test procedure. If, however, the FTC or any other authority takes action to change the procedure the strategy should then be to stretch out any discussions (both with the authorities and later at ISO) until exhaustive studies have established that an alternative procedure is in fact more relevant.

In the meanwhile it is essential that we should increase our own research into how and why people smoke: eg what the smoker needs or gets from the cigarette in terms of nicotine and other sources of satisfaction. Until we have such knowledge we shall not be in a position to judge what would be best for the industry in the longer term.

   . . .

Whatever the outcome of the various public debates on compensation and test procedures, we must aim to use our knowledge to develop products that give improved smoker satisfaction. The concept of 'smoke elasticity' can be expected to play an important role [emphasis added]. {1180.07, pp. 8–9}

The Barclay investigation was spurred by B&W's competitors' crying foul to the FTC about the test results for B&W's Barclay brand of low-tar cigarettes. Competitors charged that the Barclay cigarette was designed to be smoked one way by the machine and another way by the consumer. The resulting investigation focused FTC attention on the compensation problem for the first time and provided the agency with some of the industry's data on the problem. This increased attention did not lead to any change in regulatory approach for many years. (It was not until late 1994 that there was some visible movement on this issue. In

December the National Cancer Institute convened a meeting to examine alternatives to the FTC test method.)

BAT scientists were concerned that a governmental agency might impose a new measure for product labeling which would have an uncertain or at least initially unknown relationship to product strength and nicotine satisfaction. The company's strategy was to jawbone regulators to delay any settlement of the matter until it could be sure that any resulting labeling scheme would not upset its ability to market cigarettes effectively to its various market segments.

BAT scientists, meanwhile, continued to work on compensation. By 1984 the consensus among them, as the proceedings of a joint R&D/marketing conference indicate, was that consumers adjust their smoking behavior to achieve specific nicotine dosing. The immediate signal for gauging nicotine dose is the "impact" of the puff on the throat. The impact, in turn, is directly related to nicotine dose.

> [It] is accepted that nicotine is both the driving force and the signal (as impact) for compensation in human smoking behaviour. {1226.01, p. 56}

The 1984 Montreal conference materials also demonstrate that BAT laboratories were evaluating design features of cigarettes that influenced a parameter called "elasticity." Elasticity quantifies the ability of the consumer to affect nicotine dose through compensation (by smoking the cigarette differently). The study appeared to measure the effect of different cigarette ventilation designs on smoke composition under conditions of differing puff volumes {1226.01, p. 58}.

The fact that people smoke in ways that defeat the engineering tricks of low-tar, low-nicotine cigarettes did not become widely appreciated in public health circles or the medical profession generally until the early 1980s, when Neal Benowitz published his studies showing that consumers smoke low-yield cigarettes more vigorously than they do higher-yield ones (25). In fact, the doses of nicotine delivered from all but the lowest-yield cigarettes are remarkably similar, and those from the lowest-yield versions are far higher than would be predicted from strict comparisons of machine-measured yields. Nonetheless, until about 1983 standard primary care medical textbooks advised physicians to recommend low-tar cigarettes for patients who were unable to stop smoking (26). Indeed, the tobacco industry promoted this view (see chapter 9).

Had the results of these internal BAT studies been generally known in the mid-1970s, medical advice in this matter might have changed earlier. The fact that smokers compensate for low-yield cigarettes seriously

undermines the implicit claim that low-tar, low-nicotine cigarettes reduce the risk of harm from smoking. In 1994 Jack Henningfield and his
colleagues at the National Institute on Drug Abuse advanced a proposal
to change the way the Federal Trade Commission (FTC) requires nicotine delivery to be reported by manufacturers, so that the amounts reported will more closely reflect the actual bioavailability of nicotine to
the consumer (27).

A research conference held at Pichlarn, Australia, in 1981 focused
some discussion on the regulatory aspects of compensation.

> It is felt that the time is close when Government agencies worldwide will take
> more notice of compensation—and of the scale of the differences, for a given
> commercial product, between smoking machine numbers and the dose of
> smoke actually obtained by smokers. This issue may well go beyond the
> simple technical measurement of deliveries. If for no other reason than de-
> fence, we must pay increasing attention as to how our products—especially
> new products—are smoked by different categories of smokers. {1178.01,
> pp. 13–14}

The concern was misplaced at two levels. First, governments did not get
seriously interested in this problem for another dozen years. Second, dealing with the compensation problem in a conscientious manner requires
more than taking a merely defensive, public relations–oriented posture.

MONTEBELLO RESEARCH CONFERENCE, 1982

The first entry in the minutes for the 1982 Montebello research conference, under the heading "Subjects of Major Group Importance," is "Human Smoking Behaviour."

> More must be known about how different consumers smoke different prod-
> ucts and derive different levels of satisfaction or response therefrom. We are
> concerned with two aspects:
>
> (a)   Sensations and responses at the mouth level—which influence initial
> selection and brand loyalty.
> (b)   The pharmacological result of smoke uptake. {1179.01, p. 1}

The minutes refer to work under way in Germany on precise nicotine
dose measurements in consumers; Canadian studies of puff duplication
techniques to measure how the smoker smoked the cigarette; and work
planned in the United States at B&W on surreptitious videotaping of
smoking to measure smoking behavior in natural settings. Similarly, the
Southampton program, although it was aimed at identifying market

segments based on "smoking bahavioural characteristics," also was paying attention to "the biochemistry and pharmacology associated with
the inhalation of major smoke components" {1179.01, p. 3}. The minutes of the Montebello conference specify a design objective for new
products:

> *to enhance or maximise sensory and pharmacological sensations, ie to 'make*
> *the smoke work harder'* so as to achieve maximum sensation at a given de-
> livery level without encouraging the smoker to compensate [emphasis added].
> {1179.01, p. 3}

Once again, the R&D staffs of BAT and B&W show their understanding of the purpose of a cigarette as a nicotine delivery device. Pharmacological sensations are not only intended to occur; they are to be manipulated so that the consumer can get the desired dose of nicotine
without taking in more tar than intended.

BAT's R&D group at Southampton held a series of informal discussions on the characteristics of cigarette smoke in late 1982 or early 1983.
These discussions seem to have been sparked by recommendations made
at the 1982 Montebello conference. Colin Greig, a participant in the
Southampton discussions, compiled his notes, and C. I. Ayers circulated
them to the heads of BAT research labs in the United States, Germany,
Australia, Brazil, and Canada in February 1984 {1179.02}. Under the
heading "Physiological Consequences," Greig's notes include the following comment about nicotine:

> It is well known that nicotine can be removed from smoke by the lung and
> transmitted to the brain within seconds of smoke inhalation. Since it is the
> major or sole pharmacologically active agent in smoke, it must be presumed
> that this is its preferred method of absorption and thus why people inhale
> smoke. {1179.02, p. 10}

In short, the purpose of cigarette smoke inhalation is the absorption of
nicotine and the transport of nicotine to the brain.

NICOTINE DOSE AND "SMOKER SATISFACTION"

The R&D unit at BAT contracted for a major study of smoking in the
mid-1970s. Project Wheat was designed to measure the personal characteristics of a large group of male smokers in the community and then
to ask each smoker how well he liked or disliked cigarettes containing
different tar and nicotine deliveries {1206.01; 1206.02; 1206.03}. The
project was to rely on the sophisticated statistical technique of factor

analysis to assess what characterized different smokers' preferences. The goal was to separate smokers into various group on the basis of "inner need" to smoke (this group was thought to inhale more heavily) and "health concern." These groupings make sense only if one believes that tar is toxic and that nicotine satisfies an "inner need." The results were somewhat unclear—partly because, as it turned out, the cigarettes used in testing did not actually meet the design specifications. The matrix of "inner need" and "health concern," though, illustrates the frame of mind of the BAT scientists who approved the protocol.

Two BAT Southampton R&D reports describing methods for measuring nicotine and cotinine levels in blood and urine provide valuable insights into the important role BAT scientists thought nicotine played in smoking behavior {1208.04; 1208.05}. The first report, from May 1980, states,

> In some instances, the pharmacological response of smokers to nicotine is believed to be responsible for an individual's smoking behaviour, providing the motivation for and the degree of satisfaction required by the smoker (5, 6). {1208.04, p. 2}

The second report, from 1981, describes a technique for estimating the "whole body nicotine dose to the fat following intravenous administration." The authors' direct interest in using knowledge of the absorbed dose of nicotine as an aid in cigarette design is revealed in the report's description of the value of the new technique:

> This technique has an immediate and direct relevance for
> (i)   animal toxicity studies in the comparative assessment of cigarettes,
> (ii)   human behavioural studies in the assessment of an individual's nicotine dose in response to modification in cigarette design. {1208.05, p. 1}

Thus, the absorbed dose of nicotine is an important consideration in cigarette design.

A similar concern with the relationship of nicotine dose and product design is evident in a paper describing the conclusions of a research conference setting priorities for the R&D group at Southampton in 1984 {1210.01}. Under the category "Smoker Behaviour," a series of studies are planned, which, among other things, would explore "the efficient use of smoke nicotine through pH modification" {1210.01, p. 2}. The goal of this series of studies is described as follows:

> These studies will identify the relationship between nicotine dose and nicotine-related subjective improvement. This will further help to identify

the relationship between product acceptability and smoker satisfaction.
{1210.01, p. 2}

This comment—which ties together the terms "satisfaction," "nicotine
dose," and "nicotine-related subjective improvement"—is about affecting the structure or function of the body.

The importance of pH in fine-tuning nicotine delivery was emphasized ten years later in testimony by the head of the FDA, Dr. David
Kessler, on June 21, 1994, before the House of Representatives Subcommittee on Health and the Environment (5). Kessler reported that at
least one major cigarette manufacturer uses ammonia compounds as additives to tobacco blends, to enhance nicotine delivery in cigarette smoke
by pH adjustments. The *Wall Street Journal* has reported that UST, a
maker of tobacco snuff, uses additives to adjust the acidity (pH) of moist
snuff products (28)—a practice resulting in levels of free nicotine that
vary in accordance with their market niche (28–31).

RESEARCH AGENDA ON NICOTINE, 1983

At the 1983 research conference in Rio de Janeiro, participants developed a research agenda on nicotine itself. Here are the notes from the
minutes on this subject:

> The growing concern about compensation is focussing attention on the role
> of nicotine in the smoking process. It was agreed that we must know as much
> as possible about:
>
>> factors that affect the transfer of nicotine from leaf to smoke aerosol
>>
>> factors that influence the rate of transfer of nicotine from particulate
>> matter to the vapour phase
>>
>> the contribution of nicotine to smoke sensory characteristics (includ-
>> ing harshness and irritation)
>>
>> *the site and mechanisms of absorption of nicotine within the human
>> system*
>>
>> *the way nicotine stimulates both the central nervous system and the pe-
>> ripheral organs (eg heart and lung)*
>>
>> *the metabolism of nicotine within the body, including rates and equi-
>> librium levels.*
>
> The developing programme of research at Southampton was supported,
> albeit that *greater emphasis should be placed on direct human studies rather
> than on animals—particularly in view of recent major advances in brain phar-
> macology.* It is envisaged that much of such work will be undertaken under
> contract.

It was proposed that a senior person at Southampton should be responsible for coordinating all the relevant interest and work throughout the Group. *There is an urgent need to prepare a status review on all major aspects of the pharmacological influences of nicotine in the smoking process* [emphasis added]. {1180.07, pp. 13–14}

BAT scientists clearly regarded nicotine as a drug. The reference to the action of nicotine on the lung as well as the heart may be in recognition of the fact that the lung has an extensive network of nerve endings that can respond to nicotine and directly stimulate the brain (3). The earlier discussion on compensation made it clear that R&D felt under some pressure to get one step ahead of the regulators in test design. Here, the compensation problem was driving these scientists to look more closely at nicotine itself. The practical result of such research might be seen in testing procedures, in product design, or both.

In any case, the reason for the emphasis on nicotine in these conference minutes is the perceived need, the intention, to have a product that delivers a reliable and predictable dose of nicotine.

VIEWS OF NICOTINE IN 1984

In June 1984 a three-day technical exchange meeting on nicotine was held in Southampton. The summary of the meeting appears in a set of notes for the 1984 BAT research conference in the United Kingdom {1181.07}. The summary is reproduced below in its entirety because it shows very clearly the importance of nicotine for the normal, expected functioning of a cigarette in the opinion of BAT scientists only a decade ago.

The main conclusions reached were:—
- a) Plasma nicotine/cotinine measurements can give reliable estimates of the nicotine uptake by groups of smokers, and with suitable precautions, by an individual smoker. Many smokers appear to obtain 12–14 mg. of nicotine per day from their cigarettes.
- b) Cigarettes which have a delivery of less than 0.7 mg. of nicotine per cigarette[,] as measured on a smoking machine, do not achieve large volume sales.
- c) Providing smoke is inhaled—even shallow inhalation—95% of the nicotine is retained.
- d) Intuitively it is felt that "satisfaction" must be related to nicotine. Many people believe it a "whole body response" and involves the action of nicotine in the brain.

e)   Although many smokers appear to approach a plateau or constant
     level of nicotine in the blood, it is not known:
     (i)   whether a smoker feels the need for another cigarette when his
           blood level falls significantly below this plateau level
 or (ii)   whether the smoker is seeking the more transient peak levels su-
           per-imposed upon the general plateau level.

f)   If level in the brain is the key feature, we have little idea at present on
     the relationship between blood levels/pattern and those in the brain.

g)   An immediate sensory affect [sic] associated with nicotine is the "im-
     pact" on inhaling. Is this sensation a genuine part of the reward a
     smoker is seeking or is it a "cue," i.e. a smoker has learnt by experi-
     ence, that if he perceives a particular level of impact, he will subse-
     quently receive an acceptable degree of satisfaction.

h)   If we are to make better use in product terms of the levels of nicotine
     in smoke currently available—and even more so if we are forced to
     market cigarettes with reduced levels of nicotine—then it is important
     to significantly increase our understanding of impact/satisfaction.

There is an urgent need for experimental cigarettes in which the levels of nicotine in smoke (and smoke pH) are carefully controlled [emphasis in original].
{1181.07}

This summary indicates that BAT scientists had a sophisticated and
up-to-date understanding of nicotine and its role in smoking behavior.
The importance of smoke pH in designing an effective product at lower
nicotine deliveries is apparent. Satisfaction is described as being related
to the effects of nicotine on the body, especially on the brain, and the importance of inhalation is emphasized. This is the only place where we
have seen a definition of the term "satisfaction" offered by tobacco company personnel. In most instances the term's meaning in relationship to
the pharmacological effects of cigarette smoke must be inferred. Here it
is explicit.

The discussions held at this technical exchange were reviewed in detail at the joint R&D/marketing conference in Montreal in July 1984.
Both the notes summarizing the technical exchange and the minutes of
the discussion mention the importance of considering nicotine levels in
product design {1226.01, pp. 61–63}. The minutes note,

[An] improvement in our understanding of nicotine action is of major importance for future product development. {1226.01, p. 63}

At this same meeting, G. A. Read, Group Leader, Smoker Behaviour,
GR & DC, at Imperial Tobacco, gave a fairly technical presentation on
the constituents of smoke that affect product design, acceptability, and
smoking satisfaction. It is clear from this material, presented at a mar-

keting conference, that BAT appreciated the key role of nicotine in selling cigarettes. The talk focused primarily on the role of nicotine in smoking behavior and included slides on nicotine absorption and pharmacology. In contrast to public statements made by the tobacco companies, Read's slides note:

> strong indirect evidence for smokers smoking nicotine
>
> . . .
>
> underlying smoking maintenance through nicotine, and as a consequence nicotine probably provides the basis of smoking satisfaction
>
> in its simplest sense puffing behavior is the means of providing nicotine dose in a metered fashion {1224.01, pp. 46–47}

Read concluded by suggesting that the minimum dose requirement for nicotine to maintain smoking behavior should be determined and that product quality and satisfaction would be enhanced if this minimum dose of nicotine were provided.

THE SEARCH FOR NICOTINE ANALOGUES

The documents show that, although the tobacco industry considered nicotine a mostly harmless drug, it was concerned about the potentially harmful effects of nicotine on the cardiovascular system. For example, nicotine acts directly on the heart and arteries, and carbon monoxide in the smoke reduces the ability of the blood to transport oxygen. The industry tried to solve this problem by looking for analogues to nicotine, drugs that could mimic the effects of nicotine on the brain without affecting the cardiovascular system. Although Philip Morris pursued this approach in the 1980s (4, 32), the documents show that BAT was interested in the problem in the early 1970s.

A decade before the first research report on nicotine analogues from BAT's R&DE (Research and Development Establishment) lab, Sir Charles Ellis described the research program the tobacco manufacturers in the United Kingdom were undertaking to investigate the cardiovascular toxicity of nicotine. In his keynote address at BAT's 1962 research conference in Southampton, Sir Charles said,

> You are of course aware that smoking, by means of its nicotine content, is supposed to have an effect on the cardiovascular system. T.M.S.C. [Tobacco Manufacturers' Standing Committee] has agreed to contribute £12,000 over three years to Dr. Shillingford of the Cardiovascular Research Group of the Medical Research Council to enable them to extend their experiments to cover

the effects of nicotine. We think that it is well worth while having this work carried out by a skilled authoritative group with which we will have close contact.

It is the case that most previous work on the effects of nicotine on the cardiovascular system has been done with old techniques, and much of it is of doubtful quality. What T.M.S.C. believes is of particular importance is that Shillingford has developed entirely new techniques for analysing heart function and circulation in health and disease. These are based on observing changes in blood-flow by the use of short-lived radioisotopes which, for example, make it possible to measure the heart output every five minutes for an hour without using the old-fashioned catheter. *You will be interested to know that Dr. Shillingford accepts the existence of beneficial effects of smoking and believes that although nicotine undoubtedly affects the cardiovascular system these effects are probably quite innocuous for normal healthy people* [emphasis added]. {1102.01, pp. 19–20}

Concrete evidence of BAT's interest in nicotine analogues is documented in three research reports from the BAT Group Research and Development Centre in the 1970s {1205.11; 1205.13; 1208.03}. None of the reports indicate precisely what problem with nicotine the analogue work is designed to solve. However, when researchers for Philip Morris conducted a more extensive study of analogues in the 1980s, they were looking for compounds that had the central nervous system effects of nicotine while avoiding the cardiovascular effects (4, 32). BAT's concern with nicotine analogues may well have been based on the same considerations.

The abstract of the first of the three reports (written in November 1972) emphasizes the importance of the pharmacological actions of nicotine for smokers: "[T]he present scale of the tobacco industry is largely dependent on the intensity and nature of the pharmacological action of nicotine" {1205.11, p. 2}. The abstract emphasizes the need to develop acceptable substitutes should nicotine itself come to be regarded as unacceptable, and describes an analogue developed at Bath University through a postdoctoral fellowship supported by BAT. The summary reads as follows:

> *Should nicotine become less attractive to smokers, the future of the tobacco industry would become less secure.*
>
> Factors that could influence the attractiveness of nicotine are discussed, and it is concluded that substances closely related to nicotine in structure (nicotine analogues) could be important. Synthetic studies at Bath University have produced a compound that was shown by Bioassay Limited to have a powerful inhibitory effect on some of the pharmacological actions of nicotine.

> It is recommended that this work continue with suitable collaborators to clarify some of the possible threats to, and opportunities for, the Company [emphasis added]. {1205.11, p. 1}

Although couched in somewhat hedged terms, the introduction amplifies the sentiment expressed in the summary and further discusses the importance of the pharmacological effects of nicotine.

> *It has been suggested that a considerable proportion of smokers depend on the pharmacological action of nicotine for their motivation to continue smoking [references omitted].*
>
> *If this view is correct, the present scale of the tobacco industry is largely dependent on the intensity and nature of the pharmacological action of nicotine.*
>
> A commercial threat would arise if either an alternative product became acceptable or the effect of nicotine was changed.
>
> An alternative product could come from the pharmaceutical industry. With a socially acceptable route for administration, and with medical endorsement, the product could be successful.
>
> The effect of nicotine could be inhibited by an antagonist, and cigarettes would tend to become insipid. Such an antagonist could arise by accident or design from the pharmaceutical industry. It might be used tactically to advance that industry's alternative product, or its general use could be advocated by the anti-smoking lobby, with or without government support [emphasis added]. {1220.01, p. 2}

The concern about a "commercial threat" might be related to the work reported by Murray Jarvik earlier that year at a CTR-sponsored symposium on nicotine-blocking drugs (33). Jarvik's experiments, which had been supported by the American Cancer Society, included one on nicotine-blocking agents. He reported that a centrally acting agent called mecamylamine, which blocks the effects of nicotine in the brain, was associated with a compensatory increase in smoking in a short-term experiment. However, over time, such a blocking drug would be expected to reduce the attraction of smoking by preventing the reinforcing effects of nicotine on the central nervous system. In this way, smokers would become less and less compulsive about the use of tobacco products. Mecamylamine itself was unsuitable as a therapeutic agent because it also caused a marked lowering of blood pressure. However, Jarvik's experiment held an obvious lesson for BAT: conventional pharmaceutical companies might be able to market a safe nicotine antagonist that would prevent the nicotine in tobacco products from doing its thing. The nicotine analogue work may have been seen as a way to get ahead of this disturbing possibility.

The abstract of a second report, from 1973, indicates that the work did, in fact, continue, at least to some extent. The abstract describes the pharmacological activity of an isomer of a previously synthesized analogue {1205.13}. In this instance, the synthetic work had been performed at the School of Pharmacy of London University. The full reports are not available.

The third report, dated June 10, 1979, describes the testing of an analogue, including tests on muscle tissue {1208.03}. This may have been a screening test for cardiovascular activity, since Dr. Victor DeNoble indicated that tests of smooth-muscle reactivity had served this function in the Philip Morris research program (32). The results in this instance were not encouraging, but there seem to have been plans to test additional compounds.

THE INDUSTRY'S PUBLIC STATEMENTS ON NICOTINE

The tobacco industry has repeatedly told the public that nicotine is not addictive. Most specifically and most dramatically, at a congressional hearing on April 14, 1994, seven tobacco company CEOs—each in turn—stated that nicotine is not addictive. Thomas Sandefur, the CEO of B&W, testified, "I do not believe that nicotine is addictive."

In discussing the pharmacological properties of nicotine, the industry has largely relied on the way nicotine was discussed in the 1964 Surgeon General's report (2). This report draws a distinction between habituating and addicting drugs based on the then current understanding of the importance of tolerance and withdrawal phenomena in defining addiction. However, the report clearly states that nicotine is responsible for a variety of pharmacological actions in smokers and that the habituating nature of the process can make it difficult to stop. The addictive nature of nicotine is now well documented and widely appreciated (3). Significantly, even before the 1964 Surgeon General's report, B&W and BAT privately had concluded that nicotine is addictive.

Although industry representatives have suggested that nicotine contributes to the flavor of tobacco, the Food and Drug Administration, in its investigation of nicotine-containing cigarettes and smokeless tobacco products, found no evidence that nicotine serves such a function (6). In fact, the agency found that consumers perceive nicotine as an irritant, and that the industry uses additives to disguise the sensations which nicotine contributes to the experience of ingesting tobacco products.

The documents include an example of one industry formula for discussing the addiction question. It is contained in an undated set of questions and suggested answers (which appear to date from the early 1980s), titled "Tobaccotalk," that a B&W employee might use when questioned by people outside the industry.

Q: Aren't cigarettes addictive?

A: It is difficult to discuss addiction today because people apply the term to many different circumstances. Some people say their children are addicted to TV. The 1964 Surgeon General's report concluded that cigarettes should be classified as habituative, like coffee, and not addictive, like morphine. Many people have given up smoking. Why do some people continue to smoke who say they want to quit? Why do people continue to overeat when they say they are overweight? {2133.01, p. 5}

The exchange coaches the B&W employee on how to deal with this issue from the industry perspective. The proposed answer confuses the matter by blurring the term "addiction" to include a very broad array of activities, such as compulsive TV watching. Nicotine is addicting in exactly the same sense that heroin, cocaine, and alcohol are addicting (3). It is a drug that has powerful, reinforcing actions on the brain, and repeated use tends to produce continued use. The 1964 Surgeon General's report employed a different definition of addiction than is generally understood today. At about the same time, B&W's general counsel, Addison Yeaman, accepted, without hesitation, the fact that nicotine is addictive and that "we are . . . in the business of selling nicotine, an addictive drug" {1802.05, p. 4}.

The fact that many people have stopped smoking is no more proof that nicotine is not addictive than is the fact that many people who have been clearly addicted to other drugs, such as heroin, have stopped using them as well (3, 34). Spontaneous recovery is part of the natural history of addictions, and indeed forms the basis for public health advice about drug use. Focusing on those who have recovered from addiction ignores those who still use a substance but who would like to stop. As discussed above, in any given year about a third of smokers attempt to quit, but only about 10 percent succeed, because of nicotine addiction (3). B&W's suggested answer seeks to avoid the real question at hand.

The tobacco industry has consistently avoided talking about nicotine in its marketing campaigns. One of the documents {1203.01} shows how references to nicotine and withdrawal (a drug addiction term) were edited out of an externally prepared prospectus for a marketing campaign for a low-delivery cigarette. Around 1978 Lisher and Company, a marketing management consulting firm in New York, submitted a draft proposal for a low-delivery cigarette to B&W for review. The goal of the project was to develop cigarettes that matched the parameters suggested as desirable by Dr. Gio Gori of the National Cancer Institute, discussed in chapter 4. Before editing, the second paragraph of the proposal had read,

> Current market trends clearly indicate a major trend toward low-tar brands, although *current "ultra" low tar brands have had limited success because of their failure to deliver satisfaction/maintain an adequate nicotine level.* An ancillary concern relative to nicotine delivery is that *if a satisfying, low-nicotine cigarette were to be developed, it could represent an effective means of withdrawal with severe implications for long-term market growth* [emphasis added]. {1203.01, p. 1}

The editor changed it to read,

> Current market trends clearly indicate a major trend toward low-"tar" brands, although current "ultra" low "tar" brands have had limited success because of their failure to deliver satisfaction. {1203.01, p. 1}

All specific mention of nicotine, including the stated need to maintain an "adequate nicotine level," was excised. As originally written, the paragraph accurately reflects a concern with providing a pharmacologically sufficient dose of nicotine to consumers. The editing process concentrated all of this meaning into the euphemism "satisfaction." This is an example of the use of code words such as "satisfaction" to obscure the genuine pharmacological intent of the tobacco companies. The intent to provide satisfaction is, in this instance, clearly an intent to maintain an "adequate nicotine level." Examples such as this comprise one kind of evidence that the FDA could use to make the case that tobacco companies intend that tobacco products affect the structure or function of the body.

As discussed in more detail in chapter 7, the documents include another comment on nicotine from a public relations perspective. It appears in an attachment to a memo from Ernest Pepples, B&W's assistant general counsel, to J. V. Blalock, the director of public relations, dated February 14, 1973 {1814.01, p. 1}. Pepples asked Blalock to assemble current clippings on nine different topic areas regarding tobacco. One of those topic areas was addiction, and this is how Pepples framed the problem:

> ADDICTION—Some emphasis is now being placed on the habit-forming capacities of cigarette smoke. *To some extent the argument revolving around "free choice" is being negated on the grounds of addiction. The threat is that*

this argument will increase significantly and lead to further restrictions on product specifications and greater danger in litigation [emphasis added]. {1814.01, p. 3}

"Restrictions on product specifications" because of addiction did not become a realistic possibility for another twenty years, when the Food and Drug Administration began to show an interest in this area (4) and when lawsuits focusing on the plaintiffs' addiction began to be filed. The industry's defense is now as it has been in the past: a denial that nicotine is addictive and that the industry in any way intends the pharmacological effects that nicotine provides.

Even as this position comes to appear more and more absurd, some commentators with ties to the industry have actually argued that addiction does not impair free will (35). This argument has been used to help justify the conclusion that it would not be good public policy to raise excise taxes on tobacco products (36).

CONCLUSION

A 1973 handout for a talk by Dr. S. J. Green, who headed R&D at BAT in the 1970s, at a conference of industry executives includes the following definition of nicotine:

A pharmacologically active material present in tobacco and tobacco smoke. It can act as a stimulant or depressant depending very much upon the person and the situation. In even small quantities it is a poison but it is metabolized rapidly by humans and not stored in tissue. When smoke is inhaled the nicotine is largely retained by the smoker. {1184.01, p. 4}

There is no mention of any taste or flavor value for nicotine, only its pharmacological effects. The definition assumes that inhalation is a normal way to ingest this "pharmacologically active material."

The private papers of Dr. Green include a revealing diagram of the importance he accorded nicotine {1186.08}. It is undated, but it uses company jargon from the early 1970s. Titled "Approaches to Problems in the Association of Smoking and Disease," the schematic places "nicotine administration" at the top, as the overall goal to be achieved. The very bottom of the diagram indicates that nicotine is to be administered to the mouth, in the case of noninhalable forms of tobacco, or to the mouth and lungs if the product is to be inhaled (i.e., cigarettes).

Strategic research was to involve nicotine itself (including "dosing" issues), "alternative pharmacological agents," and "health-oriented cigarettes" (cigarettes that produce less disease). Tactical research and product development included "re-assurance" or "health-image" cigarettes and ways of responding to public health pressures such as the publication of tar and nicotine yields. "Health-image" cigarettes, as discussed in chapter 4, were intended to provide the appearance of reduced harm.

Again and again, the documents demonstrate the central importance of nicotine to the normal use of tobacco products. The role of nicotine in tobacco products is that of a pharmacological agent: B&W and BAT value nicotine not for its taste and flavor but for what it does to the brain. The dose of nicotine absorbed by the consumer is a factor to be considered in product design. Moreover, at least in the early 1960s, some B&W and BAT officials almost seemed to take pride in the addictive nature of nicotine.

Taste is irrelevant to nicotine as it is discussed in these documents. Sensory panels occasionally described in the documents were not asked to measure taste. Rather, they were concerned with the level of irritation nicotine in different forms causes, or with whether it has a certain "impact." Whereas taste is irrelevant, the documents demonstrate that inhalation is essential to the normal functioning of a cigarette. Inhalation is essential for nicotine absorption from a cigarette. It has no other purpose.

BAT's idealized cigarette was Ariel, a product designed to minimize toxic smoke components and deliver but one main active ingredient: nicotine. While not as fully laid out for BAT as for Philip Morris, the nicotine analogue program betrays the same focus: the purpose of the product is the delivery of a pharmacologically active substance to the brain—preferably a substance with lower toxicity to the heart and blood vessels. The logical goal of Project Ariel (provide a smoke-free nicotine aerosol), combined with the analogue work (find a less hazardous form of nicotine), is the creation of a product that delivers a nicotine analogue and no other active ingredient.

The public relations posture of B&W differs markedly from the internal working views expressed within B&W and BAT over the years. While the public posture has been that nicotine is not addicting and the company does not intend any of the pharmacological effects that occur, the internal writings consistently assume addiction and throughout demonstrate a keen interest in all aspects of the pharmacology of nicotine.

The contract work and the internal company research projects reviewed here have not been published in the scientific literature. Often, the work was well ahead of its time. The Battelle work in Geneva was at the cutting edge of pharmacological work on nicotine at the time. The work on smoker compensation in the 1970s preceded the main published reports by a decade. Today B&W accepts one, and only one, conclusion from the 1964 Surgeon General's report: that nicotine is a habituating, not an addicting, drug. Yet high-level executives at B&W and BAT did not accept this conclusion in 1964.

In early 1992, BAT considered whether to purchase a manufacturer of nicotine patches (37). B&W's chief attorney, Mick McGraw, objected because of the unwanted attention such a move might draw to the cigarette business from the FDA. He also felt that selling a nicotine patch to help people manage withdrawal symptoms as they tried to stop smoking would undercut the company position that people choose to smoke and that they can stop at will. In contrast to McGraw's feelings, Patrick Dunn, the head of research at the Canadian subsidiary, Imperial Tobacco, regarded the patch business as a natural extension of the cigarette business. A scientific analysis of the nicotine patch prepared by B&W staff compared the nicotine delivery rate from a cigarette with that from a patch. These candid appraisals of the nicotine patch, written in 1992, demonstrate that the perspectives on nicotine reflected in the documents from the early 1960s through the mid-1980s, which have been reviewed in this chapter, were still operative at BAT and at its subsidiaries only two years before Thomas Sandefur, B&W's CEO, told Congress, "I believe that nicotine is not addictive."

Are cigarettes drugs? Do cigarette manufacturers intend that their products affect the structure or function of the body? The documents reviewed in this chapter, taken as a whole, demonstrate that, for B&W and for BAT at least, the answer is yes. This answer, in turn, means that cigarettes made by these companies come under the jurisdiction of the FDA through the federal Food, Drug and Cosmetic Act.

REFERENCES

1. APA. *Diagnostic and Statistical Manual of Mental Disorders, IV (DSM IV)*. Washington, DC: American Psychiatric Association, 1994.
2. USDHEW. *Smoking and Health. Report of the Advisory Committee to the Surgeon General of the Public Health Service*. US Department of Health, Education and Welfare, 1964. Public Health Service Publication No. 1103.
3. USDHHS. *The Health Consequences of Smoking: Nicotine Addiction. A Report of the Surgeon General*. US Department of Health and Human Services, Public Health Service, Centers for Disease Control, Center for Health Promotion and Education, Office on Smoking and Health, 1988. DHHS Publication No. (CDC) 88-8406.

4. Kessler D. *A Statement on Nicotine-Containing Cigarettes before the Subcommittee on Health and the Environment.* Committee on Energy and Commerce, US House of Representatives, March 25, 1994.

5. Kessler D. *A Statement before the Subcommittee on Health and the Environment.* Committee on Energy and Commerce, US House of Representatives, June 21, 1994.

6. Food and Drug Administration. Proposed rule analysis regarding FDA's jurisdiction over nicotine-containing cigarettes and smokeless tobacco products. *Federal Register* 1995 August 11:41453–41787.

7. Food and Drug Administration. Regulations restricting the sale and distribution of cigarettes and smokeless tobacco products to protect children and adolescents. *Federal Register* 1995 August 11:41314–41451.

8. USDHHS. *Preventing Tobacco Use among Young People. A Report of the Surgeon General.* US Department of Health and Human Services, Public Health Service, Centers for Disease Control and Prevention, National Center for Chronic Disease Prevention and Health Promotion, Office on Smoking and Health, 1994.

9. Royal College of Physicians. *Smoking and Health. A Report of the Royal College of Physicians on Smoking in Relation to Cancer of the Lung and Other Diseases.* London: Pitman Medical Publishing Co., 1962.

10. Martini L, Ganong W. *Neuroendocrinology.* New York: Academic Press, 1966.

11. Medvei V. *The History of Clinical Endocrinology.* Pearl River, NY: Parthenon Publishing Group, 1992.

12. Grunberg N. The effects of nicotine and cigarette smoking on food consumption and taste preferences. *Addictive Behaviors* 1982;7:317–331.

13. Slade J. Nicotine delivery devices. In: Orleans C, Slade J, eds. *Nicotine Addiction: Principles and Management* (pp. 3–23). New York: Oxford University Press, 1993.

14. Armitage AK, Dollery, CT, George CF, Houseman TH, Lewis PJ, Turner DM. Absorption and metabolism of nicotine from cigarettes. *Brit Med J* 1975;4(5992):313–316.

15. Ellis C, Schachner H, Williamson D. Smoking device. US Patent 3,258,015. Assigned to Battelle, 1966.

16. Ellis C, Hughes W. Smoking devices. US Patent 3,356,094. Assigned to Battelle, 1967.

17. Slade J. *Statement before the Subcommittee on Health and the Environment.* Committee on Energy and Commerce, US House of Representatives, March 25, 1994.

18. R. J. Reynolds Tobacco Co. *Chemical and Biological Studies on New Cigarette Prototypes That Heat Instead of Burn Tobacco.* Winston-Salem, NC: R. J. Reynolds Tobacco Co., 1988.

19. Slade J. The tobacco epidemic: Lessons from history. *J Psychoactive Drugs* 1989;21:281–291.

20. Hilts P. Little smoke, little tar, but still lots of nicotine. *New York Times* 1994 November 27:1.

21. Litzinger E. Smoking article. US Patent 4,924,886. Assigned to Brown and Williamson Tobacco Corp., 1990.

22. Johnson R, Tang J-Y. Cigarette. US Patent 4,955,397. Assigned to Brown and Williamson Tobacco Corp., 1990.

23. Porenski H, Plotner R. Smoking article. US Patent 5,327,915. Assigned to Brown and Williamson Tobacco Corp., 1994.

24. Russell M, Jarvis M, Iyer R, Feyerabend C. Relation of nicotine yield of cigarettes to blood nicotine concentrations in smokers. *Brit Med J* 1980;280:972–976.

25. Benowitz N, Hall S, Herning R, Jacob P III, Jones R, Osman A-L. Smokers of low-yield cigarettes do not consume less nicotine. *N Engl J Med* 1983;309(3):139–142.

26. Warner K, Slade J. Low tar, high toll. *Am J Pub Health* 1992;82:17–18.

27. Henningfield J, Kozlowski L, Benowitz N. A proposal to develop meaningful labeling for cigarettes. *JAMA* 1994;272:312–314.
28. Freeman A. How a tobacco giant doctors snuff brands to boost their "kick." *Wall Street Journal* 1994 October 26:A1.
29. Djordjevic M, Hoffman D, Glynn T, Connolly G. US commercial brands of moist snuff, 1994: I. Assessment of nicotine, moisture and pH. *Tobacco Control* 1995; 4:62–66.
30. Henningfield J, Radzius A, Cone E. Estimation of available nicotine content of six smokeless tobacco products. *Tobacco Control* 1995;4:57–61.
31. Connolly G. The marketing of nicotine addiction by oral snuff manufacturers. *Tobacco Control* 1995;4:73–79.
32. DeNoble V. *Testimony before the Subcommittee on Health and the Environment.* Committee on Energy and Commerce, US House of Representatives, April 28, 1994.
33. Jarvik M. Further observations on nicotine as the reinforcing agent in smoking. In: Dunn W, ed. *Smoking Behavior: Motives and Incentives* (pp. 33–49). Washington, DC: V. H. Winston and Sons, 1973.
34. Robbins L. Vietnam veterans' rapid recovery from heroin addiction: A fluke or normal expectation? *Addiction* 1993;88:1041–1054.
35. Viscusi W. *Making the Risky Decision.* New York: Oxford University Press, 1992.
36. Gravelle JG, Zimmerman D. *Cigarette Taxes to Fund Health Care Reform: An Economic Analysis.* Washington, DC: Library of Congress, Congressional Research Service, 1994.
37. Schwartz J. Tobacco firm's inside debate revealed. *Washington Post* 1995 October 9:A8.

CHAPTER 4

The Search for a "Safe" Cigarette

Any work undertaken must be with a commercial or political motive as well as a scientific motive. The object is for the company to be able to say that, in the light of all available knowledge, it " . . . is doing its best to supply a 'safer' smoke."

Letter from BAT to B&W president Ed Finch, 1964 {1804.01}

INTRODUCTION

Throughout most of the 1960s, the tobacco industry was convinced that it could make cigarettes safe—that is, that it could discover the toxic components of cigarette smoke and eliminate them. In the lab the tobacco industry's scientists quietly worked on reducing the toxicity of cigarettes by various means. To this end, they developed an array of biological tests, using mouse skin painting (cigarette tar painted on the skins of mice) as the gold standard for testing carcinogenicity. At the same time, in its public statements the industry challenged the validity of this test as evidence that tobacco poses any harm to human consumers. In fact, we now know that mouse skin painting *underestimates* the total carcinogenic action of tobacco smoke. Some of the most important carcinogens in tobacco, such as nitrosamines, are in the gas phase of the smoke, not in the particulate phase that makes up the "tar" painted on the skins of mice (1). As with its research on nicotine, the secret research being conducted by the tobacco industry was at least as high in quality as the work reported in the open scientific literature at the time. Despite the importance and quality of this research, little of it was ever published in peer-reviewed scientific journals.

B&W and BAT's early work seemed motivated by a genuine concern over the health effects of smoking and a belief that, if the toxic components of cigarette smoke could be identified, these agents could be removed and a "safe" conventional cigarette created. By the late

1970s, however, the tobacco industry had largely abandoned the search and turned to a more defensive posture. This chapter describes what the documents reveal about the industry's effort to develop a "safe" cigarette. The industry did not disclose these research efforts to the public, and it was simultaneously engaged in two campaigns: an internal research campaign to develop a "safe" cigarette and an external public relations campaign to convince the public that cigarettes had not been proven dangerous to health.

As discussed in chapter 2, in the 1950s, in the wake of the rapidly growing scientific evidence that cigarettes cause lung cancer (2), cigarette companies created brands with filters and claimed that these brands gave "health protection" to smokers. These claims were not based on proof of "health protection"; indeed, some filter brands had higher tar deliveries than unfiltered products from the same manufacturer, and smoke from filter cigarettes was shown to be just as carcinogenic as smoke from unfiltered brands (3). Nonetheless, the hype worked, and by 1960 filter brands were well on their way to replacing nonfilter cigarettes in the marketplace. At the same time, cigarette companies conducted serious research to see whether they could lower the toxicity of their products.

"ZEPHYR" AND ITS CAUSES, 1957

One of the first references in the documents to the tobacco industry's effort to identify carcinogenic elements in tobacco smoke appears in a memo dated March 1, 1957, and titled "Smoke Group Program for Coming 12–16 Week Period" {1100.01}. The memo describes research under way at the BAT laboratory in Southampton, but it uses code words for lung cancer (ZEPHYR) and for the suspected carcinogens (BORSTAL and 3,4,9,10-DBP) in tobacco smoke.

> As a result of several statistical surveys, the idea has arisen that there is a causal relationship between ZEPHYR and tobacco smoking, particularly cigarette smoking. Various hypotheses have been propounded, from time to time, as explanations of this conception. The two which seem most important at present are:
>
> (i)   Tobacco smoke contains a substance or substances which may cause ZEPHYR[.]
>
> (ii)   Substances which can cause ZEPHYR are inhaled from the atmosphere, e.g. in the form of soot.
>
> Because of the way in which these causative agents are bound to the soot, they are in an inactive form; but the inhalation of compounds with solvent properties leads to the elution of the agents and their subsequent activation into a

form which readily causes ZEPHYR. This "Elution Hypothesis" may account in part for a subsidiary relationship claimed between ZEPHYR and the level of urbanisation (and consequently of atmospheric pollution). {1100.01, p. 1}

Both of the working hypotheses presented in this document assume that cigarettes are an important link in the occurrence of lung cancer. The first hypothesis is that one or more carcinogens are present in cigarette smoke; the second is that carcinogens which enter the lung from other sources are activated by their dissolution into the tar fraction of cigarette smoke as it is inhaled. Either way, cigarette smoke is hypothesized as part of the directly causal chain in the occurrence of lung cancer. The Smoke Group took these hypotheses seriously, as evidenced by their use of code words, and pursued internal studies based on these hypotheses.

As mentioned, the major suspected carcinogens are called BORSTAL (thought to be arsenic by the compiler of the 1988 chronology of B&W's smoking and health research {1006.01, p. 3}) and 3,4,9,10-DBP (thought to be dibenzo(a)pyrene).

> Until very recently the most suspected compound was BORSTAL. Most values for BORSTAL content of cigarette smoke are held to be too low to reach a biological threshold value for ZEPHYR causation, even on a basis of continued dosage; this conclusion was published by one who is, nevertheless, one of the strongest proponents of the hypothesis under discussion. Very recently, a second compound has been claimed to have been detected in cigarette smoke and this has been stated, independently, to be twenty times as active as BORSTAL. It is 3,4,9,10-DBP. This work still requires confirmation and meanwhile BORSTAL remains as the most widely suspected component in smoke and atmospheric pollution. {1100.01, p. 2}

The research plan describes examinations of cigarette combustion temperatures under different puffing parameters and analyses of smoke fractions for BORSTAL and for polycyclic aromatic hydrocarbons (PAH), of which 3,4,9,10-DBP is an example, using smoke from the "front" and the "back" of cigarettes {1100.01, p. 6}. Some of the cigarettes to be studied were to be made of tobacco leaf lamina (the conventional cigarette material) or CRS (cut, rolled stem) {1100.01, p. 6}. This plan means that the lab was looking for the presence of carcinogens in cigarette smoke and also trying to determine whether different starting materials produced different amounts of these carcinogens. This work was an early attempt to reduce toxicity of cigarettes by attempting to reduce the levels of suspected carcinogens. It fit in precisely with recommendations from experts such as Ernst Wynder that tobacco product manufacturers should seek ways to lower the levels of toxic constituents in cigarette smoke (3).

SOUTHAMPTON RESEARCH CONFERENCE, 1962

As mentioned in chapter 3, BAT held periodic research conferences so that its scientists from around the world could meet to discuss research developments and other issues facing the industry. Such a conference was held at Southampton in early July 1962. The documents include a detailed set of minutes from a major session that dealt with a wide range of smoking and health issues. These included reaction to the recently issued report of the Royal College of Physicians on smoking and health, the company's research program, and research that was being undertaken through an industry-wide consortium in the United Kingdom known as the Tobacco Manufacturers' Standing Committee (TMSC; see chapter 2). As discussed in chapter 2, the British Royal College of Physicians issued its first report on smoking and health in the spring of 1962. That report concluded that cigarettes cause lung cancer and recommended that government take "decisive steps" to control the rising consumption of cigarettes.

The Southampton conference was attended by twenty-nine executives and research scientists from BAT offices and laboratories in five countries (including the United States and Canada, which sent four delegates each) {1102.01, front matter}. The record of the conference shows that, despite its public statements contending that the evidence on smoking as a cause of lung cancer was inconclusive, the British tobacco industry was moving aggressively to examine the problem with sophisticated toxicological testing.

In addition, a special session was devoted to a major problem that had arisen in the United States about six weeks earlier, when a B&W competitor announced its development of a cigarette filter that selectively removed phenols, a group of compounds suspected of enhancing the carcinogenic activity of cigarette smoke.

The documents include a detailed set of minutes from a major session dealing with a wide range of smoking and health issues. In a keynote speech Sir Charles Ellis, an executive in BAT's Research and Development Establishment at its Millbank headquarters in London, presented an overview of the smoking and health issues faced by the company and explained how the TMSC was responding to these issues. The full text of his remarks is included in the minutes. (The parts of his comments related to nicotine were discussed in chapter 3.) Sir Charles reviewed public and scientific perceptions of the cancer issue with a variety of rationalizations, but he also outlined a well-planned, comprehensive research program designed to reduce the toxicity of cigarettes.

LUNG CANCER AND THE BRITISH ROYAL COLLEGE OF PHYSICIANS REPORT

In his speech Sir Charles tries to downplay the Royal College of Physicians' conclusion that cigarettes cause lung cancer, calling it an emotional reaction based on an incomplete examination of the data. He does, however, acknowledge that smoking causes bronchitis.

> After reading the Report of the Royal College of Physicians and the debate in the House of Lords the dominant impression I received was that of people who had reached an emotional conclusion in which they believed passionately and sincerely. This report provided the occasion for statements of faith by people who seemed to find it necessary, however, to silence their own self-criticism by repeating phrases like, "conclusive proof beyond the shadow of doubt" [,] . . . "devastating effect of the marshalling of cold scientific facts", and so on. Yet we who have been immersed in the subject for many years know that this report produced no new fact, produced no new arguments, indeed, except for the contribution of an emotional gloss, left the subject untouched. We know only too well that there are no conclusive proofs; that there are few, if any, cold scientific facts.
>
> However, emotional conclusions cannot be disregarded. They may not be right, but they are not necessarily wrong. Emotional judgments are often the basis for national thinking, and since a national attitude to smoking may be building up it is essential for us to consider what are the components in this emotion.
>
> The most important is the dread word "cancer". Most people cease to be able to reason once it is mentioned, and you will all be aware how difficult it is for doctors to overcome the reluctance of people to admit the possibility of having cancer and to present themselves for early examination. Lung cancer carries with it all of these associations, and also shares some of the aura of dread connected with tuberculosis. I can well remember how pneumoconiosis in the coal mines had much of this emotional background and was correspondingly difficult to deal with in a rational manner. *Smoker's cough is a real phenomenon and obvious to everyone*, and we should recognize that it is a factor in the emotional build-up [emphasis added]. {1102.01, pp. 3–4}

"Smoker's cough" is a symptom of lower airway irritation caused by cigarette smoke. "Bronchitis" is the clinical term that is implied by the phrase "smoker's cough." This irritation occurs as a result of smoke inhalation, which, in turn, is necessary for nicotine absorption from a cigarette (see chapter 3). Where there is a smoker's cough, there is some degree of bronchitis.

Sir Charles states that the evidence directly implicating cigarette smoking as a cause of lung cancer was epidemiological except for a single study by Blacklock (4). Blacklock had injected cigarette smoke condensates mixed with the adjuvant eucerin, a material to amplify the effects of smoke condensate, into the lungs of rats, guinea pigs, and rabbits. The animals lived out their natural lives and then were examined. Cancers were observed in six of seventy-two rats and in one rabbit.

In saying that Blacklock's work was the only biological study in the literature that addressed the question of smoking as a cause of lung cancer, Sir Charles is framing the issue very narrowly. A decade earlier, the young US physician Ernst Wynder had shown that cigarette smoke tar condensate caused cancer in a mouse skin model (5, 6). The test involved repeatedly painting smoke condensate onto the skin of mice and observing the animals over a long period of time to see whether cancers developed at the exposed site. Although Sir Charles does not mention the mouse skin–painting model as relevant to the question of whether smoking causes lung cancer, BAT was to use this very model in Project Janus (discussed below) as its gold standard for determining whether specific product modifications could reduce the dangers of smoking.

JOINT RESEARCH BY BRITISH TOBACCO INDUSTRY

Sir Charles then describes the new tobacco toxicology laboratory at Harrogate, which was to be run jointly by tobacco companies in the United Kingdom through the Tobacco Manufacturers' Standing Committee (TMSC). In the course of his discussion, Sir Charles explains the BAT board's policy on the smoking and health issue:

> *The Board recognises that this problem must be tackled from two sides, the first being medical research on the origin of lung cancer and bio-assay on the biological effects of smoke, and the second being the composition of smoke and the possibilities of modifying it.* The Board has decided that if this Company makes any significant scientific discovery clearly relevant to health it will share its knowledge with its co-members of TMSC and not seek to obtain competitive commercial advantage. The Board has therefore decided that they will whole-heartedly support TMSC to carry out and co-ordinate all research on smoking and health. TMSC will do this by itself carrying out biological work at its establishment at Harrogate and by sponsoring biological and medical work at Institutions. TMSC will depend on member companies for physical and chemical work [emphasis added]. {1102.01, p. 5}

While the BAT board made a commitment to share information on how to reduce cigarette toxicity with other tobacco companies rather than "seek[ing] to obtain competitive commercial advantage," there is no mention of making research information available either to the public or to public health authorities.

More important, as of July 1962, BAT was committed to cooperative investigations and product development when they were "health-
oriented." A "health-oriented" product, as it would later be defined at
the Hilton Head research conference in 1968, was one that reduced the
actual hazard of smoking. In contrast, a "health-image" cigarette only
appeared to provide a health benefit (see below). The fact that the company had decided to share any promising results with the industry as a
whole strongly indicates that the company now realized that its products did, in fact, present a hazard. If the company regarded the evidence
that smoking causes cancer as false, misleading, or inconclusive, it is difficult to see why it would have seen the possibility of a competitive advantage and adopted the policy that it did.

Sir Charles couches the rationale for conducting "health-oriented" research in the following guarded terms:

> *The central fact in this subject is that in sufficient doses tobacco condensate*
> *acts as a carcinogen when painted on the backs of mice, or when injected sub-*
> *cutaneously into rats.* In sufficient dose it also acts as a co-carcinogen in mouse
> painting tests. On present evidence the amount of the known carcinogens in
> smoke are insufficient to make it plausible that these experiments could be
> extrapolated to support the view that smoking is harmful to human beings,
> but at least they serve to indicate a group of substances which require intense
> investigation and which, even if we do not know why, we would be pleased
> to see less of [emphasis added]. {1102.01, p. 7}

Despite this cautious attitude toward the implications of the mouse skin
model, mouse skin painting had by this time become the test used by
BAT to examine whether a particular manipulation of cigarettes reduced the risk of cancer. Indeed, discussion later on at this research conference demonstrated the hard-nosed attitude within R&D at BAT that
the company would rely primarily on mouse skin tests in estimating the
value of any maneuver to remove toxins from cigarette smoke. Mouse
skin painting was, then, the definitive assay for cancer at BAT—even
though, in public, the tobacco industry minimized the value of data
from mouse skin–painting experiments. The public posture was that
this model was not at all relevant to a determination of whether cigarettes cause cancer in humans.

The TMSC laboratory, which was to open at Harrogate on September 1, 1962, was to be capable of running mouse skin–painting experiments at twenty-five to fifty times the size of in-house efforts. Two thousand mice were to be used in the initial experiment, instead of the forty
to eighty that were conventionally used. The start-up costs were put at

£250,000, and the annual budget was estimated to be £100,000. Research results of this and other studies were to be published as a matter of policy {1102.01, p. 33}. In determining the sample sizes to be utilized in the initial experiment, the planners had done calculations of how small a difference could be detected between the activities (i.e., carcinogenic potential) of different condensates. Sir Charles notes that the experiment at Harrogate "should with almost certainty show up a difference of 30 per cent in the two condensates and will give good information about possible differences of 15 per cent" {1102.01, p. 9}.

One of the criticisms of earlier work was that the smoke condensates used were not "fresh"; that is, they had been stored for some time prior to being painted onto the mice. People inhale "fresh" smoke, not old smoke, and any chemical changes that made the stored smoke more toxic to mouse skin might skew the results. So the first experiment conducted at Harrogate was to be a comparison of "fresh" and "stored" condensate.

Besides looking at carcinogenic and cocarcinogenic activity in smoke, Harrogate was also charged with investigating the mechanisms whereby tobacco smoke causes irritation of the respiratory passages. A cocarcinogen is a material that amplifies the action of a carcinogen but is not itself carcinogenic. This research was relevant to the work at Harrogate, rather than simply a matter for competitive improvement of consumer acceptance, for three reasons. Sir Charles notes that irritation could

[a]   cause chronic bronchitis,
[b]   be responsible by itself for carcinogenesis,
[c]   act as a co-carcinogen or promoting factor in association with specific "carcinogens". {1102.01, p. 10}

The term "chronic bronchitis" is a specific diagnosis of some importance. In 1962 British investigators of what we now call chronic obstructive pulmonary disease (COPD) called the disease "chronic bronchitis," while investigators in the United States used the term "emphysema." The term "COPD" was coined to encompass both major phenomena of the condition, the narrowing of airways and the destruction of lung tissue, so that the literature would be easier to follow. Nearly all COPD seen in the United States is caused by cigarettes (7).

At Harrogate researchers would be able to conduct two kinds of tests: (1) by looking at the proliferation of mucus-secreting goblet cells in the lung (a response to irritation), they could determine the potential of smoke to produce bronchitis; (2) by looking for hyperplasia of the epithelial cells lining the bronchi, they could determine the presence of carcinogenesis and cocarcinogenesis (the stimulation of these cells to divide is an early action of carcinogens). Harrogate was to have the capability to set up both of these experimental models and then to test specific smoke constituents in these systems.

Sir Charles emphasizes the importance of the studies on irritation with the following comments:

> I regard the attempt to probe more deeply into the cause of irritation as equally fundamental [to investigating the cancer problem]. Some smoke is irritating, *smoker's cough is a reality, and it cannot be good for health to cause this irritation whether or not this irritation has any effect on the incidence of lung cancer.* Some of you may regard irritation as so important that you are willing to make a guess and attribute it with but little evidence to a class of compounds such as aldehydes, or you may be ready to take a short cut and attempt to identify irritation by an organoleptic technique [subjective report of people exposed to potentially irritating materials]. This is a matter on which I hope you will express your views. Personally I think the TMSC policy is right; this subject of irritation is just too important to incur the danger of reaching a wrong conclusion due to a faulty technique. Once we have solved the problem of establishing a quantitative test[,] progress in identifying irritating components will be rapid. Whether their removal will be easy is another question, but to identify them will be a good first step [emphasis added]. {1102.01, p. 22}

Sir Charles also describes other work supported by TMSC outside the Harrogate facility: an examination of the relative carcinogenicity of smoke from tobacco that has been cured in different ways; a large, prospective epidemiological study on susceptibility factors (other than smoking) for cardiac and pulmonary disease among 200,000 men; a study of the carcinogenicity of aliphatic lactones (material found in plants that was thought likely to occur in cigarette smoke); an epidemiological study of lung cancer in South Africa and Australia; and the psychological work of Dr. Hans Eysenck. (Dr. Eysenck later received support through the special projects of the Council for Tobacco Research; see chapter 8.) TMSC also funded work on viruses and immunogens as causes of cancer and on the effects of tumor transplants treated in various ways in experimental animals. Taken as a whole, this work plan has a defensive tone: most of these projects sought explanations for the diseases at issue other than that they are caused by cigarettes.

After describing the overall research activities sponsored by TMSC, Sir Charles returns to the experiment on fresh versus old condensate.

> [If] fresh condensate has a smaller biological effect than old condensate we do not of course at one stroke destroy the emotional conclusion [that smok-

ing causes cancer]—in fact it remains unaltered—but we do clear the decks of a great deal of previous experimentation and smoke condensate will then be accepted as such a weak carcinogenic agent that other explanations of the association of smoking and lung cancer assume greater importance. *Conversely, and this is always a possibility, the biological effect may increase as the condensate is used fresher and fresher. This possibility need not dismay us, indeed it would mean that there really was a chemical culprit somewhere in smoke, and one, moreover, that underwent a reaction fairly quickly to something else. I feel confident that in this case we could identify this group of substances, and it would be worth almost any effort, by preliminary treatment, additives, or filtration, to get rid of it. We should have brought the problem out into the open where it could be attacked.* I feel sure you will give your full support to this experiment [emphasis added]. {1102.01, p. 21}

Sir Charles's willingness to accept the possibility that something intrinsic to cigarette smoking could cause cancer—and that, once identified, this "group of substances" could be removed—reflects a greater level of scientific openness than the tobacco industry has evidenced in recent years.

Ultimately, the experiment showed that "fresh" condensate (twenty-four hours old) actually had *more* carcinogenic activity than "old" condensate (one week old) (see below) {1105.01}.

THE BAT RESEARCH PROGRAM

BAT's intramural research activities, Sir Charles explains, are devoted mainly to a detailed investigation of the physics and chemistry of tobacco smoke.

> Now, as regards work in our own laboratories on chemistry and physics. Our objective must be to prepare ourselves as fully as possible to utilize any result the moment it appears from these biological and medical experiments. In effect, this means that we would like to know the origin of all the compounds that we currently think may be important, whether they are wholly or partially distilled from the tobacco or formed in some of the pyrolytic reactions, and at what temperatures. We might then hope to be in the position of being able to enhance or suppress certain classes of compounds by either pre-treatment or additives once we knew which compounds had to be so influenced.
>
> This of course is precisely what we have been doing and are doing, and in my opinion progress is excellent. {1102.01, p. 24}

These comments indicate that a goal of R&D at BAT in 1962 was to reduce the toxicity of its cigarettes as rapidly as possible.

Sir Charles concludes his conference remarks with the following analysis and exhortation:

We must admit that the threat to our industry is serious and very real, and it is of little help to us that it is based on an emotional guess and not on reasons. I believe we are now starting on a sound programme of investigation that in a few years will make it possible to see the situation and judge the future much more clearly. I hope to-day's discussion will start your active participation in this particular section of Group Research, and that the measures we propose will enable it to continue and grow. {1102.01, p. 25}

Unfortunately, this optimistic view that cigarette toxicity could be largely eliminated through research and engineering proved to be wrong.

Participants at the conference also discussed the feasibility and development of a safer cigarette. It emerged that BAT knew how to make a cigarette with low levels of what was regarded at the time as the major carcinogen (benzpyrene) but had not marketed it. There was concern about how to make claims for safer products that would not indict other products, and there was a keen appreciation of the difference between product innovation for public relations purposes and product innovation to reduce the hazard of the product. Finally, there was an appreciation of the spirit of sharing and comity among the British companies as regards "health-oriented" innovations in contrast to the competitive turn that had just emerged in this area in the United States.

The following exchange, during the discussion following Sir Charles's talk, illustrates the tension that knowledgeable spokesmen for tobacco companies were under at the time, because they were denying the scientific evidence that smoking is dangerous while, at the same time, they knew that the evidence was sound and that internal studies such as mouse skin–painting experiments were consistent with the publicly available results.

<u>Mr. Reid</u> suggested that no industry was going to accept that its product was toxic, or even believe it to be so, and naturally when the health question was first raised we had to start by denying it at the P.R. level. But by continuing that policy we had got ourselves into a corner and left no room to manoeuvre[.] [I]n other words *if we did get a break through and were able to improve our product we should have to about-face, and this was practically impossible at the P.R. level. If we could ease the approach a bit, then when we did make positive contributions we could at least say so without having to crawl behind the door.*

   Mr. McCormick did not quite agree that we in this country had got ourselves into that position, although it might be true of other countries [presumably, the United States]. *We had more room to manoeuvre because, whatever we had said initially, in the last year or two we had been prepared to admit that there was a working hypothesis which ought to be examined. The fact that we had started with a donation to the MRC* [Medical Research Coun-

cil] *had indicated that we thought there might be something in it. But it was*
very difficult when you were asked, as Chairman of a Tobacco Company, to
discuss the health question on television. You had not only your own busi-
ness to consider but the employees throughout the industry, retailers, con-
sumers, farmers growing the leaf, and so on, and you were in much too re-
sponsible a position to get up and say: "I accept that the product which we
and all our competitors are putting on the market gives you lung cancer",
whatever you might think privately [emphasis added]. {1102.01, p. 45}

THE PHENOL CRISIS

On May 22, 1962, the P. Lorillard Company precipitated a crisis within
the cigarette industry: it announced that it had introduced a modification to the Micronite filter of its Kent brand that selectively removed 90
percent of the phenols from mainstream smoke (8). (The filter Lorillard
had announced for Kent had been produced in collaboration with Dr.
Ernst Wynder of the Sloan-Kettering Institute for Cancer Research.) The
fallout from this announcement was still being felt in July, and the phenol problem was a major topic of discussion at BAT's 1962 research conference in Southampton.

The phenols were regarded as irritants and probable cocarcinogens.
The irritating effects of phenols were thought to account for paralysis of
normal ciliary function in the tracheo-bronchial tree that cigarette smoke
causes. The cilia, little hairs that line the windpipe, help cleanse the lung
by moving mucus up to the throat. As reported in the *Wall Street Jour-*
nal, Lorillard's public relations firm issued a statement claiming that
"studies on the cilia in frogs show that the workings of the cilia are un-
affected by smoke from Kents with the new filter. . . . Smoke from another brand of filter cigarette, it claims, slowed the cilia down by 67 percent, while smoke from an unfiltered cigaret slowed action of the cilia
by 85 percent. There is no mention made [by Lorillard's public relations
firm] of any research or theories on the possibility that phenols may be
cocarcinogens. The statement also claims that in smoke from an unfiltered cigarette there are about 105 micrograms of phenol. By comparison, it claims, there are 35 micrograms in a filtered cigarette, 24 micrograms in an old-style Kent and 12 micrograms in Kents with the new
filter" (9). Lorillard's announcement, then, meant that it sought a competitive advantage from a product that seemed to offer a genuinely
"health-oriented" benefit.

Ernst Wynder had made numerous contributions to the scientific understanding of cigarettes and disease in the 1950s and 1960s, initially at

Washington University and then at the Sloan-Kettering Institute. He participated in major epidemiological and laboratory studies of smoking and health. In the mid-1950s he developed the mouse skin–painting model that was to become the cigarette industry's standard for assessing the carcinogenicity of cigarette smoke condensate.

In testimony before Congress in 1957, Wynder had pointed out that the cigarette filters of the day were not selective. That is, they did not remove toxins to any greater degree than they removed harmless smoke components (3). He also criticized some cigarette manufacturers for blending the tobaccos in their filter cigarette brands so that they produced smoke with higher levels of tar than came from the nonfilter brands of the same manufacturer. The year before Lorillard's announcement, a paper Wynder and Hoffman had published in the journal *Cancer* had drawn attention to the fact that the phenolic fraction of cigarette smoke had cocarcinogenic activity (10). This finding provided a rationale for seeking the selective removal of phenols.

The problems that the new Kent filter created for BAT—and, particularly, B&W—are reflected throughout the general proceedings of the Southampton conference {1102.01}. The matter was of such urgency and importance that a special session at the conference was devoted to the problem, and a full transcript of this session, including both the presentations and the discussion, was made {1102.02}. The mood at this session suggested that BAT was about two years behind Lorillard in the development of selective filtration. In his opening remarks at this session, Sir Charles Ellis acknowledged the profound embarrassment the BAT scientists had felt as well as the challenge that lay before them.

> Gentlemen, we must all recognise that it is natural for our Boards to wonder why scientists of another Company should have brought to their Board's attention the possible importance of the problem of the selective filtration of phenols and that we ourselves unfortunately did not. I suspect that this has already been mentioned in their discussions and they are now awaiting anxiously for the next surprise to burst upon them. It is precisely to avoid such unpleasant situations that they provide themselves with expensive research establishments. Let us admit that it would be both natural and reasonable for our Boards to think in this way and irrespective of whether they do or do not, as may be the case, there is definitely something for us to answer. I personally feel this responsibility very keenly for I am in as good a position, if not better, than anyone to know the facts and to guess trends. If there were to be any kicks to be distributed I think they should first land on me. I suggest that this morning anyone should feel free to job [sic] backwards and say what in their opinion should have been done. If this involves the suggestion that someone should have done some-

thing different or acted more quickly then let it be said openly and frankly—straight speaking—we are all friends.

Now the reason for raising this point in rather a direct manner is because of the overriding importance of making our Group Research a successful reality—a reality which can grapple with situations like this. Obviously, it can be successful Group Research if it expresses joint opinions of you all acting as equals with equal responsibilities. I hope our discussions this morning will help that onwards. {1102.02, pp. 1–2}

These opening remarks were followed by presentations by H. D. Anderson from Millbank, who gave an overview of the situation; by T. M. Wade, Jr., who presented the problem from the B&W perspective; and by Mr. Laporte, who commented on the problem from a Canadian point of view. In his presentation Anderson emphasized the political importance of Lorillard's going public with the connection between phenol and ciliatoxicity, since the impairment of ciliary activity was, in his view, "implicated in the cancer problem" {1102.02, p. 8}.

How important is phenol? There are two sides to this—the scientific side and the political attitude. Let's be quite certain about this: *the political implications have at the moment by far the greater importance* and they have been summed up very adequately in a letter from Add [Addison] Yeaman, the lawyer at B. & W. Now that Lorillards have come right out into the open and made it publicly known that the [sic] connection between phenol and cilia activity, and because cilia activity goes back a long way and has been implicated in the cancer problem, the argument would run like this—I quote from Yeaman's letter:

"1.   The uninhibited movement of the cilia tends to eject from the lung (or impede entering into the lung) particulate matter.

"2.   It is known that phenol inhibits the action of the cilia.

"3.   It is known that phenol occurs in the inhaled smoke.

"4.   It is now known that phenol content of the smoke can, by use of certain additives in the filter, be very substantially reduced.

"Query: *In this state of knowledge is it negligence on the part of the cigarette manufacturer either*

(a)   *to fail to remove phenols, or,*

(b)   *to fail to warn consumers of the product of its potential danger?"* [italic emphasis added]. {1102.02, p. 8}

Yeaman was suggesting that B&W had legal vulnerability if it did not act to remove phenols or warn smokers of the problem. Of course, these discussions took place before the advent of warning labels, which, ironically, have had the effect of largely protecting the industry from liability under a failure-to-warn theory.

The phenol crisis presented a real-world example of the competitive problems that would arise if a tobacco company were to develop a "safe" cigarette—most notably, that all other cigarettes would be admittedly more dangerous. The potential liability issues were formidable (see chapter 7).

In his presentation Tom Wade, of B&W research and development, complained about the absence of a cooperative approach in the United States.

> This is a typical example of too little, too late. This situation of ours [B&W's] is somewhat different from yours [BAT's] over here as it is now proven that certain elements of the industry will go it alone, rather than through T.I.R.C, in spite of the fact that they are members of the T.I.R.C. That leaves us in a very awkward situation in the States. Of course, we don't know the level of activity of phenols or the importance of them, but the Reader's Digest can make a powerfully good case of this; in all practical purposes they are anti-tobacco to begin with—thanks to their association with our boyfriend (Wynder). Secondly, it increases the circulation [of the Reader's Digest] by having a good scare . . . , and on top of that, they are very much insulted at the United States Government and the Federal Trades [sic] Commission in particular for having stopped all kinds of reference to fil-tration in terms of total tar; we can talk about the foolish side if we want to, taste and flavour and so on, but the implications from the medical stand-point are being carried by the Reader's Digest in opposition to the Federal Trades [sic] Commission. . . .
>
> We have gone through to the battle of the total tar and we are now in the battle of the phenols—tomorrow it will be something else. Of course Wyn-der does not believe that a cigarette will ever be completely safe. {1102.02, pp. 15–16}

The *Reader's Digest* had a long history of publishing articles about smoking and health, and since the mid-1950s it had published impor-tant articles about the relative tar and nicotine deliveries of various fil-ter and nonfilter cigarettes. In 1955 the Federal Trade Commission put a stop to the most obvious health claims in cigarette advertising. Refer-ences to "health protection" and to "reduced irritation" disappeared and were replaced by what Wade calls "the foolish side," an emphasis on taste and flavor. Wade's complaint, in part, was that although the FTC had barred the manufacturers from making the most flagrant health claims in their cigarette advertising, the *Reader's Digest* was still pub-lishing articles on the relative benefits of various cigarette brands in terms of tar delivery (11). These articles were, inevitably, detrimental to some particular companies' brands, and the companies could not respond in their advertising.

The phenol crisis illustrates the complex environment in which the R&D scientists operated. Most important, it illustrates the fact that the tobacco companies' scientific agenda was set by competitive and public relations needs as much as by scientific priorities.

INDUSTRY-WIDE RESEARCH IN THE UK, 1965

A report of a site visit in June 1965 to tobacco industry research facilities in England by Dr. R. B. Griffith, head of R&D at B&W, provides a glimpse at what had happened in the three years since the Southampton research conference. Dr. Griffith presented a report in person to high-level B&W executives on July 1, 1965, two days after his return. This presentation is summarized in a "Report to Executive Committee," marked "STRICTLY CONFIDENTIAL" {1105.01}.

Dr. Griffith reported that the first set of mouse skin–painting studies from the Tobacco Research Council laboratory at Harrogate was scheduled for publication within the year. The results demonstrated once again that tobacco smoke condensate is carcinogenic to mouse skin. Contrary to hopes expressed at the Southampton research conference in 1962 {1102.01}, fresh condensate was found to be actually *more* carcinogenic than old condensate. Griffith notes,

> *Scientists with whom I talked were unanimous in their opinion that smoke is weakly carcinogenic under certain conditions and that efforts should be made to reduce this activity* [emphasis added]. {1105.01, p. 2}

Griffith stops short of saying that this "weakly carcinogenic activity" commonly leads to cancer in humans. By this time, statistician Sir Ronald Fisher, a consultant for the British tobacco industry, had conceded that epidemiological evidence established that there was a real association between smoking and lung cancer (12).

"Most people" Dr. Griffith spoke with in the United Kingdom were also worried about the potentially adverse impact of the reports from Harrogate {1105.01, p. 2}. At least one person expressed concern "that the Harrogate report may bring about some type of industry regulation by agencies of the British government" {1105.01, p. 2}. Moreover, "The personal opinion was expressed that the Harrogate report, and the possible repercussions in England, would have a significant impact on the American tobacco industry" {1105.01, p. 2}.

At the same time, industry scientists at Harrogate were actively working on ways to reduce the toxicity of smoke by various means. They had found, for example, that a charcoal filter and a PEG (polyethylene glycol)-treated cellulose acetate filter substantially reduced carcinogenic activity when equal weights of tar were tested. These results offered some hope of a safer cigarette.

The Harrogate lab was being doubled in size, and new machinery for the manufacture of condensate and smoke was under development. The lab staff was seeking the ability to process tobacco and to make its own cigarettes, but the R&D staff at BAT (Southampton) and at Imperial Tobacco (Bristol) were concerned that the Harrogate lab might thereby become too independent of the sponsoring tobacco companies.

The Imperial Tobacco laboratory at Bristol was in a rapid growth phase as well. (Imperial Tobacco was, and is, one of the largest tobacco companies in Great Britain.) Dr. Griffith notes:

> Their entire laboratory facilities are operating on a "crash" basis on the smoking and health problem and activity was evident at the Director level. Two more floors are already planned for their new smoke research facilities (less than two years old) and every project in their new process development facility was concerned with this research. *Their approach seems to be to find ways of obtaining maximum nicotine for minimum tar.* Approaches being used include:
>
> (a)   *P.E.I.* [polyethyleneimine] *treatment of filters*
> (b)   *Nicotine fortification of cigarette paper*
> (c)   *Addition of nicotine containing powders to tobacco*
> (d)   Alteration of blends
>
> I was told that they were making moves to be in a position where 30% of their production could be dual filter production by June 1966. Arrangements had been made with Cigarette Components for production of P.E.I. treated filter cigarettes which will be submitted for biological testing this August [emphasis added]. {1105.01, p. 2}

The Imperial scientists at Bristol were approaching the problem by concentrating on boosting nicotine dose to achieve a lower dose of tars. As discussed in chapter 3, PEI, when used as a filter additive, boosts free nicotine delivery {1205.03}. This research strategy is consistent with the view that people smoke in order to receive a dose of nicotine. The real task, then, was to reduce the delivery of other combustion by-products that cause cancer.

The German tobacco industry was developing a lab similar to the one at Harrogate. In addition, BAT had arranged for biological testing at Battelle in Frankfurt, Germany, while Imperial Tobacco had made similar arrangements with a private lab in England. Dr. Griffith felt that these latter two operations would be used for commercial purposes. The Battelle operation was a branch of the same industrial laboratory that had conducted BAT's nicotine research in Geneva a few years earlier (see chapter 3). Battelle's work on tobacco carcinogenesis for BAT was known within the company as Project Janus (see below).

Ed Finch, the president of B&W, had been away when Dr. Griffith presented his report to the executive committee on July 1. Dr. Griffith briefed Finch upon the latter's return. A July 19, 1965, memo from Dr. Griffith to Finch, with copies to J. G. Crume and to the general counsel, Addison Yeaman, reviews this meeting {1106.01}. In this memo Dr. Griffith indicates that, in his opinion, the adverse information from Harrogate—that fresh condensate is more carcinogenic than old condensate—will not provoke a "significant" public reaction but might precipitate government intervention. Therefore,

> The company should take steps to place itself in best possible position to minimize chances of government intervention by
>
> (a)   Having at least one brand on market which is "safest" possible cigarette on basis of knowledge to date.
>
> (b)   Obtaining biological test data to indicate the degree to which the cigarette is "safer." {1106.01, p. 1}

The memo continues,

> In the discussion of these points it was agreed that a modified LIFE [brand of cigarette] would represent the best company approach to a "safer" cigarette and that work on such a cigarette should be started as soon as possible. Approaches discussed were:
>
> 1.   Filter. AVALON type with acetate mouthpiece treated with P.E.G., bondex charcoal center section and paper treated with Polyethylene Imine (P.E.I.) or potassium carbonate next to tobacco.
>
> 2.   Tobacco. Blend changes will probably be required and it is possible that fermentation may be used to improve smoking qualities and decrease biological activity. A fermented burley blend was considered one possibility. {1106.01, p. 1}

The filter modifications were those that research at Harrogate had indicated would reduce carcinogenic activity of smoke condensate. The PEI additive increases the proportion of free nicotine. Potassium carbonate was used to reduce benzpyrene levels {1109.01, p. 2}. (By 1967, though, it was suspected that, despite the reduction in resulting benzpyrene level, potassium carbonate treatment resulted in *increased* carcinogenicity in mouse skin tests.)

Dr. Griffith also argues that B&W should have its own biological testing program, preferably based in the United States. Moreover, B&W should maintain control over the publication of any results, doubtless to avoid other instances of the expected embarrassment from the publication of the Harrogate results:

> Changes in biological activity must be measured by a reputable organization willing to make the results public only upon request. {1106.01, p. 2}

The memo closes on an unresolved note:

> No decisions were made and the question of biological tests was tabled for further discussion at a later date. {1106.01, p. 2}

There is no evidence in the documents that Dr. Griffith ever got his wish that B&W conduct biological testing as part of product development in this country.

REPORT ON SOUTHAMPTON RESEARCH, 1967

The documents include a detailed report on research activities at BAT's Southampton facility as of July 1967, two years after Dr. Griffith's visit to England {1109.01}. Dr. Robert R. Johnson from R&D at B&W had spent two weeks in residence at BAT's Southampton facility, and the file note summarizes his findings.

> Current studies on the design of "safe" cigarettes fall into several main approaches. These are (1) synthetic tobacco substitutes, (2) cigarettes incorporating a large percentage of air-cured tobacco, (3) smoking products delivering smoke with a high nicotine/tar ratio, and (4) selective filtration. Ancillary research is also proceeding in areas of biological testing, human smoking patterns and smoke absorption, and smoke analysis. The supposed paramount importance of nicotine is evident in almost all of this research. {1109.01, p. 1}

Five years after the phenol crisis, selective filtration work had become a major function of the Southampton laboratory. The lab was also exploring a variety of additives and modifications to tobacco, including changes in the tobacco blend to reduce toxicity. Nicotine pharmacology was under study, and methods were being developed to look for nitrosamines, the most potent carcinogens in tobacco and tobacco smoke. Some work continued on Ariel (discussed in chapter 3), but in the main the emphasis of this wide-ranging but integrated research effort seems to have been on finding ways to make conventional cigarettes safer.

Ed Finch, CEO of B&W, read Dr. Johnson's report carefully enough to raise a question about it with Dr. Griffith {1110.01}. Why did "tumorigenicity" increase even though the 3,4-benzpyrene content of smoke had been reduced after treatment with potassium carbonate {1109.01, p. 2}? In his memo to Finch, Dr. Griffith explains that benzpyrene is by no means the only, or even the most, carcinogenic compound in cigarette smoke.

> Actually, the data from the initial Harrogate experiment would indicate that the benzpyrene fraction can account for, at most, one third of the [carcinogenic] activity of the total condensate.
>
> I personally feel that far too much attention has been given to 3,4-benzpyrene and other polycyclic hydrocarbons in England and elsewhere and not enough attention has been given to other materials which are probably of greater importance. {1110.01}

The more industry scientists learned about the toxicity of cigarettes, the more complex the problem seemed to become.

MONTREAL RESEARCH CONFERENCE, 1967

At the research conference held in Montreal in October 1967, participants discussed, among other topics, the applicability of mouse skin painting in their research.

> The meeting agreed that it would be worthwhile to make a cigarette with lower biological activity on mouse skin painting, provided this did not adversely affect the position with respect to irritation and other factors. It was recognized that this implied certain assumptions about the relevance of mouse skin painting. However, it was agreed that it was unlikely this test would be replaced by cheaper, shorter and more meaningful tests for the next few years. In the light of this, the biological testing of new cigarettes must only be applied to those which have already satisfied the requirements of taste, cost, etc., and which are, therefore, considered viable commercial products. {1165.02, p. 3}

The participants agreed, then, that a less hazardous product must be similar enough to existing products that consumers would readily move to using it. Reduced toxicity in mouse skin painting was desirable, but secondary to marketing considerations. They considered a possibly "more meaningful" test, an inhalation test, but dismissed it because it was unlikely to become available.

> The difficulties associated with inhalation studies were discussed and it was agreed that in the likely event that no satisfactory inhalation test could be found, it would be necessary to make an intuitive judgement based on cellular biochemical studies. {1165.02, p. 4}

Public statements from the industry have often pointed to the paucity of studies showing lung cancer from tobacco smoke inhalation as evidence against a causal link. In contrast, these company scientists did not look on the lack of an inhalation model as evidence of the lack of a causal link. Rather, they saw it as a technical problem. They were prepared to make an "intuitive judgement" about the toxicity of specific materials in the absence of such a test.

The likely impact of the publication of results from independent research groups was also discussed. Specifically mentioned were programs at the University of Kentucky and at the Environmental Health Unit at Research Triangle in North Carolina. The minutes note,

> [T]he fact that they will[,] of necessity, publish their results should lead to a reconsideration of our own policy on publishing and it was agreed that where results which we had obtained were likely to be covered by such publication, we ourselves should publish first. It was also agreed that we should cooperate in such programmes as far as possible. . . .
>
> It was felt that Kotin's work [at the Research Triangle facility] could well provide the occasion for the cooperation of the American industry at the scientific level, preferably without any involvement of the company lawyers. It was mentioned that these programmes could also be supported by the industry, perhaps at the expense of contributions to CTR [Council for Tobacco Research] or AMA [American Medical Association]. {1165.01, pp. 5–6}

The minutes acknowledge that research results from R&D ordinarily were not published but should be published in this instance to ensure that the company would receive credit for results that were going to become public in any case.

The expressed wish that scientific exchange could take place without lawyers is interesting, as is the preference for channeling B&W resources for external research away from the public relations–driven outlets of the CTR and the AMA. As described in chapter 8, lawyers were heavily involved in most tobacco industry–sponsored research. These comments seem to indicate friction between the scientists and the lawyers; later minutes from research conferences demonstrate that the scientists came to accept the lawyers' supremacy as a matter of fact.

HILTON HEAD RESEARCH CONFERENCE, 1968

A dozen company scientists from various countries, including Sir Charles Ellis and Dr. R. B. Griffith, attended the 1968 research conference, held at Hilton Head, South Carolina. The conclusions reached during the proceedings on a wide range of topics were summarized by the conference chairman, Dr. S. J. Green of BAT, in a six-page set of minutes {1112.01}. The documents also include a thoughtful letter to Dr. Green in which

B&W's technical manager, Dr. R. A. Sanford, comments on these minutes {1112.02}. The mood that comes through the conference report is one of cautious optimism. The R&D labs seemed to be making incremental but important progress in developing the capacity to make cigarettes that had reduced activity in biological tests but still would deliver nicotine (see chapter 3).

Dr. Green's minutes and Dr. Sanford's letter describe the contrasting concepts of "health-image" and "health-oriented" cigarettes {1112.01, p. 2}. This discussion goes to the heart of the company's approaches to the problems posed by the toxicity of their products. In the official conference summary, Dr. Green expresses the consensus of the delegates on this subject.

> Research staff should lay down guide lines against which alternative products can be chosen in everyday operations. *Although there may, on occasions, be conflict between saleability and minimal biological activity, two types of product should be clearly distinguished,* viz:
>
> a)   A *Health-image* (health-reassurance) cigarette.
>
> b)   A *Health-oriented* (minimal biological activity) cigarette, to be kept on the market for those consumers choosing it [emphasis added]. 1112.01, p. 2}

In his letter to Dr. Green, Dr. Sanford suggests this clarification of the discussion and the consensus:

> We find [this conclusion] confusing. Would it be better to say "A new product development might give undesirable biological test results, and the research staff should lay down guidelines insuring, in context of present understanding, a new product would have *no greater activity in biological testing* than current products. Preferably, the new product would give lower values. It was also recognized that there are two types of health products possible and that they should be distinguished.
>
> a)   *Health image (health reassurance cigarette)* such as a low tar–low nicotine cigarette which the public accepts as a healthier cigarette and
>
> b)   *Health-oriented cigarette* which has minimal biological activity; for example, one which would yield a near zero reading in a mouse skin painting test"? [emphasis added]. {1112.02, p. 1}

The term "biological activity" is a euphemism for toxicity and, especially, for carcinogenicity.

The "health-image" cigarette meets public relations needs, while the "health-oriented" cigarette serves a public health function (2). This interchange suggests that the company's scientists believed that low-tar and low-nicotine cigarettes conferred few, if any, actual benefits on the smoker, and that these products were mainly a marketing device because the public "accept[ed]" the view that these cigarettes were less toxic (see chapter 2). Also striking is Dr. Sanford's remark that, in the opinion of those at the conference, any future product should have no greater biological (carcinogenic) activity than existing ones. This consensus is, of course, an implicit recognition of the fact that cigarettes are actually toxic.

The minutes summarize other key conclusions of the Hilton Head Conference:

1.   It is clear that a number of features of cigarettes can modify the biological activity of smoke condensate. These include the incorporation of PCL [processed cigarette leaf] and CRS [cut, rolled stem], the form of the smoking vehicle, the type of tobacco, the presence of additives and the volume of puff taken in smoking the cigarette. These factors will become increasingly important when future cigarettes are designed.

2.   *The biological results are also indicating the importance of both* [cancer] *initiators and promoters in smoke and this lead should be followed up vigorously in the biological research.*

3.   Studies in instant condensate are showing a biological activity towards mouse-skin of the same order as that of stale condensate, suggesting that the biological activity is not time-dependent. The clear possibility of producing cigarettes with reduced mouse-skin biological activity therefore becomes of greater importance and a research solution to the whole problem is more likely.

4.   There was general agreement that a cigarette with such reduced mouse-skin biological activity should be produced; other biological features, e.g. irritation, ciliastasis, must also be satisfied simultaneously [emphasis added]. {1112.01, pp. 1–2}

A number of other topics received attention during the discussions— among them, the development (at BAT's contract lab in Frankfurt) of reliable short-term tests to screen for carcinogenic activity; the merits of a noninhalable cigarette to protect smokers from developing emphysema, bronchitis, or cardiovascular diseases, conditions that depend on the inhalation of cigarette smoke for their development; the possibility of making a less irritating cigarette by lowering the proportion of nicotine compared to tar in the smoke (a filter from Germany, identified as the R6-acid filter, is mentioned in this connection); and the possible reduction of carbon monoxide levels in mainstream smoke through filtration or tobacco rod modifications with reconstituted tobacco. While these ideas apparently were not major focal points of product development at the time, their discussion reveals that BAT scientists thought that cigarette smoke inhalation was related to a number of diseases in addition to lung cancer and that nicotine was an irritant in cigarette smoke.

The conference participants' commitment to making cigarettes less dangerous, as measured by bioassay, is clear in the following conclusions:

13.   Following discussion of the specific examples, it was agreed that no synthetic smoking material can be considered for product development unless the biological activity of its condensate is less than that of modified tobaccos or PCL. Despite the disappointing results reported by Montreal and Southampton on the Bell and Laing modified cigarettes—with an axial channel through a tobacco column of increased packing density—it was agreed worthwhile to attempt to acquire the patent for a reasonable sum, because it represents an alternative approach to cigarette design, in which B-A.T. already has some patent protection [i.e., Ariel].

14.   The adoption of an objective to make cigarettes which yield condensates with lower biological activity (but which must sell on their ordinary qualities) reduces the degrees of freedom in terms of taste, acceptability, economics, etc. in cigarette design. Because of its importance in smoker preference, there is a need to expand the systematic examination of the effects of casings and flavours on the flavour and aroma of cigarette smoke.

It was agreed it would be unreasonable to hold up the introduction of a new development of a significant nature until it had been proved conclusively to be of lower biological activity. Provided that available short-term tests had been passed, and the development was judged to be in the right direction, the meeting agreed that the development could well be introduced subject to the immediate initiation of long term testing procedures. {1112.01, pp. 4–5}

The invention referred to in paragraph 13 may be described in a US patent issued in 1971 and assigned to B&W (13). The patent, filed a few weeks before the conference, describes an article that arranges tobacco in a cigarette-like device around a central core. The core contains material capable of removing toxins such as polycyclic aromatic hydrocarbons from the smoke. The tobacco is lit. As puffs are taken, tobacco smoke is channeled through the central core on its way to the consumer.

Finally, the conference report includes a reminder of the need to increase communication among the laboratories. There is also a veiled reference to limits on communication for some information because of "special legal agreements." This restriction may be a reference to trade secrets or, perhaps more likely, to efforts to insulate B&W from receiving reports that might be embarrassing for it to have in its R&D files (see chapter 7).

The various changes in organisation were outlined and their effects in terms of communication links [between laboratories at the several operating companies] were discussed. It was concluded that there is still a need to strengthen these links in addition to personal visits, but it must be recognised that there can be occasions when these must be restricted to certain channels because of special legal agreements entered into by individual companies. {1112.01, pp. 5–6}

KRONBERG RESEARCH CONFERENCE, 1969

Nine delegates from various affiliated companies, including delegates from England and from Kentucky, attended the 1969 research conference, held in Kronberg, Germany. The draft agenda {1113.01} covers a range of topics similar to those discussed at the Hilton Head conference: (1) reports of ongoing research projects, including Hilton (an inhalation experiment at Battelle), Lokstedt, and Janus (mouse skin painting to test for cancer); (2) discussions of nicotine pharmacology, carbon monoxide, solids in smoke, nontobacco materials, reconstituted tobacco, coumarin, black-fat tobacco, PEI, and "the current safest cigarette"; (3) product development; (4) process R&D, including leaf tobacco developments, freeze-drying, tobacco treatments, additives, reconstituted tobacco, and microbiological flora.

The minutes of the meeting include a lengthy discussion of the biological testing program. A major conclusion of this discussion is expressed as follows:

> The conclusion of the Conference was that at the present time the Industry had to recognise the possibility of distinct adverse health reactions to smoke aerosol:
> (a)   Lung Cancer
> (b)   Emphysema and bronchitis
> and present and future bioassay tests could usefully be classified according to their applicability to one or other or to both. {1169.01, p. 3}

The careful wording here is in keeping with industry dogma, but the statement is, nonetheless, far more forthright than the Zephyr document of the previous decade. A yet more frank assessment was to appear in the minutes of these meetings in the 1970s (see below). Despite this wording, the relative frankness of the comments on smoking and cancer in these minutes led to a strong letter (discussed in detail in chapter 7) from David Hardy at the law firm of Shook, Hardy, and Bacon to DeBaun Bryant, B&W's general counsel, warning that such admissions could lead to serious liability problems for the company {1840.01}.

Participants also discussed the mouse skin–painting experiments at Harrogate and the relative value of short-term biological tests as compared to mouse skin–painting studies. Cooperative industry studies in the United Kingdom had revealed important differences in carcinogenic activity between two preparations of tobacco condensate:

> This appears to be a significant alteration in mouse-skin bioassay reaction brought about by an alteration in tobacco composition. {1169.01, p. 1}

Unfortunately, though, a difficulty had arisen in specifying the precise compositions of the two condensates, so it was not clear how to replicate the finding or what changes to make in blending to carry this result further. The participants suggested that those in charge of this work should get in touch with the University of Kentucky to explore ways in which conventional strains of tobacco could have such marked differences.

The conferees endorsed fractionation experiments at Harrogate to see what subfractions of condensate act as promoters and initiators of cancer. Mouse skin painting remained the standard for carcinogenesis:

> In the foreseeable future, say five years, mouse-skin painting would remain as the ultimate court of appeal on carcinogenic effects. {1169.01, p. 4}

At the same time, short-term biological tests, such as a test of hyperplasia (an abnormal increase in the number of cells), were of interest both for their potential to act as predictors of mouse skin–painting results and as indicators in their own right of important toxicities of tobacco smoke. The conferees agreed, though, that there would be no consensus on what the results of short-term tests meant: any interpretation of short-term bioassay results as predictive of carcinogenic potential was "the responsibility of the user" alone {1169.01, p. 4}. Meanwhile, the tobacco industry's public position was that mouse skin painting is an unreliable way to test whether cigarette smoke causes cancer.

BIOLOGICAL TESTING COMMITTEE DISCUSSIONS, 1970

The Biological Testing Committee at Southampton provided oversight, review, and direction for the BAT toxicology research program. BAT-funded contract research as well as work funded by the UK industry group as a whole was discussed at these meetings. Committee membership usually consisted of BAT scientists in the United Kingdom, but individuals from other BAT companies in the UK industry group occasionally were present. Minutes from some of the meetings held between 1968 and 1977 are available in the documents. The minutes involve technical issues and it is often difficult to understand what is being discussed apart from the context. However, the general subject is the experiments on various product modifications and innovations to learn what maneuvers might lower the carcinogenic potential of cigarettes.

Two notes, one concerning inhalation, from a meeting held in May 1970 (the eighteenth meeting of this committee), and one on carbon monoxide, from a meeting in October of the same year, are included here as examples of these discussions.

The minutes of the discussion of inhalation tests read,

> There was an extensive discussion of inhalation tests. Dr. Sanford [B&W], Dr. Fordyce [UK] and Mr. Wade [Canada] urged that BAT should be actively engaged in inhalation tests in the near future. It was agreed, however, that at present an inhalation test which led to the production of cancer and which could be used for the comparison of different cigarettes was not available. Dr. Green [UK] suggested that the development of these tests could be left to the industry [cooperative laboratory at Harrogate]. With regard to shorter-term tests, [the Imperial Tobacco Company laboratories at] Huntingdon were obtaining encouraging results on the mouse-irritancy screen, a goblet cell test and a macrophage test. Dr. Bentley suggested that these should be available within about 12 months. It was agreed that BAT should wait for these tests to be developed rather than attempt to duplicate the work at the present time. Similarly, the development of the "monkey-smoking" programme at Huntingdon would be followed with great interest. {1164.06, pp. 3–4}

In its public statements, B&W was insisting that the evidence did not support the hypothesis that smoking caused cancer {2110.06, pp. 6–10}. Here, a group of BAT scientists clearly stated their expectation that an inhalation test would be developed that "would lead to the production of cancer" and expressed an eagerness to have such a test available as a tool for comparing different cigarettes. Thus, the issue was a comparison of how different cigarettes caused cancer, not whether smoking caused cancer. In addition, the industry position was that even a successful inhalation test showing cancer causation in animals would not be indicative of cancer causation in humans. Yet the BAT scientists embraced animal inhalation tests for this very purpose. In the meantime, they continued to use mouse skin painting for purposes of evaluating human toxicity.

The brief mention of work under way at Imperial's laboratory in Huntingdon reflects an information-sharing arrangement between BAT and Imperial. The agreement covered exchanges of research results on smoking and health issues as well as on leaf characteristics, agronomy, and machinery evaluation {1171.02}. The documents do not contain any information about the monkey-smoking work, but chapter 3 discusses a series of experiments at Imperial on the pharmacology of nicotine; monkeys were used as subjects in these experiments.

Carbon monoxide was discussed at a committee meeting in October 1970.

> It was considered that it was still very important to reduce the level of carbon monoxide in cigarette smoke. It is a known poison present in relatively large amounts and, despite the lack of success in developing a suitable filter, efforts should be continued. {1164.06, p. 4}

As will be described later, carbon monoxide was to continue to be a problem. However, as time went on, the nature of the problem became more one of public relations and the avoidance of regulatory oversight than the reduction of toxicity for its own sake.

HEALTH VERSUS PUBLIC RELATIONS, 1970–1982

ST. ADELE RESEARCH CONFERENCE, 1970

The group research conference for 1970 was held in November at St. Adele in Quebec {1170.01}. The group consensus about the potential for achieving a "safe" cigarette was significantly tempered in 1970 compared to conclusions the group had reached in 1967. According to the 1970 minutes, the 1967 meeting had concluded,

> The smoking and health problem *is amenable* to a research solution. This is a significant change in thinking and is a direct result of research [emphasis added]. {1170.01, p. 1}

By 1970 the conference participants (nearly the same group of individuals) reached a different conclusion:

> The smoking and health problem *is at least partially amenable* to a research solution [emphasis added]. {1170.01, p. 1}

Underlying both statements is the assumption that constituents of tobacco products have toxic effects. The statements represent an important shift between 1967 and 1970 in the degree to which BAT scientists believed there was a technical fix for the problem of smoking-induced cancer and other diseases.

CHELWOOD RESEARCH CONFERENCE, 1972

The minutes of the 1972 conference, held at Chelwood, England, include a specific statement of the "main objective" envisioned for R&D at the Southampton facility.

The main Southampton objective was stated 'To design cigarettes which are preferred by smokers either generally or in significant special cases. The products are to conform to policy requirements with respect to composition and biological activity.' The main criticism was not with the objectives but that these might be too difficult to achieve. {1171.02, p. 2}

A comment later on in the minutes, following the presentation of a paper by Dr. Green, the head of the Southampton laboratory, suggests what a measurable goal for an acceptable level of biological activity might be.

> One suggestion was that our aim should be to provide smoking pleasure accompanied by risk no greater than that with comparable habits, such as alcohol. This may already be the position achieved in some countries. {1171.02, p. 5}

New products, first of all, had to be commercially successful. Hazard reduction was couched in relative terms. This stance acknowledged both the reality of the hazard and the practical impossibility of eliminating it.

DUCK KEY RESEARCH CONFERENCE, 1974

Twelve delegates from five countries, including the United Kingdom and the United States, attended the 1974 research conference, held at Duck Key, Florida {1125.01}. Discussions concerned work on tobacco substitutes (see below), smoker compensation to achieve a consistent nicotine intake (see chapter 3), puffed (expanded) tobacco, carbon monoxide, caffeine as an additive, selective filtration, sidestream smoke (see chapter 10), and the financing of research, among other topics.

Puffed (expanded) tobacco was being investigated in Germany and Austria. The problem was that cigarettes made of expanded tobacco yielded fewer puffs per cigarette. In expanded tobacco, the layers of the tobacco leaf tissue are forced apart by physical pressure provided by the rapid vaporization of a liquid (such as freon) or solid (such as carbon dioxide in the form of dry ice) that has previously been saturated into the leaf. Expansion increases the volume per unit weight of tobacco. Cigarettes made of expanded tobacco reduce tar delivery because there is less fuel in a given volume if some of it has been puffed up. Carbon monoxide in smoke was recognized as a problem, but available means to reduce CO (such as a lithium hydroxide process) tended to increase the levels of polycyclic aromatics and to increase "tumorigenic activity." The direction of future combustion studies at Southampton was to be directed toward controlling both CO and polycyclic aromatics. Caffeine was noted to reduce "tumorigenic activity" of smoke condensate, but concern was expressed about the public relations problems that the use of caffeine as an additive might engender {1125.01, p. 3}.

Product development throughout the company in 1974 centered on "selective filtration and constant puff by puff deliveries." Constant deliveries are most important pharmacologically, since the customer then gets a predictable dose of nicotine with each inhalation. When cigarettes were merely cured, cut leaves wrapped in paper, the product was uneven and nicotine deliveries unpredictable (14). With technological innovations introduced in subsequent decades, cigarettes became much more consistent products. In this connection, a program within BAT of systematically analyzing commercial and technical information on Philip Morris products from around the world was mentioned as worth continuing.

Advertising restrictions attracted discussion. At the time, the only actual restrictions were on broadcast advertising. However, broader restrictions were feared. The conference summary notes,

> With increasing restrictions in advertising, there will be less opportunity for the creation of brands in traditional ways (imagery) but an increasing requirement for products to have new visible, demonstrable or detectable attributes. {1125.01, p. 4}

The Duck Key conference highlights the priority that R&D continued to place on making cigarettes safer. Issues of smoker compensation and environmental tobacco smoke appeared for the first time in this series, and a major portion of the conference report was devoted to the search for tobacco substitutes, which is treated in a separate section (see below).

MERANO RESEARCH CONFERENCE, 1975

At the 1975 conference, held at Merano, in northern Italy, much of the discussion centered on tobacco substitute materials such as Cytrel and New Smoking Material (NSM) (see below). The conferees expressed concern that the tobacco substitutes might themselves contribute to the toxicity of cigarettes, resulting in a greater toxic impact than that of regular cigarettes.

> The implications of the initiation-promotion hypothesis [of carcinogenesis] on the risks of smokers changing to cigarettes containing substitutes was discussed. It was agreed that this was important and that the mouse skin painting experiment proposal for TRC [the industry research group in the UK] (the so-called cross over experiment) should be supported. If it was not

agreed at TRC to undertake this experiment it is recommended that consideration should be given to B.A.T. undertaking these or similar experiments. {1173.01, p. 3}

The conference participants recognized that the "smoking and health" issue was never going to go away.

The meeting agreed that the earlier conclusions that cigarette smoking is now irreversibly associated with health issues is still valid. {1173.01, p. 3}

Moreover, the assembled BAT and B&W scientists recognized that their potential contribution could never offer more than a partial solution to the problem. Apparently, some in the group felt that the R&D group had, however, understated its role in prior statements.

It was felt by some members that the assumption that there would be no R & D 'breakthrough' in smoking and health had been misinterpreted in some ways. It was emphasised that this does not mean that there are unlikely to be important R & D contributions. It is believed that considerable and continuing progress will be made leading to a progressive series of product improvements. {1173.01, p. 3}

Technical improvements would never make a cigarette safe; the only credible goal was to make the product less dangerous.

The R&D objectives in the "smoking and health area" were explicitly set forth. These objectives represented a decided departure from the optimism of the 1960s, when it seemed that smoking might be made safe, and revealed a predominantly reactive, defensive posture.

The immediate objective is to provide a scientific contribution in those territories where pressures in relation to smoking and health require such a capability. This function is carried out locally where adequate R & D establishments exist and from G.R. & D.C. [Group Research and Development Centre at Southampton] in their absence. Specific services include:

1.   Design of products having attributes dictated by the attitude of local health authorities, e.g. control of smoke constituents considered harmful.

2.   Advice [to management] regarding the health implications of product design and constituents.

3.   Interpretation [for management] of smoking and health discoveries.

4.   Assessment of health implications and availability of materials and processes under development and purported to have a bearing on the smoking and health issue, e.g. N.T.M.s [new tobacco materials].

As a longer range, and perhaps never ending, objective R & D has a goal of developing products that respond positively to scientific information having relevance to smoking and health.

. . .

Until such time as assay methods already developed, or to be developed, are given authoritative endorsement by medical experts, the longer range work will remain as basic research. {1173.01, p. 5}

The immediate goal was to provide assistance to management in responding to public relations and regulatory demands. The provision of a less dangerous product for its own sake was relegated to a secondary role.

SYDNEY RESEARCH CONFERENCE, 1978

The minutes of the 1978 research conference, held in Sydney, Australia, reflect the acceptance by BAT and B&W scientists that smoking causes serious disease. Moreover, they expressed hope that the generation of low-tar cigarettes already on the market would prove to be far safer than those having higher-tar deliveries.

The first conclusion of the meeting affirmed the *absence* of any scientific controversy on smoking and health.

There has been no change in the scientific basis for the case against smoking. Additional evidence of smoke-dose related incidence of some diseases associated with smoking has been published. *But generally this has long ceased to be an area for scientific controversy. . . .* The meeting affirmed that cigarettes acceptable on all counts can probably be achieved by research and, indeed, may in fact be available [emphasis added]. {1174.01, p. 1}

This frank statement stands in marked contrast to the industry's public posture that a substantial controversy still existed.

Near the end of the minutes from this meeting, a discussion of less dangerous cigarettes includes an important epidemiological definition of what such a product would be.

Cigarettes of substantially reduced biological activity (SRBA) can be made by product modification and will continue to present a range of marketing opportunities. *By SRBA is meant cigarettes where epidemiology would show no greater incidence of disease for smokers than non-smokers.* But there remains a need for credible biological tests to facilitate developments. Credibility will continually evolve but could be provided by outside independent medical and scientific advice.

As indicated in Note 1 [quoted above], we may already have an SRBA cigarette and *it may be worth studying epidemiologically the current smokers of low tar products over the next decade.* But until this evidence is available alternative products should be developed. To do this, research must provide a continuing basis for cigarette formulation and design for related process needs and better understanding of smokers' behaviour. Defensive research will need to be provided for as far ahead as can be seen and this may well include social aspects [emphasis added]. {1174.01, pp. 6–7}

While the industry was publicly insisting that incidence of disease, as measured in epidemiological studies, is not a valid measure of disease causation, the BAT scientists privately adopted incidence of disease as the measure of degree of biological activity against which to evaluate the success of efforts to make a "safe" cigarette. There is no scientific controversy here. Cigarettes cause serious diseases.

The companies' scientists were saying that biological testing is only used as an indirect measure of what really matters—namely, whether customers of tobacco companies get sick and die more often than people who do not smoke. The official dogma, in contrast, is that epidemiology can never be used to reach conclusions, and that there is no animal model that proves causation. The absolute standard for measuring success of the R&D effort to make a less dangerous cigarette is whether fewer people get sick from smoking the supposedly SRBA product. In fact, the goal is that the SRBA smoke not cause any detectable excess incidence of disease. Unfortunately, the low-tar cigarettes that the group hoped were SRBA devices have not turned out to be substantially less hazardous than other cigarettes (7).

This passage sharply illuminates what is perhaps the most distressing aspect of the tobacco problem. Scientists at B&W and BAT were intent on developing a safe product. At the same time, tobacco products known to be dangerous were being continually produced by their employers and sold to the public. Even when the scientists believed (wrongly) that they might have developed a safe product, it was marketed for only a special segment of the market. That is, products known to be dangerous were kept on the market, whereas those thought to be safe were introduced only as niche brands. Moreover, the supposedly safe brands had not been adequately tested and therefore had not been proven safe. The tests that counted, the results of epidemiological studies of the companies' customers, were necessarily post-marketing research that would take many years to complete.

LONDON RESEARCH CONFERENCE, 1979

The R&D conference held in London in the fall of 1979 was notable for the brief discussion in the minutes of the biological testing program.

> The expenditure at Southampton on biological testing represents a significant portion of the total R&D expenditure (£0.54m internal and £0.37m external out of £5.3m gross total). Before agreement can be reached on the details

on any proposed programme of work, it was thought essential to have established the current Board policy on research on smoking issues e.g. (a) for early warning, (b) as evidence of a responsible attitude by the Group, (c) as the basis for future positive support to Group products. {1176.02, p. 9}

At the time, then, BAT was spending £910,000 per annum on its biological testing program through the Southampton facility. As the references to "early warning" and "responsible attitude" indicate, the scientists regarded the value of the work as mainly defensive; possible product improvements based on this work seemed of secondary importance. This emphasis may simply have reflected their realization that a "safe" cigarette was not an achievable goal and that the company had other pragmatic reasons to do work in this area.

PICHLARN RESEARCH CONFERENCE, 1981

The 1981 research conference was held in Pichlarn, Austria, in August {1178.01}. Smoker compensation, the tendency for consumers to smoke low-delivery products more vigorously than higher-delivery products (see chapter 3), was a theme that came up in several places. For instance, the strategic objective for filters referred to "human smoking patterns."

> To develop novel filters and novel filter technology aimed at the development of marketable low-tar products, paying particular regard to human smoking patterns. {1178.01, p. 3}

Similarly, in the discussion of carbon monoxide in cigarette smoke, "human smoking pat[t]erns"—that is, the way people actually smoke, in contrast to the way machines smoke—also are mentioned:

> Though the political relevance of medical opinion on the importance of CO [carbon monoxide] varies between countries, it was agreed that GR&DC should continue to seek means of reducing the CO/tar ratio of the main types of products. Before any such products are offered commercially, it would be advisable that they should have been examined in the context of human smoking pat[t]erns. . . .
>
> It is felt that the time is close when Government agencies worldwide will take more notice of compensation—and of the scale of the differences, for a given commercial product, between smoking machine numbers and the dose of smoke actually obtained by smokers. This issue may well go beyond the simple technical measurement of deliveries. If for no other reason than defence, we must pay increasing attention as to how our products—especially new products—are smoked by different categories of smokers. {1178.01, pp. 13–14}

Compensation, recognized by BAT and B&W scientists in the early 1970s, threatened to undermine the potential benefits of well-intentioned improvements in cigarette design. Instead of dealing with this threat as a problem in toxicology, however, company scientists seemed more pressed by its regulatory implications.

MONTEBELLO RESEARCH CONFERENCE, 1982

The minutes of the 1982 conference, held at Montebello, Canada, acknowledge that smoking and health problems had not been solved despite a quarter century of work on them. The following notes summarize discussions under the heading "Smoke Quality."

> Despite intense research over the past 25 years, the biological activity of smoke remains a major challenge. In particular, it is not known in quantitative terms whether the smoke from modern low and ultra-low delivery products has a lower specific biological activity than that from previous high delivery products. Nor is it clearly established (other than in broad terms such as sheet and stem) what are the main factors that influence biological activity. In the UK, the Independent Scientific Committee is calling for information on the quality of smoke from modern products, but the formulation of an appropriate research programme will prove extremely difficult and will need very careful planning. The US Surgeon General has previously also drawn attention to the general need for a better understanding of biological activity.
>
> In a survey of the current US scene, the broad area of smoking and health (less hazardous cigarette, additives, self-extinguishing cigarette [to reduce the risk of cigarette-caused fires]), the possibility was identified that a competitor could in the future well make competitive capital out of health-related attributes, eg low nitrosamines or even a biological index.
>
> The Canadian contribution to the Group Biological Programme, which is closely co-ordinated with GR&DC [Group Research and Development Centre], will concentrate on factors that might influence mutagenic [cell changing] activity:
>
> (a)   Different tobacco types including sheet.
> (b)   Smoking regime—human vs standard smoking machine.
> (c)   Product design features.
>
> The research at McGill University, which is funded by the Canadian Tobacco Manufacturers Council, will also contribute to Group knowledge. {1179.01, pp. 4–5}

This passage acknowledges that BAT and B&W scientists did not know "in quantitative terms" whether the innovations they had pioneered were effective in lowering the biological activity of the products. Pressure from public health quarters continued unabated. Especially troublesome was the presence of nitrosamines, extremely potent carcinogens in tobacco. Nitrosamines also presented a possible competitive problem if another company made claims about low nitrosamine levels.

Concerns about nitrosamines are further emphasized in the outline of work to be undertaken in the following three years (1983–85). Since nicotine and other nicotinic alkaloids in tobacco combine with nitrates to form the tobacco-specific nitrosamines (15), removal of nitrates from tobacco (thereby reducing levels of this precursor of nitrosamines) was regarded as a priority {1179.01, p. 15}. A related investigation would try to determine whether "certain nitrogen-containing components [nitrates and proteins/amino acids {1164.26, appendix F}] are major precursors of smoke mutagenicity" {1179.01, p. 16}.

In addition to these veiled references, the specific discussion about nitrosamines is summarized as follows:

> There was support for the identification of this [nitrosamines] as a new Work Area. It was emphasized, however, that the approach should be two-pronged, ie:
>
> (i)   Understanding the routes by which nitrosamines in whole smoke are formed, and possible modification thereof by additives etc.
>
> (ii) Selective removal of nitrosamines.
>
> Before starting experimental work on the environmental analysis of nitrosamines, the past work of Wynder and Hoffman, Philip Morris and the German Verband should be fully appraised. {1179.01, p. 17}

Stems, otherwise valued for their relatively low tar production, were high in nitrates and so could potentially contribute to nitrosamine formation. During the late 1970s and early 1980s, many patents were issued to tobacco companies on ways to remove nitrates.

BAT'S RESEARCH PROJECTS, 1960s–1980s

PROJECT JANUS

BAT did not rely solely on the UK industry-wide cooperative lab at Harrogate for its long-term toxicology program. In 1965 it set up a contract operation of its own, called Project Janus. Project Janus was winding down in 1977 {1164.23}, but continued at least into 1978. BAT contracted with Battelle-Institut Frankfurt am Main to conduct long-term mouse skin–painting experiments as part of BAT's product development program. This was another branch of the same laboratory that had conducted the nicotine projects Hippo I and Hippo II (discussed in chapter 3) a few years earlier. Battelle hired a staff of between twenty and twenty-seven people for Project Janus and built a special building to house it {1138.03}. Battelle undertook a wide variety of studies under Project Janus. The core activity was mouse skin painting, and different ideas were tested to examine the toxicity of specific cigarette components and of different proposed modifications. In addition, Battelle developed a variety of short-term biological tests under this project.

The selection of projects initially seems to have been decided by the priorities of the BAT staff in the United Kingdom. Early on, before the project had even started, Dr. R. B. Griffith of B&W expressed concern that the initial testing was entirely related to British-type 100 percent flue-cured cigarettes and ignored the blended cigarette typical of the US market {1105.01}. B&W did, however, contribute materials for a variety of Janus experiments. The preparation of samples for testing at Harrogate and at Frankfurt consumed a good bit of time at the Southampton lab in the late 1960s {1138.01, p. 3}, but B&W was also involved in this work {1143.01}.

A glimpse at how Southampton contributed to Janus comes from an undated, two-page fragment of an annual report from about the late 1960s to the early 1970s {1138.01, pp. 3–4}. The lab's work is categorized into "(a) the reduction in biological activity, and (b) the understanding of consumer acceptance." The report indicates,

> *Additive-treated tobacco and sheet materials show considerable merit biologically, indicating that tobacco can be altered advantageously.* It would appear that the tobacco type and the processing it receives may be the major factors. . . . The formulation of non-tobacco materials has also been undertaken.
>
> The investigation of additives to reduce aromatic polycyclic hydrocarbons has continued. Several have been found to be effective, and two have sufficient commercial potential to warrant detailed study regarding levels and methods of addition [emphasis added]. {1138.01, p. 3}

The preparation of samples for Project Janus testing at the Battelle facility in Frankfurt and at the Tobacco Research Committee (TRC) lab at Harrogate (TRC was the successor to TMSC) consumed a substantial amount of effort.

The results of a study of the toxicity of inhaled tobacco smoke at the Battelle laboratory are discussed in a 1972 report {1152.01}. Groups of male mice were exposed to the smoke of one of two cigarette types; their fertility then was compared to that of a group of mice that had not been exposed to smoke and to each other. Sexual activity was less in the experimental groups than in the controls, and the controls had a higher fertility rate than the smoke-exposed groups.

In 1967 Janus testing had established that the additive potassium carbonate, even though its use resulted in lower benzpyrene levels, was associated with higher rates of tumor formation in mice {1109.01, p. 2}.

Part of the Project Janus research plan in 1968 was to test the effects of different levels of cigarette ventilation on condensate carcinogenic activity and to test processed cigarette leaf (PCL) as a substrate {1112.01}.

In an overview of Janus mouse skin–painting experiments prepared in April 1971 {1138.04; 1163.13}, E. B. Wilkes summarized results from six different experimental test preparations. The rates of tumor production at the lowest of the three doses tested for each preparation are presented here in order of the size of the effect {1138.04, pp. 5–6}:

Condition	% Tumors at 25 mg dose
PCL, based on CN102 lamina and Canadian stem binder	16.9%
Flue-cured lamina (CN102) and Canadian Stem (as CRS), in equal portions	31.1%
"Typical" U.S. K.S.F.T. [king size filter tip] cigarette	33.6%
Flue-cured blend (CN102), lamina only	47.7%
Yeast treated flue-cured lamina (CN102), strand widths 30, 60 and 120 c.p.i. [cuts per inch]	59.1%
Flue-cured lamina (CN102) control for B6; strand widths 30, 60 and 120 c.p.i.	62.2%

By late 1971, however, BAT was expanding its options for toxicology testing. A progress report on Project Janus for 1971, written by a BAT scientist, notes that BAT expects to set up its own laboratory facilities within a year {1163.10}. Moreover, this new lab would concentrate on inhalation studies. The new inhalation work would feature precise control and measurement of the retained dose from different cigarettes. Nevertheless, the author of this report continues to expect that a role for mouse skin–painting experiments will remain.

> [I]t is anticipated that mouse-skin painting experiments will be continued at Battelle and[,] although the demands are reducing[,] the next long-term test has already been planned. Future requirements are somewhat less certain but it is likely that such tests will be required for the examination of new technical developments in the reconstitution process and the incorporation of different materials or additives in the process. {1163.10, p. 10}

A Project Janus experiment on the effect of different puff volumes on tumorigenicity was reported by the Battelle lab to BAT in 1973 {1138.02}. At issue was whether cigarette smoke condensates taken at puff volumes of 10, 25, and 50 ml were equally potent when the same amounts (50 mg) were applied to mice in the standard manner. While the eventual rate of tumor formation was similar in all three groups, there was a clear dose-response relationship in the time of appearance of tumors. The 10-ml puff volume was associated with the most rapid appearance of tumors, the 25-ml puff volume was intermediate, and the 50-ml puff volume was associated with the most gradual onset of the appearance of tumors. In this experiment, the carcinogens in the condensates seemed to be in higher concentration in the tar from the smaller puffs than the larger puffs. Combustion may have been more complete in the later stages of the larger puffs, resulting in a dilution of carcinogens from the first part of the puff. The report describes the results as showing a dose-response relationship. The presence of a dose-response relationship is very strong scientific evidence that the material being tested, in fact, causes cancer.

Janus, which continued for more than a dozen years, made major contributions to BAT's understanding of safe cigarette strategies. It utilized long-term and short-term assays to help the R&D staff make decisions about product design. Even though the work led at best to only marginal improvements in cigarettes, the goal of the work was always clear: to help make cigarettes less toxic. To achieve this goal, BAT was willing to support a large contract research operation in Frankfurt from 1965 until at least 1978.

PROJECT RIO

A review of BAT's biological testing program was held at Southampton in May 1983 {1164.26}. The notes on this meeting contain the first reference in the documents to Project Rio, a project designed to organize the company's research on cigarettes having reduced biological activity. Additional information about Project Rio is found in the report of the Rio de Janeiro research conference held in August 1983 {1180.07}. (Chapter 7 discusses the concern that B&W lawyers had about the possible discovery of Project Rio by lawyers for plaintiffs in products liability lawsuits.)

Three distinct components were recognized in Project Rio:

(a)   Phase I would be the design of low activity cigarettes in the 5–10 mg [tar] range, using existing technology and tests.

(b)   Phase II would be the further investigation of such cigarettes with additional tests, possibly after their introduction onto the market. Within the additional tests it is likely that there would be a requirement for a long-term study: Dr. F. J. C. Roe recommended that an inhalation study would be preferable, providing a viable test procedure was available.

(c)   A further stage in the development of low activity products could be envisaged, involving more speculative procedures such as the adventitious addition of materials to cigarettes. However, *the work associated with the development and evaluation of such cigarettes would be substantial and might pose problems similar to those faced by the pharmaceutical industry* [emphasis added]. {1164.26, p. 1}

The work was to be done through the laboratories in Hamburg, Montreal, and Southampton. The first two parts of the project sound very similar to the things that the R&D group had been involved with over the past generation. The third, though, was something of a departure: the use of additives to reduce biological activity. The document mentions one such possibility: Vitamin A.

The current status of Vitamin A as an anti-cancer agent should be reviewed in the context of the possible addition of Vitamin A (or some derivative) to tobacco. {1164.26, p. 2}

Such a proposal would make sense only if one believed that tobacco causes cancer. Compounds related to Vitamin A found in food had been related to reduced cancer risk, and this information was coming to public attention around this time. However, the use of such cancer-reducing materials as additives "might pose problems similar to those faced by the pharmaceutical industry" {1164.26, p. 1}. The reference here appears to be to FDA regulation.

Toward the end of the 1980s, a B&W marketing executive, Douglas Keeney, left the company to start a new company, CA Blockers. CA Blockers was set up to market a cigarette that used an additive, N-Bloctin, which promised to reduce the consumer's exposure to nitrosamines. The product, Spectra, was regulated as a drug by the FDA because of the implied health claim (2). The FDA regarded N-Bloctin as a drug, since it was intended to reduce the absorption of carcinogens from tobacco smoke, and the agency declared that any product containing N-Bloctin was also a drug. Therefore, it exerted jurisdiction.

By August 1983 the R&D scientists at BAT had decided against actively pursuing Vitamin A as an additive. The decision was based on the results of a literature review, which led to the conclusion "that Vitamin A (and closely related compounds) does not present an opportunity for the cigarette industry directly to influence human response to smoke" {1180.07, p. 4}.

A fear expressed during the discussions about Project Rio in the initial 1983 concept paper was that competitors might publish a ranking of cigarette brands according to the results of mutagenicity tests such as the Ames test. (The Ames test uses bacteria that because of a defective gene are unable to make a particular nutrient that is lacking in a specially prepared growth medium. A mutation at this gene locus can permit the bacteria to grow in the deficient medium. The relative mutagenicity of a test material—such as cigarette tar—can be estimated by the rate at which the material induces mutations that permit the bacteria to grow.)

> The possibility of competitors producing a biological ranking of brands e.g. based on Ames test data is real and we should be in a position to respond to such a situation. {1164.26, p. 2}

It is interesting that this threat was seen as coming from other tobacco companies and not from a source such as the *Reader's Digest*, which had previously caused such problems with its publication of tar and nicotine yields. Clearly, in a country such as the United States, the only competing company that would publish such a list would be one whose product had the least Ames mutagenic activity. In other words, the competitor would have to be a start-up company such as CA Blockers. Nonetheless, the concern that someone else might develop a brand-specific table of mutagenic activity led to a plan to evaluate the Ames test mutagenicity of company brands and those of competitors in selected countries from around the world {1180.07, pp. 3–4}. This work would actually have enabled BAT to publish a biological index table. The work was to be completed on this initial testing by mid-1984.

Project Rio was to be the company's major biological research activity for the 1984–86 period {1180.07, p. 18}. While the work would concentrate on the Ames test, the minutes reflect an attitude of caution about "over-dependence" on this single measure; "more direct tests" were preferred if possible.

Preliminary results from Project Rio are summarized in the minutes of the biological conference held at Southampton in April 1984 {1181.06}.

> The Ames is the main screening assay and from the results to date it is clear that:
>
> (i)   *Cigarette <u>brands</u> can be readily distinguished. This is in contrast with the earlier mouse skin painting results. An unfortunate side-effect is that the sensitivity increases the probability of an Ames League Table*

appearing. A further unfortunate examination is that, to date, it is not uncommon for BAT brands to have a higher result than those from the opposition.

(ii)   Important fractionation work in Montreal indicates that the Ames activity is associated with the basic materials in cigarette condensate. Again, this is in contrast to the mouse skin painting results, where the bulk of the activity resides in the neutral fraction. Any response to this observation must wait until the initial work in Montreal has been completed.

(iii)   Initial results indicate that reduction in circumference [of the cigarette] reduces activity.

(iv)   Early results from Hamburg indicate that the addition of casings and flavours can increase the Ames activity. Observations from Montreal suggest that certain other casings bring about a reduction in Ames activity.

(v)   Ventilation brings about an increase in mutagenicity which with Canadian cigarettes was not significant. German cigarettes however showed a significant increase. It could be important to evaluate changes in design features with a number of cigarette types as the interaction with the tobacco blend could well be important.

(vi)   Montreal is to produce a review examining variations in design parameters and mutagenicity.

Clearly we need tests in addition to the Ames test and Southampton is obtaining encouraging results with an enzyme induction assay. There was general agreement that the work should be actively pursued. Similarly it was agreed that the "yeast system" showed promise as a useful assay and should be followed up.

The eventual need for a long-term bioassay, preferably based on inhalation, was considered. The significance of such a test to the tobacco industry was discussed, particularly if the animals used were pre-treated with a known initiator such as radon. No firm conclusions were reached but it was agreed that Southampton should explore the feasibility of a long-term assay [italic emphasis added]. {1181.06, pp. 1–2}

BAT scientists had been able to stratify cigarette brands according to Ames activity, but not with mouse skin painting. The constituents of cigarette smoke responsible for the Ames test activity seemed to be different from those associated most strongly with carcinogenesis in the mouse skin–painting model. This result suggests that these were additional constituents of tobacco smoke with negative health effects.

A joint R&D/marketing conference held in Montreal in July 1984 included a report on Project Rio from the Montreal lab {1226.01, p. 85}. The report presents data showing that changes in smoker behavior (compensation effects) could alter Ames test results.

Traditionally, mouse skin painting has been used as an indicator of biological activity. Recently, short term tests such as the Ames mutagenicity test have also been used to determine biological activity. With the increases [*sic*] use of short term tests, there has been, within the BAT group, discussions focussing on the possibility of legislative bodies using the Ames or other short term tests to assess the "tar quality" or arriving at biological league tables. Project RIO is an example of BAT's response to a potential need for a reduced biologically active product.

   . . .

In all cases, the biological activity of the human generated smoke condensate was compared to standard machine smoking condensate.

   . . .

These results appear to indicate the following:

1)   that human smoking does influence biological activity relative to standard conditions.

2)   certain aspects of human smoking behaviour affect the biological activity of the smoke condensate more than others.

Further studies will revisit this area and investigate in more detail:

1)   those aspects of human smoking behaviour that appear to be most influential with regards to biological activity.

2)   whether these aspects can be modified through product design. {1226.01, pp. 85–86}

The study compared human and machine smoking of two Imperial Tobacco Ltd (Canada) brands, Matinée Extra Mild and duMaurier Light King Size. Matinée had a greater level of "specific biologic activity under human smoking conditions"; that is, Matinée smoke had a higher level of activity per microgram of smoke. In contast, deMaurier had a higher level of activity than Matinée when the data were examined on a "total" (per cigarette) basis. Human smoking profiles had greater "specific" and "total" biological activity associated with them than did the machine standard {1126.01, from overheads used in the presentation}. These data seemed to confirm the study hypothesis that human smoking behavior differs from machine-based smoking enough to be of practical importance.

All in all, Project Rio seemed to leave unresolved problems that had plagued the search for a safe cigarette from the beginning. The Ames test offered a credible short-term assay, but it measured different things from the mouse skin test that had been the standard for decades. The focus at this late stage, three decades on, was still on developing a good assay, when the technological difficulties involved in reducing toxins to safe levels while still delivering a satisfying smoke remained formidable. The whole matter was further complicated by the fact that people do not smoke like machines.

The bleak prospects for making meaningful progress on this front are reflected in the five themes for R&D found in the minutes of a Group R&D meeting at Wallingford, England, in September 1985 {1182.01}.

   i.   Product/smoke quality to be as good as, and preferably better than, competitors.

   ii.   Develop technology to be the lowest cost producer and others necessarily of a longer term nature.

   iii.   Produce a recognised step forward on the S&H [smoking and health] issue.

   iv.   Remove concern for passive smoking by various initiatives including superior products.

   v.   Develop alternative products. {1182.01, p. 2}

Progress toward a safe cigarette had become the third objective, was regarded as a long-term objective, and had been diluted to the point that a reasonable goal was seen as merely offering management a "recognised step" in this direction.

SHORT-TERM BIOLOGICAL TESTS

In order to develop a cigarette that was less prone to cause cancer, BAT scientists needed an assay procedure to test out various possible product modifications. Mouse skin painting was BAT's standard test for carcinogens, but it required up to two years to get the results of a single experiment. This built-in delay and expense made rapid progress impossible. Accordingly, Sir Charles Ellis suggested that BAT develop a battery of short-term tests for use in-house. In January 1964, coinciding with the publication of the US Surgeon General's report, Sir Charles wrote Richard P. Dobson at BAT headquarters, recommending that BAT develop a set of short-term toxicological tests for the use of B&W {1103.02}.

Sir Charles suggested that Battelle, the contract research organization that did other work for BAT on both nicotine pharmacology (Project Hippo) and carcinogenicity of tobacco smoke (Project Janus), or some other organization be engaged to set up the ciliastasis test. He wanted to use it in assessing cigarette brands selected by B&W. In addition, he wanted to develop two other tests from among the five suggested, or to develop other sorts of short-term bioassays. The proposed testing program seems to have been mainly for the benefit of B&W. It is unclear why the work was to be done at Battelle rather than in-house, except that Battelle was shortly to do the company's mouse skin–painting work to evaluate carcinogenic potency of cigarette smoke under the Janus project. Having the toxicology work done in an overseas, outside laboratory also provided B&W a buffer against discovery in legal proceedings (see also the section headed "Specific Strategies to Avoid Discovery" in chapter 7).

In his letter Sir Charles speculates that having such a battery of tests available would be of similar importance to conventional quality control:

> If this project were to prove feasible it might lay the basis for a continuing health monitoring service on our cigarettes analogous to the Quality Control practised for physical characteristics. The work would be quite distinct from the researches into the relation between smoking and lung cancer which is carried out on a co-operative basis by T.R.C. [at Harrogate]. {1103.02, p. 3}

A week later, in Louisville, Tom Wade of R&D at B&W wrote an analysis of this memorandum for Ed Finch, B&W's president {1103.01}. A copy was hand-carried to Mr. Dobson of BAT when he was in New York on the following day. Wade endorses the concept of rapid tests without commenting on the technical feasibility of the specific proposals made by Sir Charles. Wade also blurs the distinction between tests to look for carcinogenic potential and tests for immediate toxicity. He concludes, "Naturally the whole purpose back of this is to get a reasonably rapid method to determine differences" {1103.01}.

The documents do not include further information on this attempt to establish short-term biological testing within BAT's research establishment. Nearly three years later, though, in October 1966, an internal progress report on a research project at the Southampton lab demonstrated that there was by then active work on the development of short-term assays. In this case the goal was the development of a short-term test that would predict carcinogenic activity {1107.01}.

By November 1968, as a memo from Dr. R. A. Sanford, technical manager of research at B&W, to J. W. Burgard (with copies to the company president, general counsel, and the director of research and development) indicates, the contract lab operated by Battelle in Frankfurt, Germany, had achieved some success with a short-term test that measured hyperplasia in mouse skin as a predictor of malignant transformation {1111.01}. The test required only eight days to perform. It measured thickening of the skin on the backs of mice exposed to the test materials. This test had shown agreement with the mouse skin–painting test in most of the following situations:

> The addition of certain PCL's, Celanese synthetic materials, or certain additives to the blend reduces biological activity rating.

Filters containing charcoal, cellulose acetate, PEI (polyehtyleneimine), or paper do not affect tumorigenic results.

With the exception of one result, increasing puff volume progressively from 10 to 50 ml reduces activity.

U. S. cigarettes are less active [i.e., less capable of inducing cancerous changes in the mice] than English varieties. The addition of either burley or up to 50% CRS [cut, rolled stems] to flue-cured tobacco reduces activity. {1111.01, p. 1}

Dr. Sanford suggested that some experimental versions of Viceroy be submitted for testing in this system and that it be used in connection with an upcoming project called Project Hilton {1111.01}. Project Hilton was to be an inhalation study under the management of Battelle, with the goal of looking at the short-term toxicity of tobacco smoke in animals.

By the middle of December, Dr. Sanford had received clearance to send samples to Europe for the hyperplasia test {1112.04}. He sent current versions of Kool and Viceroy, the same brands with 28 percent WTS (water-treated system), and Life filters and Life filters without PEI (poly-ethyleneimine) but with a Viceroy tobacco rod. The mention of Life filters without PEI suggests that the normal filter for Life contained this additive, an ingredient that was known to increase the proportion of "extractable nicotine" in cigarette smoke {1205.03}. It had not, however, reduced tumorigenic activity of smoke condensate {1111.01}. By 1968, then, B&W had at its disposal a short-term bioassay that correlated reasonably well with the standard test for carcinogenesis, mouse skin painting.

Notes on the 1974 Duck Key, Florida, research conference refer tersely to a short-term bioassay test that the BAT lab in Germany had developed.

BAT (Germany) NMFI test is proving of significant value in rapid prediction of mouse skin activity. We propose not to make this test available to competitors at this time since it might be of considerable commercial advantage [emphasis in original]. {1125.01, p. 2}

This assay was the subject of a research report from the BAT affiliate in Canada three years later. A 1977 research report from Imperial Tobacco Limited (Canada) details the possible use of a test called "the nitromethane fraction index (NMFI)" as an indicator of "biological activity" {1129.01}. The NMFI test was designed to be an inexpensive and quick test that predicted carcinogenicity in mouse skin. The test involved the extraction of cigarette smoke in a way known to concentrate polycyclic aromatic hydrocarbons; this smoke fraction was then mixed with egg albumin, and the resulting degree of binding by fluorescence was determined. The degree of binding in turn showed a correlation with the biological activity of the smoke.

The test had been developed at the BAT lab in Germany and also was in use at Southampton. The test was found to be reproducible and to correlate well with the results of mouse skin–painting carcinogenicity tests conducted under the Janus program. Despite some reservations, the report recommends the routine inclusion of the NFMI test among the tests done "in future projects where there is a possibility of a change in the biological activity of the smoke" {1129.01, p. 4}. The report emphasizes that the NMFI test is for internal use only; it is not to be shared with other companies. In this context, the term "biological activity" is used as a euphemism for "carcinogenic activity." The development of this test is one more example of how the company knew its products caused cancer, and tried to do something about it, while publicly denying this fact.

US "SMOKING AND HEALTH" PROJECTS

SELECTIVE FILTRATION: THE FACT CIGARETTE

Selective filtration, the approach first legitimized in 1962 by Lorillard's new filter for its Kent brand, is the focus of several of the documents. B&W developed the Fact brand of cigarette around a filter designed to selectively remove certain volatile compounds, such as acetaldehyde and acrolein, from cigarette smoke (16). Introduced in 1975, Fact was on the market for only a few years.

In November 1977 B&W contracted with Celanese Fibers Company to analyze the vapor phase constituents of Fact in comparison with the following competing brands: L&M Flavor Lights (Liggett), Real Menthol (RJR), Merit (Philip Morris), and Kent Golden Lights (Lorillard). The Celanese report, dated January 1978, includes analyses of fifty-four different vapor phase constituents for the five different brands {1130.01}. The results for acetaldehyde, acrolein, nitrogen oxide, and cyanide are highlighted with handwritten marks in the results table. The Fact brand had lower values than the competition for acetaldehyde and for cyanide, but it ranked second highest for nitrogen oxide. Acrolein was not measured for Fact. The documents do not indicate what use was to be made of these data. Perhaps they were simply an internal check to see whether the competition had introduced filter additives that had effects similar to those found for Fact cigarettes; perhaps they were obtained to justify possible advertising claims of selective filtration.

In 1979 B&W commissioned a survey of physicians to learn whether they would be responsive to claims of reduced gases in cigarette smoke (see chapter 9).

THE TOBACCO WORKING GROUP

The Tobacco Working Group (TWG) was a federally supported project, launched by the National Cancer Institute (NCI), with the purpose of developing a less hazardous cigarette. The documents show that the tobacco companies participated in the meetings of the TWG and attempted to influence the group's work. At first, the tobacco industry attempted to convince the members of the TWG that cigarettes are not dangerous. When this strategy failed, the industry gained unexpected assistance from Dr. Gio Gori, deputy director of the National Cancer Institute's Division of Cancer Cause and Prevention and chairman of the TWG. Gori publicized the idea that less hazardous cigarettes could be created. Gori's proposal ultimately became an embarrassment for the federal government, which was focused on getting smokers to quit, but was a boon for the tobacco industry. The tobacco industry took advantage of Gori's proposal in its marketing of low-tar and extra-low-tar cigarettes.

On February 8, 1973, the Department of Health, Education and Welfare issued a charter for the TWG, which made it a formal and multidisciplinary group consisting of researchers from academia, the government, and the tobacco companies. The group had actually begun meeting informally in 1968 to discuss generally research related to smoking and health, cancer, cardiovascular disease, and respiratory disease {1400.01}. The 1973 charter specified that the purpose of the group was to "identify the criteria and prescribe methods for the development of a less hazardous cigarette, and other methods to decrease the smoking hazard" {1402.02, p. 1}.

The TWG was chaired by Dr. Gori; the other members were "selected on the basis of their personal qualifications in the field of smoking and health, cancer, cardiovascular [disease], and respiratory disease" {1402.02}. In addition to academic and government researchers, the research directors of Liggett & Myers, R. J. Reynolds, Lorillard, and Philip Morris participated in the TWG meetings {1401.02}. The documents clearly show that the main purpose of tobacco companies' participation in the TWG was not to share information but, rather, to keep the tobacco industry informed about government policy and research direction and to attempt to influence such policy.

A B&W file memorandum dated March 15, 1973 {1400.01}, describes
a meeting of a subcommittee of the Tobacco Institute's Committee of
Counsel and the research directors of the tobacco companies at which
they agreed that they would probably not be able to influence Gori's work
on the "safe cigarette." Because of this lack of influence, the scientific directors were instructed to distance themselves from the TWG because it
could reflect badly on the industry. The file memorandum states:

> It was generally felt that *there is no chance that the tobacco industry can in-*
> *fluence the Government to cut back on the proposal made by Dr. Gori for*
> *the Tobacco Working Group.* If the industry makes a counter-proposal, it
> would be but for the record only.
>
>   . . .
>
> After careful consideration of the views of the members of the Tobacco In-
> stitute staff with regard to the public relations and political effects of the pub-
> lic withdrawal from TWG [in original document CTR is crossed out and re-
> placed with TWG], it was concluded that the research directors cannot
> withdraw. *We should take steps to give the industry as much protection as is*
> *possible and at the same time remain in the Tobacco Working Group* [em-
> phasis added]. {1400.01}

To give the tobacco industry as much protection as possible from any
TWG statements suggesting that cigarettes are dangerous, the memorandum describes a three-point plan:

> 1.   When called by Gori, scientific directors decline to concur with or com-
> ment on Gori's recommendations. . . . Dr. Gori *should also be informed that*
> *the scientific director does not accept the premise that smoking is harmful.*
> 2.   Scientific directors will informally try to persuade Gori to eliminate or
> modify those proposals which are propaganda-oriented, rather than scien-
> tific—e.g., cessation clinics.
> 3.   Subcommittee of Committee of Counsel [a Tobacco Institute committee
> consisting of the chief counsels of the member companies] (with representa-
> tion from ranks of scientific directors) re-examine previous letters from sci-
> entific directors to TWG stating their roles [emphasis added]. {1400.01}

Other documents show that the tobacco industry carried out the plan.
Throughout the documents related to the TWG, the tobacco companies
repeatedly state that they were just observing and were not fully participating in the meetings. A May 31, 1973, letter from I. W. Hughes (research director at B&W) to Gori states:

> At the risk of repeating myself, I see my role as making available my knowl-
> edge of cigarette design and chemistry of tobacco and smoke, and not par-
> ticipating in approving the many research proposals proposed by the TWG

and outside of my area of expertise. *Finally, I would reiterate my view that my participation should not be construed as agreeing with the premise that cigarettes are hazardous or contribute to the development of human disease* [emphasis added]. {1400.02}

It is interesting that representatives of the tobacco industry were now making a distinction between the animal studies and *human* disease.

Friction between the tobacco industry's researchers and other researchers in the TWG is described in an October 10, 1974, memo from Horace Kornegay of the Tobacco Institute {1907.01}. Kornegay reports an incident in which Dr. Phillippe Shubik, a member of the National Cancer Advisory Board, criticized industry-employed members of NCI's Tobacco Working Group by saying, "you [the industry-employed members] will go down in history denying facts well-known to the scientific community" {1907.01, p. 1}.

The September 10–11, 1974, meeting of the TWG concluded with a discussion by Gio Gori on the scientific foundation of the safe cigarette program:

> In the projection of the future [it] is unlikely that Heart and Lung Institute will put much support in TWG in the development of safer cigarettes. On the other hand, the TWG work should not only be limited to reduced nicotine and tar, but at the same time should examine the other phases including CO [carbon monoxide], NOx [oxides of nitrogen], etc., which may cause other health problems. . . .
>
> Dr. Gori presented a rough draft of a policy statement which will serve as a guide for the TWG program. He presented a flow chart which indicates three stages of screening for the development of a safer cigarette. The first stage is mouse skin painting; the second stage is inhalation by hamsters or rats; and the third stage is dog (beagle) and/or humans if possible. {1401.02, p. 5}

As the TWG's work on developing a less hazardous cigarette began to be reported in the lay press, the tobacco industry took a proactive role by attempting to prevent publication of comments suggesting that tobacco is dangerous. Both Dr. I. W. Hughes (research director at B&W) and Dr. A. W. Spears (research director at Lorillard) commented on press releases that Gori sent to them in late 1975 regarding research to develop a less hazardous cigarette. The statements in the press releases were made by the directors of the National Institutes of Health's National Cancer Program, the National Cancer Advisory Board, and the National Heart, Lung and Blood Institute. The tobacco industry evidently convinced Gori to cancel at least one press release. The original press releases referred to three upcoming reports from the TWG (to be released

January 1976): (1) a report on the first set of experimental cigarettes; (2) a report on the second set of experimental cigarettes; and (3) a report on an in vitro bioassay of cigarette smoke from experimental filters. The release contained the following statements that disturbed the industry:

> Evidence gathered by research efforts throughout the work indicts cigarette smoking in over 300,000 premature deaths each year in the United States alone.
>   . . . calling upon the tobacco industry to adopt newly developed techniques to make cigarettes less hazardous . . . {1404.08, pp. 1–3}

> Because some people are unable or unwilling to quit, the cigarette industry should strive to offer the smoking public cigarettes that minimize the risk to the smoker. {1404.09, p. 1}

Hughes evidently sought advice from Ernest Pepples, general counsel for B&W, about how he should respond to the press releases. Pepples responded to Hughes's request as follows:

> It is the classic "pig-in-a-poke" [referring to the fact that the three reports are unpublished].
>   . . .
> [T]he TWG members from the industry need to dissociate themselves from the releases and any underlying materials which allegedly support the releases.
>   . . .
> At bottom I think you should come off saying to Gori that such activity as these releases abuses the industry members of the TWG. It is a bad way to treat them. It makes continuing cooperation difficult or impossible. {1404.10, p. 1}

Hughes's letter to Gori (unsigned) states:

> I have no choice but to urge you to try and convince the people concerned not to use them [the press releases]. . . . from earlier discussions with you regarding the drafts of the publications you considered it important not to draw any firm conclusion from the work done to date. . . . The whole attitude of the press releases in contrary to this. . . . I certainly would dissociate myself from the releases. . . . Lastly, I feel that such releases abuse my membership of the TWG. {1404.03, pp. 1–2}

Horace Kornegay, president of the Tobacco Institute, also commented on Hughes's response to the press releases:

> Dr. Hughes' views are sound and, hopefully, they will be persuasive with Gori to be more careful in drafting news releases which purport to report on scientific work. {1404.01}

Spears's comment to Gori (December 18, 1975) states:

> I am surprised and disappointed by the dramatic nature of the language, over-interpretation of the data and what I consider to be false statements. . . .
> The press materials state that newly developed techniques and scientific evidence indicate that 'without question less hazardous cigarettes can be made today.' Less hazardous with respect to what? . . .
> Another statement asserts that 'people are unable or unwilling to quit.' I am unaware of any information that suggests people are unable to quit smoking [emphasis in original]. {1404.07, pp. 1–2}

Spears also says, "Based upon our recent telephone conversation, I understand that it is unlikely that there will be a press release from NCI along the lines of the material which you previously forwarded" {1404.06}.

After this press release incident, Pepples urged (in a January 19, 1976, memo) Dr. Hughes to keep his distance from the TWG.

> I recommend you decline the proffered appointment [to formally join the TWG] and ask to continue in your present capacity—auditing, but not voting, present but not participating. {1405.01}

In October 1976 the TWG's safe cigarette project did make the press. An October 29 article in the *Louisville Courier-Journal* reported on a speech made by Gio Gori at the National Academy of Sciences in which he talked about safe cigarettes and the numbers of cigarettes that could be smoked without causing cancer (i.e., safe smoking standards) {1408.02}. A letter from Pepples to H. A. Morini of BAT comments on the *Courier-Journal* article and expresses the tobacco industry's concern about the safe cigarette project:

> It must be kept in mind, however, that Gori is a man who claims to be building a better mousetrap with Government funds. Accordingly, he must continue pointing out that the mice are a hazard. . . . The issue would seem now to be whether "safer" smokes should be legislative or the free market system should be permitted to operate. {1408.01, pp. 1–2}

An attached written statement made by Gori, entitled "Etiology and Prevention of Smoking Related Disease," outlines the rationale for his safe cigarette program:

> It is unrealistic to expect a society of nonsmokers in a short time period. . . . Tobacco use cannot be abolished easily; therefore, alternative solutions for disease prevention are necessary. Two such solutions are the selective removal of toxic elements from smoke and the reduction of total smoke

intake. . . . The technology required to reduce hazardous components in cigarette smoke has been established, . . . the tobacco industry is beginning to
utilize these procedures. Consumer acceptability of low hazard cigarettes can
lead to intake limits that could make the resulting risk of disease virtually un-
detectable. These limits are defined as the smoke intake dose that would result in approximately the same disease risk for a smoker as for a nonsmoker.
{1408.05, p. 1}

Gori later sent a paper entitled "Less Hazardous Cigarettes[:] Current Manufacturing Advances, 1977," written by Gori and Cornelius
Lynch of Enviro Control, Inc., to the tobacco industry for comment
{1408.08}. (Enviro Control was the main contractor with NCI for the
safe cigarette project {1403.01}.) The paper describes how cigarettes
have been made less hazardous, compares them by brand name, and recommends brand switching to achieve "critical values" of smoking, below which smoking is safe:

These critical values may serve as intermediate goals for a smoker who is intent on reducing his smoking habit through progressively less hazardous
smoking stages.

       . . .

    The incorporation of these and other state-of-the-art advances, coupled
with flavor acceptability characteristics, has resulted in commercially
available cigarettes that can properly be termed less hazardous. {1408.08,
p. 6}

In other words, Gori was recommending that smokers switch to low-tar
brands in lieu of recommending that they quit.

On August 22, 1977, in a letter to Gori, I. W. Hughes commented on
this paper.

The purpose, then, of your supplying the draft to me and of my commenting
on it is not to rehash our differences in the smoking and health area, but
merely to see whether, given these differences, a paper of the kind you propose would serve to advance the scientific debate.

    For the reasons listed below, I feel that it would not:

    1.   As scientists, we have to be careful to avoid having the fruits of our
labor used in an unwarranted manner by the public or by various pressure groups whatever their persuasion. . . . I cannot help but believe that
the tables in your paper, especially since they list brand names, will be mis-
applied to the detriment of both sides of the smoking issue.

    2.   It is the nature of man to seek simplistic solutions to complex prob-
lems. . . . It is inevitable that the pulp press will, unfortunately, continue
to oversimplify and distort scientific data, drawing conclusions where only
caution and more study is warranted. In my opinion, your paper—con-

taining as it does, specific brand names—will be used to suggest a standard which is both misleading and dangerous.

3. . . .Table I lists average yields [of low tar and nicotine brands] over a twelve-year period on a <u>sales-weighted</u> basis. Surely, this is being unfair to the industry. It reflects smoker predilections rather than the industry's admittedly substantial effort in this area. . . .

4. Brown & Williamson, for its part (and I believe this is true of the other companies in the industry)[,] has deliberately stayed away from enticing non-smokers to smoke while the controversy over possible health implications rages. Could not your paper, as presently written, have the unintended and unwarranted effect of encouraging non-smokers to take up the custom [emphasis in original]? {1412.01, pp. 1–2}

It is ironic that a tobacco industry employee was worried about encouraging smoking. The main thrust of Hughes's letter, however, indicates that he was worried about the tobacco companies' using Gori's data to get into marketing wars for low-tar cigarettes.

The TWG was officially terminated on August 12, 1977 {1411.01}. However, The TWG continued to meet "unofficially" {1411.03}. The tobacco companies may now have been eager to continue their participation in the TWG so that they could remain informed about the development of less hazardous cigarettes. Such information would help the companies gain a competitive edge in the low-tar cigarette market.

In mid-1978 Lisher and Company, a marketing management consultant, submitted a draft proposal for a "low delivery project" to B&W {1203.01}, in line with emerging recommendations from the NCI under Gori. This proposal illustrates that the tobacco industry viewed Gori's work as useful for marketing purposes but was concerned about calling cigarettes "safe." The editing of this draft with regard to nicotine was discussed in chapter 3. The draft's statements on smoking and health issues were also edited. The following sentence was in the original draft:

The parameters of a "safe" cigarette have been defined by Dr. Gori of the Federal Government, although his definition of "safe" is believed to be as yet largely unrecognized by the medical community at large. {1203.01, p. 1}

The edited version reads:

Within the past several years, Dr. Gogio Gori of the National Institute[s] of Health has discussed guidelines for the potential reduction of selective cigarette smoke components. {1203.02, insert card}

The word "safe" was systematically excised at three other places {1203.01, pp. 2, 3, 4}:

The phrase "Dr. Gori's (and other Government Agencies') parameters of safety" is edited to delete the last two words.

The phrase "low tar/safe" is changed to "low tar."

The phrase "a safe and satisfying cigarette" is changed to "a Gori-type, satisfying cigarette."

Gori's support for the concept of a "safe" cigarette and a "safe" level of smoking became increasingly controversial. Gori left NCI in 1980 and became director of the Franklin Institute's Health Policy Center {1415.01}. Since 1980 Gori has been a paid consultant to the tobacco industry and testifies on the industry's behalf on issues related to smoking and health (17).

TOBACCO SUBSTITUTES

In the late 1960s and early 1970s, many in the cigarette industry thought that the use of tobacco substitutes in cigarette blends would substantially reduce the toxicity of cigarettes. Consequently, various possible substitutes were tested for tobacco-like qualities on the one hand and for reduced toxicity—especially for reduced activity in mouse skin–painting experiments—on the other. Products containing tobacco substitutes were briefly marketed in Germany and in the UK, but they did not become established in either market.

Tobacco substitutes posed special problems for American cigarette companies because of the legal environment in the United States. Putting nontobacco material into the blend as a tobacco substitute would likely have raised a variety of awkward questions in the United States. To the extent that the substitute material replaced tobacco in a cigarette, the product would be less a tobacco product and more a drug, an article intended to prevent disease. This substitution, in turn, would have raised the risk of FDA scrutiny and would have drawn the attention of attorneys specializing in products liability matters.

On October 22, 1973, William Shinn of Shook, Hardy & Bacon sent the general counsel of B&W, DeBaun Bryant, a copy of a June 2, 1973, editorial from *Lancet*, a British medical journal {1124.05}, concerning a tobacco substitute that had been developed {1124.04}. The editorial described New Smoking Material (NSM), a product developed in Britain by Imperial Tobacco Ltd. (ITL) and Imperial Chemical Industries, Ltd. (ICI), as a less toxic, wood pulp–based, tobacco substitute for cigarettes.

ITL research, as reported in this editorial, had shown that NSM "is less irritant to animal tissues and less carcinogenic for the skin of mice." ITL and ICI were building a factory to manufacture NSM, and the editorial writer speculated that if a government committee found NSM less hazardous than tobacco, the material might one day entirely replace tobacco in cigarettes. While the editorial recognized the importance of nicotine for the appeal of smoking, it did not point out the necessity of adding nicotine to an all-NSM cigarette.

Shinn may have sent Bryant the editorial in anticipation of a meeting between Ed Finch, B&W's CEO, and Malcolm Anson, ITL's CEO, in Louisville in the first week of November. Anson also met with the general counsel for B&W and the company's director of research. Following his return to Bristol, Anson wrote Finch a letter commenting on the concerns expressed by the B&W executives about substitute smoking materials.

> You and your colleagues gave me some fairly unmistakeable messages on the subject of substitute smoking materials, and on the more general political and scientific aspects of the smoking and health question. This did not entirely surprise me because I know that American manufacturers approach this matter from a different legal and philosophical background, but it was very helpful to me to be exposed to the arguments at first hand, and I now have a much more vivid picture of the considerations which are upper most in your minds when these issues are raised. This is extremely helpful and I very much hope that we shall continue this kind of dialogue at regular intervals.
>
> I particularly noted the reservations which you expressed concerning the National Cancer Institute [NCI]. I entirely understand your desire for us to be discreet but equally as I explained we shall not wish to forego making what capital we can out of any pronouncements which NCI may produce. {1124.01, pp. 1–2}

While ITL and its competitors did not put cigarettes containing tobacco substitutes on the market until 1977 (awaiting an official blessing of the British government through its Hunter Commission), Courtaulds, a small domestic British tobacco company, jumped the gun by test-marketing a brand called Planet in November 1973. The launch was greeted with substantial criticism in the press questioning whether Planet was "safer" and asking "safer than what?" {1124.03}. The criticism illuminated the potential difficulties that would confront the industry in trying to introduce a "safer" cigarette. The industry's interest is documented in a packet of press clippings {1124.03} that G. C. Hargrove of BAT's Millbank office sent to the CEOs of BAT subsidiaries around the world on November 8, two days after the introduction of Planet {1124.02}.

The BAT R&D conference at Duck Key, Florida, two months later (January 1974) shed additional light on the thinking within the company about tobacco substitutes. The first conclusions of the conference involved the substitutes.

1.   The decision that B-A.T. would not use non-tobacco materials without a demonstrable advantage on health grounds has proved particularly effective in influencing Amcel [the maker of a tobacco substitute] developments— and since I.T.L. at that time concurred, probably in influencing the development of N.S.M. The interpretation by R. & D. of "demonstrable advantage" was a reduction in specific activity for smoke or condensate by most or all relevant biological tests available. It is now recognised that the development of the non-tobacco materials and their possible "acceptance" by medical authorities may change the position. Also the non-tobacco materials may become commercially very attractive on supply and price grounds.

It is therefore now proposed that, although reduction in specific activity across the board would be most attractive and reduction in specific activity on key tests desirable, in the absence of significant behavioural differences, reduction in activity per cigarette (in all relevant tests) should now be accepted as sufficient for alternative smoking materials, both tobacco and non-tobacco.

2.   New smoking materials now under development include N.S.M., Cytrel, N.C.F. (Batflake and B. & W. version), Ecusta, Sutton Research, Reemtsma (BASF), Gallahers, Rothmans, Brinkmann and Courtaulds. No information is available on Reynolds and Philip Morris in this field. The front runners are N.S.M., Cytrel, Courtaulds, with Batflake having advantages for taste and cost. Since Courtaulds material is being tested biologically, they appear to have failed so far to make a good cigarette and yet could be on big scale production before any others; B-A.T. should talk to Courtaulds if this can be arranged . . .

3.   American Celanese have informed us that the proposed short tests by the Hunter Committee are sebaceous gland, hyperplasia, rat trachea, lung cell activity, macrophage, ciliastasis, mytochondria, mutagenicity, teratology and Goblet cell. Long term tests are mouse skin, rat inhalation, and possibly dog inhalation. It will be interesting (possibly alarming) if this list proves correct when Hunter outlines his proposals to the U.K. industry for the first time on February 8th.

Estimated cost to cover [test and bring to market?] four Cytrel 324 and 361 variants is over $1 million p.a. [per annum] for 5 years. {1125.01, pp. 1–2}

In early 1974, then, tobacco substitutes played a substantial role in BAT's R&D effort, and there was at least some sharing of information among a variety of companies outside of the United States. Reduced toxicity, as measured in a variety of short- and long-term tests, was the goal. While the UK government–sponsored Hunter Committee might insist on a large battery of tests, at the least, BAT agreed with the principle that the value of a tobacco substitute was primarily its lower toxicity in such tests in comparison to tobacco itself.

A glimpse at BAT's internal R&D effort for its own version of a tobacco substitute, Batflake, is contained in the summary of a Southampton research report {1127.01}. The document, dated July 2, 1975, relates preliminary results of inhalation toxicology testing of cigarettes containing various proportions of Batflake Mark II compared to British-style cigarettes containing 100 percent flue-cured tobacco.

> The study reported here involved preliminary range finding work to fix exposure conditions, a dosimetry experiment, measurements of respiratory function of animals and an extensive pathological examination, particularly of the respiratory system. {1127.01, p. 1}

The report indicates that the exposure system actually delivered cigarette smoke to "all parts of the respiratory system" of the rats and was similar for all the experimental cigarettes. Nasal filtration, often considered an obstacle in rodent experiments, "did not occur to a very significant extent" {1127.01, p. 1}. Carbon monoxide levels were similar in all groups. Smoke exposure led to reduced body weight and to an increase in the weight of heart, lung, and trachea. Lung and trachea weight increase was inversely related to the proportion of Batflake in the cigarette; Batflake also provided some protection against increases in heart weight.

> Most rats survived to termination and the inhaled smoke caused:
> 1. Squamous metaplasia in the larynx.
> 2. Hyperplasia and keratinisation in the larynx.
> 3. Goblet cell hyperplasia in the bronchi.
> 4. Goblet cell hyperplasia in the nasal cavity.
> 5. Increased macrophage activity in the lung. {1127.01, p. 2}

The presence of Batflake in the cigarette reduced the degree of effects 2, 3, and 5 in proportion to the amount of Batflake added. However, squamous metaplasia of the larynx was seen in every rat exposed to smoke, regardless of the proportion of Batflake in the cigarettes. So, by mid-1975 BAT had evidence from its own laboratory that cigarettes made with Batflake as part of the blend were less toxic than conventional cigarettes.

The Hunter Committee, chaired by Professor (later Lord) Robert Hunter, advised the Secretary of State in the United Kingdom on tobacco issues. In particular, its focus was on tobacco product testing and on research on less hazardous smoking. In 1975 the committee gave tobacco substitutes a lukewarm, preliminary endorsement:

The product may be no more dangerous to health than a similar product containing tobacco only and could prove to be less injurious. (18, pp. 95–96)

In July 1977 Imperial, Gallahers, and Rothmans (other competing British tobacco companies) launched a dozen versions of cigarettes made with tobacco substitutes, either NSM or Cytrel. Health groups and the Minister for Health criticized these products as unsafe because they still delivered substantial doses of toxins. Their sales were minuscule—in part because the public health community criticized them as unproven half measures—and they were withdrawn within a few months (18).

So, in the end, the concerns at B&W about the risks posed by tobacco substitutes were much ado about nothing. However, the episode illustrates the company's fear that steps taken publicly to make cigarettes safer would expose the harmfulness of the basic product and therefore constituted a great risk. The tobacco substitute story also illustrates the fact that the essential ingredient in tobacco products is not tobacco: It is nicotine.

ABANDONING THE SEARCH

By the late 1970s the tobacco industry had all but abandoned its search for a "safe" cigarette. The industry's scientists had found it much more difficult than at first anticipated to identify and remove the toxic elements from cigarettes. Perhaps more important, however, tobacco industry lawyers were becoming increasingly concerned about government regulation and litigation.

SEA ISLAND RESEARCH CONFERENCE, 1980

BAT's 1980 research conference was held in Sea Island, Georgia. The documents contain a list of proposed topics for the meeting, along with the comments of Dr. R. A. Sanford, then vice president of research and development at B&W {1132.01}. Sanford rated the various topics on a scale of 1 to 3 (1 = top priority; 2 = definite interest; 3 = little or no interest). He gave the lowest priority to topics such as short-term biological assays and studies of smoke irritation, topics that had dominated discussion at earlier conferences.

Dr. Sanford actually *discouraged* additional toxicological testing, as his comment on short-term bioassays indicates:

We need evaluation of *externally* developed methods for critique. We don't want GR&DC [that is, BAT itself] to develop methods [emphasis added]. {1132.01, table}

He has this to say about irritation and inhalation of smoke:

Dangerous area. Please do not publish or circulate. *No more work needed on biological side* [emphasis added]. {1132.01, table}

The initial enthusiasm for toxicology work to refine and perfect the product had been abandoned. In contrast, the areas ranked as top priority included the topics nicotine, basic combustion research, sidestream research, flavor research, and ventilated cigarette technology.

Sanford's choice of priorities suggests that by the early 1980s the tobacco industry had dramatically changed its focus: instead of trying to understand and eliminate the carcinogens and other toxins in tobacco smoke, it was now trying to avoid developing any potentially damaging knowledge of its products. Short-term bioassays remained of interest, but only if they were developed extramurally, possibly because of concern about the potential for discovery through litigation. By 1980 the R&D staff at B&W had seemingly come to regard continued research on the inhalation toxicology of tobacco smoke as potentially hazardous to the company.

RESPONDING TO THE MARKET, 1985

The deemphasis of reduced toxicity as a primary factor shaping cigarette design at B&W is illustrated in an April 1985 letter from E. E. Kohnhorst, manager of the B&W Development Center {1136.01}. He wrote J. A. B. Kellagher of BAT (Millbank) in response to correspondence that Kellagher had sent to B&W about carbon monoxide reduction technology. The letter praises work that Kellagher had shared with B&W about a project that correlated "the more difficult sensory attributes to the smoke deliveries," a project that would be relevant "for cigarette designs in parts of the world where carbon monoxide (CO) delivery in cigarettes is under pressure of statutory regulation." Carbon monoxide is a colorless, odorless poison gas that binds to blood and reduces its ability to deliver oxygen to the body; the carbon monoxide in tobacco smoke is one element that damages the cardiovascular system.

Kohnhorst notes that there was no such pressure to lower CO deliveries of cigarettes in the United States, even though by the late 1970s the

Federal Trade Commission's "tar" tables included a listing for CO. As Kohnhorst points out, "the CO delivery of Marlboro KS [king size] in 1979 was 15.5 mg/cig. and today it runs on an average 15.2 mg/cig." Consequently, Kohnhorst explains,

> Within B&W, we have rarely attempted to develop new products specifically designed to deliver low CO, except perhaps a prototype of FACT that was kept ready on a turn-key basis in the event of a marketing need for such product. This was done through a combination of filter ventilation, cigarette paper permeability, and appropriate cigarette paper additive. Needless to say, such need did not arise. {1136.01, p. 1}

Although the addition of shredded dried stems (SDS) to B&W's tobacco blends in the fourth quarter of 1985 would incidentally lower CO yield by 10 percent with a 12 percent level of stem addition, the reduction in CO yield was not the company's primary purpose in using the additive:

> Its benefit is process simplification, increased yield, reduced manufacturing cost, improved cigarette physical properties, and results in reduced CO generation.
>
> . . .
>
> Beyond these plans, the emphasis at B&W is on product amelioration. The major part of our resources is devoted to understanding what contributes to the harshness of cigarette smoke. Improvement of our products to achieve superiority over competitive products is a more pressing need. Therefore, *I do not see involving ourselves in designing products with the limited objective of reducing CO in the near future unless marketing needs dictate otherwise* [emphasis added]. {1136.01, p. 2}

Kohnhorst is blunt in telling Kellagher that B&W has more pressing things to worry about in product design than reducing a toxic constituent—beating the competition on mildness. This attitude markedly differed from that taken by BAT scientists in the 1960s, when they were trying so hard to reduce the "biological activity" of cigarettes.

CONCLUSION

In 1957 the BAT research department used code words like "Zephyr" for lung cancer and for the carcinogens thought responsible for lung cancer. At the 1962 Southampton research conference, there had been an enormous display of optimism and hope about the possible development of a safe cigarette. Sir Charles Ellis declared that, if cigarettes actually cause cancer, industry scientists would find a way to fix the problem.

Throughout the 1960s reports of industry-sponsored R&D activities brimmed with energy and enthusiasm for getting on with solving the problem. The problem proved intractable, however. Certainly, it is a technically difficult problem to solve. In addition, any genuine solution contained an inescapable admission of harm from conventional products. By 1973 B&W was unwilling to participate even a little bit in work on tobacco substitutes. By 1980 an R&D scientist at B&W regarded work on tobacco smoke inhalation as "dangerous." In 1985 a B&W executive declared that the only product innovations of interest were those that gave a competitive advantage. If, by chance, they also reduced toxicity, that was a bonus, but it was not a reason to make the change.

While the internal R&D work shifted over the years from a gallant acceptance of the challenge to a cynical acceptance of an inevitably harmful product, the external posture of the company remained defiant. Publicly, the smoking and health question remained an open one, a controversy. Privately, the controversy was not whether Viceroy, Kool, Raleigh, and Belair are dangerous. The controversy was over what to do about the danger. For many years the companies tried, privately and quietly, to make things better. As it became evident that a safe cigarette was not achievable, the industry turned to creating a false controversy about the scientific evidence that smoking is dangerous.

REFERENCES

1. Fischer S, Spiegelhalder B, Preussmann R. Tobacco-specific nitrosamines in commercial cigarettes: Possibilities for reducing exposure. In: O'Neill I, Chen J, Bartsch H, eds. *Relevance to Human Cancer of N-Nitroso Compounds, Tobacco Smoke and Mycotoxins* (pp. 489–492). Lyon: International Agency for Research on Cancer, 1991.

2. Slade J. The tobacco epidemic: Lessons from history. *J Psychoactive Drugs* 1989;21:281–291.

3. Wynder E. *Testimony before the Subcommittee of Legal and Monetary Affairs*. Committee on Government Operations, US House of Representatives, 1957.

4. Blacklock J. An experimental study of the pathological effects of cigarette condensate in the lungs with special reference to carcinogenesis. *Brit J Cancer* 1961;15:745–762.

5. Wynder E, Graham E, Croninger A. Experimental production of carcinoma with cigarette tar. *Cancer Res* 1953;13:855–864.

6. Wynder E, Hoffman D. *Tobacco and Tobacco Smoke*. New York: Academic Press, 1967.

7. USDHHS. *Reducing the Health Consequences of Smoking: 25 Years of Progress*. US Department of Health and Human Services, Public Health Service, Centers for Disease Control, Center for Chronic Disease Prevention and Health Promotion, Office on Smoking and Health, 1989. DHHS Publication No. (CDC) 89-8411.

8. P. Lorillard announces a new cigaret filter; keeps goals a secret. *Wall Street Journal* 1962 May 23:7;2.

9. Lorillard's new filter said to stem from test on phenols' ill effects. Firm says filter enables cilia to expel, unimpeded, particles from frogs' breathing canals. *Wall Street Journal* 1962 May 28:16;2.

10. Wynder E, Hoffman D. A study of tobacco carcinogenesis: VIII. The role of the acidic fractions as promoters. *Cancer* 1961;14:1306–1315.

11. Miller L, Monahan J. Facts we're not told about filter-tips. *Reader's Digest* 1961 July:71–78.

12. Fisher RA. Dangers of cigarette smoking. *Brit Med J* 1957;2:297–298.

13. Thornton R. Smoking articles. US Patent No. 3,614,956. Assigned to Brown and Williamson Tobacco Corp., 1971.

14. Federal Trade Commission. *Findings as to the Facts and Conclusions. In the Matter of P. Lorillard Company, a Corporation.* Federal Trade Commission, 1958. Docket No. 4922.

15. Hoffmann D, Lavoie E, Hecht S. Nicotine: A precursor for carcinogens. *Cancer Letters* 1985;26:67–75.

16. Litzinger E. Tobacco smoke filter material. U.S. Patent 3,828,800. Assigned to Brown and Williamson Tobacco Corp., 1974.

17. Otolski G. Cigarette firms find unlikely ally in adversary. *Louisville Courier-Journal* 1994 August 10:A6, A10.

18. Taylor P. *The Smoke Ring: Tobacco, Money, and Multi-national Politics.* New York: Pantheon Books, 1984.

CHAPTER 5

Public Relations in the "Safe" Cigarette Era

Doubt is our product since it is the best means of competing
with the "body of fact" that exists in the mind of the general
public. It is also the means of establishing a controversy. . . .
If we are successful in establishing a controversy at the public
level, then there is an opportunity to put across the real facts
about smoking and health. Doubt is also the limit of our
"product." Unfortunately, we cannot take a position directly
opposing the anti-cigarette forces and say that cigarettes are a
contributor to good health. No information that we have
supports such a claim.

"Smoking and Health Proposal," B&W, 1969?
{2111.01, pp. 4–5}

INTRODUCTION

During the 1950s and 1960s B&W and BAT came to realize that cigarettes cause cancer and other diseases and quietly researched how to
make a cigarette that would deliver nicotine without the carcinogens
and other dangerous chemicals in tobacco smoke. At the same time,
they worked to counter growing awareness of the dangers of smoking among members of the scientific and medical community as well
as the general public, often hiding the tobacco industry's true role in
these efforts.

GETTING OUT THE "FACTS"

The documents include what appears to be a fragment from a 1967
employee handbook on how to answer questions about the company's products. A section titled "Smoking and Health" consists of a
brief introduction by B&W's president, Ed P. Finch {1801.02}. Finch
tells his readers:

Keeping accurately informed on the smoking and health controversy is an increasing problem. Many assertions are being made which tend to condemn smoking and the tobacco industry. Headlines carry these assertions as "news." Unfortunately, the other side is sometimes overlooked.

And there is another side to the controversy! The following section states and gives factual replies to 10 of the most common assertions. From these, I hope you will gain a better insight into our position as a part of a viable and responsible industry. I also hope you will add your voice in support of the soundness of our cause. {1801.02}

Six of the ten assertions are available in the documents {1801.03}. In each case the assertion has been chosen and crafted to permit a plausible-sounding rejoinder. By dealing only with peripheral issues, the response to the assertion avoids confronting the real scientific information known at the time about the relationship between cigarettes and disease. For example,

ASSERTION: "People who smoke are select prospects for cancer and other diseases."

FACT: People who do not smoke suffer from all the diseases that have been selectively linked with smoking. Ten to 20 per cent of lung cancer, for instance, occurs in non-smokers. {1801.03, p. 1}

This "fact," although true, sidesteps the uncomfortable truth that people who smoke are more than ten to twenty times more likely to get lung cancer than people who do not smoke. It is grossly misleading in its selection of information.

Another example deals with the attributable risk of death from cigarettes.

ASSERTION: "300,000 adult smokers die prematurely each year because of cigarette smoking."

FACT: No one can accurately make that statement, because there is no valid supporting evidence. The Assistant Surgeon General, when the 1964 Surgeon General's Report was issued, said the Report "Might be as misleading as it was informative" to try to calculate "the total number of excess deaths causally related to cigarette smoking in the U.S. population." In other words, the Advisory Committee acknowledged that any such excess deaths could not be "accurately estimated." {1801.03, p. 2}

Again, the "fact" sidesteps the real issue. The Advisory Committee concluded that a substantial number of smokers were dying prematurely each year. Instead of responding to that fact, the response quibbles about whether a precise body count can be calculated. The tobacco industry still relies on this technique. James Johnston, CEO of the R. J. Reynolds Tobacco Company, in his testimony to Congress in April 1994, claimed that there is no list of dead people that adds up to the number of people who allegedly died because of cigarettes (1).

Some of the "assertions" were simply set up to invite an important-sounding rejoinder.

ASSERTION: "All doctors are convinced that smoking is dangerous."

FACT: Doctors are by no means unanimous in condemning smoking. There are many who have expressed publicly their unwillingness to accept statistical evidence as scientific proof of a causal relationship between cigarette smoking and human disease. For example, some of the country's most eminent men of medicine and science—from such renowned institutions as Bellevue Hospital, Columbia University Medical School, Yale University Medical School, and New York Medical College—have testified before the U.S. Congress that the charges against tobacco remain unproved. {1801.03, p. 2}

As described in chapter 8, many of the "eminent scientists" so often quoted by the tobacco industry were on the industry payroll, often without public disclosures of this fact. The scientists not only received support for research but also were paid to provide testimony favorable to the industry, to perpetuate controversy about the health effects of smoking and, more recently, passive smoking.

SELLING DOUBT

Following publication in 1964 of the first Surgeon General's report, *Smoking and Health* (2), concern over tobacco skyrocketed among the public and government policy makers, particularly at the Federal Trade Commission (FTC), which has the authority to regulate cigarette advertising. After an initial period of uncertainty around the release of the Surgeon General's report (see the "Grave Crisis" section in chapter 2), the tobacco industry started an aggressive campaign to create controversy about the scientific evidence that smoking is dangerous and to defend the "right" to smoke. While some of these efforts were overt, many of them were covert, with the industry operating quietly through public relations firms to secure publication of articles from seemingly neutral sources that supported the tobacco industry's position. The documents illuminate four of these efforts.

YOU MAY SMOKE

In 1966 a book titled *You May Smoke*, which questioned the health dangers of smoking, was published in England. Although the author, C. Harcourt Kitchin, wrote this book on his own, the British cigarette company Carreras Tobacco bought seven thousand copies. Tiderock Corporation, a public relations firm working for B&W, approached Kitchin to publish an American version that would debunk the 1964 US Surgeon General's report, with research assistance from American tobacco companies {2101.02}. On August 16, 1967, Kitchin wrote to Rosser Reeves of the Tiderock Corporation outlining what he could do.

> I have given a little thought to that [writing an American edition of *You May Smoke*]. The book is obviously written first for British consumption, though with the idea in mind that it might find an American publisher. *To try and disguise it as an American book* would, I am sure, fail. We can, however, introduce material, and make changes, to make it more acceptable, and less "foreign", to the American reader. Although the Surgeon General's report is fuller, and far more technical, than the report of the Royal College of Physicians, it contained no new research and no conclusions that had not already been drawn.
>
> What I think I can do, if I can find the necessary material, is to put more emphasis on arguing against the Surgeon General's report than, at present, against the British one, and to base the arguments upon American, rather than British statistics and research. If the book is to be republished anyhow, I think it will be more convincing to make these changes through the body of the script than, as you first suggested, to write additional chapters.
>
> With this in mind I have listed and attached a few first thoughts on the sort of additional information I shall need, much of which I think is not available in this country. *It may be that I could get some of it from my friendly tobacco manufacturers or from the Tobacco Research Council, but I hesitate to invite questions on why I want it* [emphasis added]. {2101.03, pp. 1–2}

Kitchin published the US edition of *You May Smoke* (3). In the prologue to the book, Kitchin explains why he wrote it. As a moderate smoker, he had been disturbed by the early reports that smoking could cause lung cancer. When the Royal College of Physicians released its first report on smoking and health in 1962 (discussed in chapter 2), however, he began to sense "a slight scent of propaganda." His own book, Kitchin states, "seeks neither to encourage smoking nor to debunk the reports. It is an attempt to look at the evidence through the eyes of an ordinary member of the general public who neither rejects the possibility that smoking may contribute to lung cancer nor is blinded by propaganda or fear" (3, p. xi).

At the end of the book, Kitchin concludes that more research is needed to prove that smoking is truly harmful to health; in the interim, he suggests, smoking in moderation probably is not too bad.

> May you smoke? The answer is for you and for you only. . . . If you enjoy your smoking, as opposed to the chain smoker who is seldom conscious of having lit the cigarette that is staining his fingers, you may decide that the answer lies in moderation. If you examine the statistics carefully you will find little condemnation of that. (3, p. 176)

Scientific studies have shown, however, that Kitchin's theory regarding moderation was wrong. The more you smoke, the more likely you are to develop diseases such as lung cancer and heart disease. Even if you smoke only moderately, your risk is still elevated above normal.

Nowhere did Kitchin mention that he had been aided by the tobacco industry to write *You May Smoke* for a US audience, or that some of the information quoted was provided by tobacco industry representatives.

BARRON'S EDITORIAL

Following publication of the Surgeon General's report in 1964, several states and the Federal Trade Commission began to move to require warnings on cigarette packages and, possibly, on cigarette advertisements. There was also talk of severely restricting or even ending cigarette advertising (4). The tobacco industry aggressively fought advertising restrictions, both at a public relations level and at a political level in Congress. In 1965, however, Congress passed the federal Cigarette Labeling and Advertising Act, which first required warning labels to be placed on cigarette packages, but preempted the states from taking any action of their own in this area. It contained an automatic review after three years. Although the tobacco industry quietly acceded to the Congressionally mandated placing of warning labels on cigarette packages, which it preferred to regulation by the Federal Trade Commission, because such labels offered protection from products liability lawsuits, it aggressively fought other parts of the legislation and mounted a strong public relations campaign against the regulation of its products generally.

For example, on October 18, 1967, the industry made use of one of its public relations tools when it ran newspaper ads, prepared by Tiderock, featuring a reprint of a front-page editorial from *Barron's* (figure 5.1). The editorial, as reprinted in the advertisements, criticizes the 1964 Surgeon General's report, *Smoking and Health*, and attacks government efforts to control tobacco.

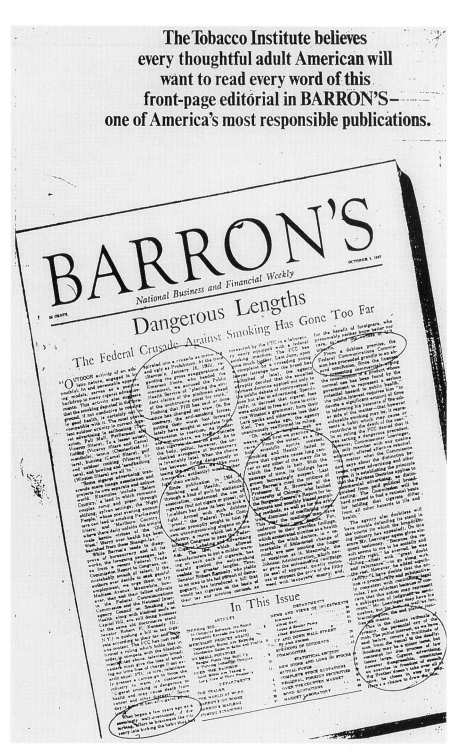

Figure 5.1. Advertisement run by the Tobacco Institute in 1967 based on *Barron's* editorial atacking government actions to control tobacco.

What began a few years ago as a seemingly well-intentioned, if disturbing, effort to brainwash the citizenry into kicking the habit thus has spiraled into a crusade as menacing and ugly as Prohibition. At the time (*Barron's,*— January 18, 1965), regarding the gross exaggerations of Emerson Foote [a former advertising executive], who headed the movement, we accused the Public Health Service of "placing the strident claims of the pitchman ahead of the unobtrusive quest for truth." Nothing that PHS has said or done since has changed our view. On the contrary, the anti-smoking forces, putting their worst foot forward, lately have sought to escalate from persuasion to coercion. As inveterate non-smokers, we freely concede that cigarets do one no good. As to the body politic, however, the unchecked arrogance of bureaucracy is invariably fatal. When the choice lies between living dangerously or toeing the party line, we (like most Americans, evidently) would rather fight than switch. [The phrase "rather fight than switch" was later popularized in a cigarette advertisement.]

Since publication in 1964 of "Smoking and Health," which through a kind of guilt by statistical association, condemned the use of cigarets (but not cigars or pipes), officialdom has done its best to pick a fight. Armed with such dubious "proof," the Federal Trade Commission promptly sought to foist its own uncompromising slogans on the industry, a move which led a more tolerant Congress to pass the Federal Cigaret Labeling and Advertising Act.

. . .

"Oh what a tangled web we weave when first we practice to deceive." From the outset, as a few bold scientific spirits insisted, "Smoking and Health" failed to prove that cigarets cause lung cancer or any other of the many ills to which the flesh is heir. With the passage of time, its findings have grown increasingly suspect. *Last year* Barron's *cited the critique of Professor K. A. Brownlee of the University of Chicago, who faulted the Surgeon-General's Report for inadequate and possibly biased sampling methods, as well as for the arbitrary dismissal of conflicting views.* This year the medicine men have undercut their own dogma. For, contrary to their previous findings, which exonerated nicotine as a health hazard, the witch doctors, in a remarkable if little-noted change of mind, are now pointing the finger of suspicion at it.

Meanwhile, the Johnson Administration, which never gave the anti-smoking campaign its seal of approval, quietly continues to support the price of the filthy weed with taxpayers' money and, for the benefit of foreigners, who presumably neither know better nor care, to extoll the virtues of U.S. tobacco.

. . .

This is the classic rationale of tyranny, the perennial cry of the mob. The public interest, as we have said before, covers a multitude of sins, from the venal to the deadly. Smoking may be a minor issue, but contempt for due process of law looms large. Cigaret advertising, however disagreeable, constitutes an exercise in freedom of speech. Big Brother doesn't take over all at once, he closes in step by step. Here's a chance to draw the line [emphasis added]. {2120.08}

Emerson Foote had been chairman of the McCann-Eriksen agency, where he had handled the Lucky Strike cigarette account, and now headed the National Interagency Council on Smoking and Health, which was pressing for anti-tobacco education, including a warning label in cigarette advertising.

In a letter dated October 26, 1967, J. W. Burgard, B&W's vice president for advertising, marketing research, and public relations, wrote to Tiderock's Rosser Reeves:

> The *Barron's* ad turned out very well. To me, perhaps the most important thing about this ad was that for the first time we have gotten the industry to take a step forward together, and it was a great opportunity to get them together. I would hesitate, however, to attach too much importance to what could be accomplished by the repeated exposure of such an ad. {2101.06, p. 1}

Reeves responded:

> I agree with you that the *Barron's* ad turned out very well. I <u>also</u> agree with you that we should not attach too much importance to what can be accomplished by the repeat exposure of one ad. One advertisement is really one raindrop in a rainstorm . . . and we need more than a rainstorm, we need a hurricane.
>
> I also agree with you that the main issue is to make widely known the facts relative to scientific research on the subject of smoking and health.
>
> Before we ran the *Barron's* ad we had Ted Bates and Company do 2,000 interviews among smokers and nonsmokers in 20 top markets. (So far as I know this is the first research that has ever been done on what the public thinks about this controversy.)
>
> The results were somewhat shocking:
>
> 1.   The public at large thinks the Government <u>should</u> assume an active role in warning people against cigarettes. Two-thirds in fact believe that the Government has not done enough.
>
> 2.   The majority are convinced cigarette smoking causes health problems.
>
> 3.   The majority believe that cigarette advertising is bad.
>
> On the other hand:
>
> 4.   The public is opposed to legal prohibition of the sale of cigarettes.
>
> 5.   The public believes that it's up to the individual to make his own decision about smoking.
>
> 6.   The public believes cigarette manufacturers are not to blame.
>
> 7.   Forty percent of the public believes the manufacturers should argue their case in public.
>
> We are giving the *True* article [discussed below] much thought. What we do with it will be woven into our complete program which we hope to present privately to the Senator [probably Earle Clements, a former Kentucky

senator with strong ties to the White House, who was president of the Tobacco Institute] within the next ten days and to all of the Tobacco Institute
within the next three weeks [emphasis in original]. {2101.07, pp. 1–2}

This interchange illustrates the thoroughness with which the tobacco industry was approaching its public relations effort. Not only did it quietly generate support, which was then represented as "independent," but
it also used this material in paid advertising.

THE *TRUE* MAGAZINE ARTICLE

The publicity regarding the dangers of smoking was accelerating in the
popular press following publication of the Surgeon General's report. In
January 1968 an article entitled "To Smoke or Not to Smoke—That Is
Still the Question," by Stanley Frank, a widely read *sports* writer, appeared in *True* magazine. Frank stated that he had reviewed the evidence
and found it contradictory and inconclusive; he concluded that "the hazards of cigarette smoking may not be so real as we have been led to believe." The tobacco industry's role in generating and disseminating this
article and other articles is summed up in the instructions to the law firm
hired to analyze the Brown and Williamson documents (see chapter 1):

> TRUE AND NATIONAL ENQUIRER ARTICLES: Documents discussing the *True* and
> *National Enquirer* articles. Joseph Field, a public relations agent for Brown
> & Williamson, arranged for Stanley Frank to write a smoking and health arti-
> cle entitled, "To Smoke Or Not To Smoke—That Is Still The Question." The
> article was published in the January 1968 issue of *True*. Tiderock, TI's [To-
> bacco Institute's] public relations agency, arranged to run an advertisement
> promoting the article. Tiderock also purchased and distributed reprints of the
> article. Stanley Frank later wrote a similar article entitled, "Cigarette Cancer
> Link is Bunk" for the *National Enquirer* under the pen name Charles Golden.
> John Blalock was one of the Brown & Williamson employees involved.
> {1001.01, p. 13}

Frank did not disclose that he worked for Hill and Knowlton, the public relations firm that created the Tobacco Industry Research Committee and the Tobacco Institute {1902.05} (see chapter 2); that he had been
paid on behalf of the tobacco industry to write the article; or that tobacco interests had reviewed the article prior to publication (4). Tiderock Corporation also played a role in creating and placing the *True* article. This information was later revealed in a series of investigations by
the *Wall Street Journal, Consumer Reports,* and US Senator Warren
Magnuson (D-WA).

The role of the tobacco industry at the highest levels in the generation and dissemination of Stanley Frank's article in *True* magazine is outlined in detail in a confidential memo dated March 28, 1967, from J. V.
Blalock, director of public relations at B&W, to Addison Yeaman, then
B&W vice president and general counsel:

> According to Joe Field, *True* Magazine has asked Stanley Frank for a formal
> outline of his projected article. This is tantamount, except in the rarest of
> cases, to a guarantee of publication.
>
> *We will receive a copy of the outline. If it is unfavorable, we can exert suf-
> ficient influence to change the "tone" before the final article. I need not em-
> phasize, however, the strategic importance of the proper guidance of Frank
> prior to the writing of the outline. We are assured by Joe that Frank has the
> desired point of view.*
>
> They both intend to talk again this week to Ed Jacob [a lawyer at Jacob
> and Medinger] in order to amplify the Roswell Park angle. Perhaps you will
> want to alert Ed to this intention. Certainly, this can be an extremely impor-
> tant part of the article.
>
> As to our financial agreement:
>
> *We will pay Frank $500.00 for his time and expenses in preparing the
> article.* This is a firm obligation whether he sells it or not.
>
> If *True* buys the article, our full obligation is satisfied. The magazine
> pays $1,750.00 for material of this type.
>
> Should *True* turn down the article, and Frank does not subsequently
> sell it to another publication, *we will pay him $1,250.00 to make up the
> difference between our guarantee of $500.00 and the anticipated maga-
> zine payment of $1,750.00* [emphasis added]. {2101.11}

Not only did Tiderock place the article with *True*, but it paid the author
and guaranteed him his fee in the event that the deal fell through with
True. The fact that this article was essentially a work for hire for the tobacco industry was not disclosed. The tobacco industry distributed
600,000 copies of the *True* magazine article with a letter from "the editors" to physicians, the media, and business and political leaders without any public acknowledgment that the tobacco industry was distributing it or that tobacco interests had a financial relationship with the
author. Not until this arrangement was exposed by the media did the
public become aware of it (4).

USING THE SAME TECHNIQUE IN THE 1990S

The tobacco industry's practice of reprinting "independent" articles and
statements that favor its position has continued into the present. The
subject matter, however, has largely shifted from active smoking to pas-

sive smoking. For example, after the Environmental Protection Agency released its 1992 report concluding that environmental tobacco smoke is a known human carcinogen that causes lung cancer in adults and respiratory problems in children, the tobacco industry reprinted articles that criticized the report (5). R. J. Reynolds ran a full-page ad in the nation's major newspapers with the headline "If We Said It, You Might Not Believe It" (figure 5.2). The ad featured an article by Jacob Sullum, at the time managing editor of *Reason* magazine, which had originally appeared in the *Wall Street Journal* and was highly critical of the EPA report. A longer article by Sullum, originally published in *Forbes Media Critic*, was featured in advertisements by Philip Morris. Philip Morris paid for four straight days of full-page ads to reprint Sullum's article in its entirety (figure 5.3).The result has been that the public has received far more exposure to criticisms of the EPA report than it has to the report itself. None of these advertisements disclosed the fact that Sullum's employer, The Reason Foundation, received a $10,000 donation from Philip Morris or that Sullum received $5,000 from R. J. Reynolds for the rights to use his writings in its advertising campaign (6–9).

Similar attacks have been directed against the federal Occupational Safety and Health Administration, for considering rules to protect non-smokers in the workplace; against the Food and Drug Administration, for considering the regulation of cigarettes as drug delivery devices; and against the prospect of higher tobacco taxes.

PUBLIC RELATIONS EFFORTS AND THE AMA

Tiderock also played a role in helping to coordinate Brown and Williamson's efforts to influence the American Medical Association's (AMA) position on smoking. Unlike most of the health community, the AMA did not actively oppose the tobacco industry in the 1960s. Instead, it generally worked with the tobacco industry, both to perpetuate the scientific "controversy" about smoking and health and to keep federal regulation to a minimum (10). On November 10, 1967, J. W. Burgard wrote Rosser Reeves:

> Enclosed is a copy of the memorandum I mentioned during our phone conversation. This is an attempt to summarize the comments made to me during the AMA meeting last week. I will not elaborate on the memorandum since I think the trend of the comments is self evident. *In view of this, I think we should give immediate attention to the possibility of running ads stating, in effect, that there is no scientific evidence of a causal relation*

Smoke & Mirrors: EPA Wages War On Cigarettes

By JACOB SULLUM

Smoking is everywhere under attack. This week a House subcommittee considered the Smoke-Free Environment Act, which would ban smoking in almost all indoor locations except residences. New York is poised to join many other cities across the country, including Los Angeles and San Francisco, that have recently enacted sweeping restrictions on smoking. In the past year, Vermont, Maryland and Washington State have also adopted smoking bans, as have major public employers including the Defence Department.

This flurry of antismoking activity is driven largely by a 1993 report from the Environmental Protection Agency that declared environmental tobacco smoke (ETS) to be "a known human lung carcinogen." Testifying in favor of the Smoke-Free Environment Act last month, EPA Administrator Carol Browner noted that "in the year since publication of the EPA report...we have seen a rapid acceleration of measures to protect non-smokers in a variety of settings."

Most supporters of such measures probably believe that the EPA report presents definitive scientific evidence that exposure to ETS causes lung cancer. But those who have taken a closer look have come to believe that the EPA twisted the evidence to arrive at a predetermined conclusion. The overriding motive was to discourage smoking by making it less acceptable and more inconvenient. Indeed, the main benefit that Ms. Browner claims for the Smoke-Free Environment Act is its expected impact on smokers.

Yet coercing people for their own good still raises a few hackles in this country, so paternalists need to offer some additional justification. That's why they've been pushing the idea that smoking endangers innocent bystanders. The problem is, the evidence for this claim is weak, inconsistent and ambiguous. The EPA's report seems designed to conceal that problem.

The agency's most blatant trick is to use an unconventional definition of statistical significance. Epidemiologists generally call an association between a risk factor and a disease "significant" if the probability that it occurred purely by chance is 5% or less. This is also the standard that the EPA had always used for risk assessment. Yet for the report on ETS, the agency abandoned the usual definition and called a result significant if the probability that it occurred by chance was 10% or less. This change in effect doubles the odds of being wrong.

Even according to the broader definition, only one of the 11 U.S. studies that the report analyzes found a statistically significant link between ETS and lung cancer (according to the usual definition, none of them did). To bolster the evidence, the EPA combined data from these 11 sources into a "meta-analysis," a technique originally intended for randomized clinical trials. UCLA epidemiologist James Enstrom says using meta-analysis with retrospective case-control studies, such as those examined by the EPA is "fraught with dangers," because the studies are apt to differ in the way they define smokers, the types of lung cancer they include and the confounding variables they consider, and so on.

In any event, the EPA's conclusion – that being married to a smoker raises a woman's chances of getting lung cancer by about 19% – is justified only according to the looser definition of statistical significance chosen especially for these data. By the conventional standard, the meta-analysis does not support the claim that ETS causes lung cancer.

Furthermore, the EPA excluded from its analysis a large U.S. study published in the November 1992 American Journal of Public

Health that did not find a statistically significant link between ETS and lung cancer. Had this study been included, the meta-analysis might not have yielded a significant result even by the relaxed standard.

Despite what a July 1992 article in Science described as "fancy statistical footwork," the EPA was able to claim only a weak association between ETS and lung cancer. With a risk increase as low as 19%, it is very difficult to rule out the possibility that the association is due to other factors. In 1991 Gary Huber, professor of medicine at the University of Texas Health Science Center, and two colleagues examined the 30 ETS studies discussed by the EPA in it's report. "At least 20 confounding variables have been identified as important to the development of lung cancer," they wrote in Consumer's Research. "No reported study comes anywhere close to controlling, or even mentioning, half of these."

Furthermore, to come up with its estimate of 3,000 additional cancer deaths a year, more than two-thirds of which are supposedly due to exposure outside the home, the EPA relied on several controversial assumptions. It assumed that cotinine, a nicotine metabolite, is a reliable measure of ETS exposure. Yet nicotine is present in a number of foods, and the report itself concedes that "cotinine is not an ideal biomarker for ETS." The EPA also assumed that lung cancer risk is directly proportional to ETS levels and that no level of ETS can be considered safe. Yet dose-response relationships vary from one substance to another, and many scientists believe that a carcinogen has to be present at a certain level before it can do any harm.

Given these and other controversies employed by the EPA, it is difficult to avoid the conclusion that policy has dictated science in the case of ETS. This approach may be politically effective in the short-term, but it is ultimately self-defeating. By compromising the standards and methods of science, the experts also undermine their claim to authority.

Mr. Sullum is managing editor of Reason magazine.

© Jacob Sullum, 1994. Mr Sullum is not associated with the tobacco industry. His opinion is his own. This was an opinion editorial published in The Wall Street Journal.

IF WE SAID IT, YOU MIGHT NOT BELIEVE IT.

Figure 5.2. R. J. Reynolds advertisement based on Jacob Sullum's article attacking the EPA report on environmental tobacco smoke.

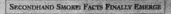

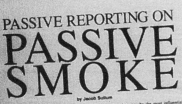

Figure 5.3. First of four full-page advertisements Philip Morris Tobacco ran reprinting Jacob Sullum's article in full during 1994.

between smoking and lung cancer. Do this in a test market, as you originally suggested, to see what the reaction of the people and the various segments of the people are to a campaign.

In considering this, *I hope you will also give some thought to an idea which intrigues us at Brown & Williamson of considering in such an ad not only the frontal attack on a causal relation but the "disclaimer" that smoking is an adult habit, or something to that effect. We feel that the combination of the two could well give the ad believability that an attack on the health relationship alone would not have.* At the same time, it would let the public know the industry does not encourage smoking among teen-agers [emphasis added].
{2101.09, p. 1}

This campaign apparently was designed to maintain the AMA's neutrality and to encourage the AMA to issue statements that could be used by the tobacco industry as part of its broader public relations campaign. It succeeded (10).

RESISTING GOVERNMENT REGULATION: ADVERTISING CAMPAIGNS

The documents describe several advertising campaigns planned by B&W and other tobacco companies in 1969 and 1970 to counter the increasing threat of government regulation. The first of these campaigns, developed by B&W, was Project Truth, which contained purely political material. Although it was aimed at the public generally, it was intended primarily to influence opinion leaders. Another campaign developed by B&W included political and health messages along with brand advertising. A third campaign, proposed by R. J. Reynolds, and intended to include the participation of all the major cigarette companies, involved the production of a series of spots to be used on prime-time network television. Still another television campaign, intended as an alternative to the R. J. Reynolds idea, was proposed by B&W's advertising agency. Although these campaigns were diverse in design, they had in common the industry's desire to go directly to the public in order to defend itself against the growing body of scientific evidence demonstrating the dangers of smoking.

PROJECT TRUTH

In late 1969, at the same time that Brown and Williamson's internal scientific staff was working to reduce the toxicity of cigarettes, its advertising agency, Post-Keyes-Gardner, was developing copy for Project Truth, highlighting themes designed to undercut the scientific evidence that smoking is dangerous. In contrast to the original "Frank Statement" advertisement in 1954, which announced the creation of TIRC and asserted a commitment to a scientific investigation of smoking, the Project Truth advertisements shifted from science to the "rights" arguments.

This advertising campaign was designed to equate any attack on the tobacco industry with an attack on freedom itself. The intent was to create a public backlash against criticism of the tobacco industry by instilling the fear that regulation of the industry would deprive smokers of their individual rights and deprive the industry of its right to operate freely in the marketplace. Rather than focusing on the reality of a powerful industry fending off the feeble attempts of an overmatched government to put some restraints on its sale of a dangerous and addictive product, the ads portrayed the industry as beleaguered and struggling to protect everyone's freedom against an overbearing government. Themes similar to the ones used in this advertising campaign continue to be used by the industry, most notably in its response to the regulation of smoking in the workplace and public places.

The excerpts quoted below are strikingly similar to much of the industry's advertising in the mid-1990s. For example, the industry continues to use hyperbolic language, such as "malicious" and "lynched," to describe government efforts to regulate tobacco use, and it continues to play on the fear that if these efforts succeed, similar efforts could be directed elsewhere. Also, the industry continues to compare proof of the health dangers of smoking with trivial matters, as a way of detracting from the seriousness of the issue. And many of the "buzzwords"—such as "scare-tactics," "freedom," "legal product," "truth," "free speech," "fair play," and "free and responsible enterprise"—are constantly used today in the industry's public relations efforts.

HEAD: Who's next?

COPY: The cigarette industry is being maliciously, systematically lynched. Who is to say it won't happen elsewhere?

As an advertising agency, we view the problem subjectively because we're proud to represent the Brown & Williamson Tobacco Corporation. Yet we view the problem objectively, because we're alarmed to witness the lynching of free speech in the marketplace and the American system of free enterprise.

Ten years ago, there was a cancer scare over the wax in milk cartons. And over using iodine to get a suntan. These theories were about as valid as the one that says toads cause warts.

And they're about as valid as today's scare-tactics surrounding cigarettes. Because <u>no one has been able to produce conclusive proof that cigarette smoking causes cancer</u>. Scientific, biological, clinical, or any other kind.

It's more than cigarettes being challenged here. It's freedom.

We will continue to bring to the American people the story of the cigarette and any other legal product based upon truth and taste.

We believe that free speech and fair play are both the heritage and promise in our society of free and responsible enterprise [emphasis in original]. {2110.01}

Twelve years before this statement was written, and five years before the Royal College of Physicians issued its first report, the eminent British statistician Sir Ronald A. Fisher, writing as a consultant to the Tobacco Manufacturers' Standing Committee in the United Kingdom, declared that the *association* between smoking and lung cancer was unequivocally proven (11). Fisher made a sharp distinction between association and causation. All that remained to be worked out, in his view, was the nature of the relationship. Do cigarettes cause lung cancer? Does lung cancer cause smoking? (Sir Ronald did not think this possible and dismissed it.) Does some third factor lead to both smoking and to lung cancer? Sir Ronald asserted that the obvious conclusion could not be reached until this last possibility had been thoroughly studied and either affirmed or negated. He proposed that genetics, one's constitution, might explain a predilection to smoking *and* to lung cancer. For the next thirty years, the tobacco industry contrived to fashion this wisp of a hypothesis, the "constitutional hypothesis," into the whole cloth of a scientific controversy (12). The effort never had much credibility, but it permitted the industry and its allies to make loud protestations about the lack of "conclusive proof." Of course, since one cannot conclusively prove a negative, there is always a way to argue in favor of the constitutional hypothesis, regardless of how much evidence piles up in favor of the conventional way of thinking. Those who want to believe that smoking does not cause cancer then have something to believe in.

This campaign was also to include a challenge to the scientific community to "prove" that scientific evidence supports the link between smoking and disease. The back cover of a proposed ten-page booklet, *The Truth,* would read:

ONE MILLION DOLLAR OFFER

For 20 years, the cigarette industry has remained silent while its product has been viciously, maliciously, unjustifiably attacked.

Despite the claims of anti-cigarette forces, no one has produced conclusive proof that cigarettes cause cancer. Biologically, scientifically, clinically or otherwise.

> We will pay one million dollars in cash to any individual, group, organization, or government source who can prove scientifically, beyond all doubt, that cigarettes cause cancer during the next 12 months.
>
> A panel of eminent physicians and scientists will be appointed by Johns Hopkins Medical School to determine the conclusiveness of any claims submitted. {2110.03}

Since it is impossible to prove anything "beyond all doubt," there was little risk that the million dollars would actually be awarded.

Two years later, in 1971, B&W put together a twenty-eight-page briefing paper for its hometown newspapers, the *Louisville Courier-Journal* and the *Louisville Times,* titled "The Smoking/Health Controversy: A View from the Other Side" {2110.06}. The arguments are demonstrably false (11, 13–15), yet they were presented as "Project Truth" to the local newspapers. The contrast between the public posture and the private policies of the company is most vividly illustrated by the statement made in Project Truth about the validity of mouse skin–painting experiments.

> Much of the experimental work involves mouse-painting or animal smoke inhalation experiments. In mouse-painting, smoke condensates are painted or dropped on the backs of mice, and cancerous skin tumors have been produced in this manner.
>
> <u>However, these condensates are artificially produced under laboratory conditions and, as such, have little, if any, relation to cigarette smoke as it reaches the smoker.</u> Further, the results obtained on the skin of mice should not be extrapolated to the lung tissue of the mouse, or to any other animal species. Certainly such skin results should not be extrapolated to the human lung [emphasis in original]. {2110.06, pp. 6–7}

As discussed in chapter 4, B&W had made cigarette product design decisions based on precisely this animal model since the mid-1960s. At the time, mouse skin painting was the standard the industry used for testing tobacco smoke condensate for carcinogenicity.

USING CIGARETTE ADS TO COUNTER HEALTH INFORMATION

In August 1969 J. W. Burgard wrote to R. A. Pittman, B&W's senior marketing supervisor, requesting that he

> undertake a special assignment of drawing up a proposed campaign, to be conducted by B&W, which would bring the industry side of the smoking and health controversy to the attention of the general public . . .
>
> It will . . . be necessary to work closely with the brand managers and the agencies to marry such a campaign with product advertising. It goes

without saying that each step of this must be thoroughly researched and you will need to call upon the Market Research Department for help in this area. {2111.02, p. 1}

This campaign was to be quite different from Project Truth, which involved straight political advertising aimed at opinion leaders. These ads were to be aimed at the general public and would attempt to associate specific cigarette brands with the message that smoking is not dangerous. The first ad, for Kool cigarettes, included a statement on "the other side of the smoking and health controversy" from a white paper {2111.02, p. 5}. Philip Morris used a similar approach in 1994 and 1995 as a way of protesting restrictions on smoking in enclosed workplaces and public places. In an advertising campaign for Benson & Hedges cigarettes, various ads depicted smokers on an airplane wing, smokers at their desks high up on the outside walls of tall office buildings, and smokers in a convertible taxi. The political message was "Smokers have to fight for indoor smoking areas."

In his memo on the proposed campaign, Burgard instructs Pittman:

I think you should approach this the same as if we were introducing a new brand on the market. You must first develop the product and sell the idea to corporate management, and after it is thoroughly researched submit a specific campaign for approval. What we are contemplating is novel, and the management of the company is going to have to be assured that it is the right thing to do. Certainly, the work done with the initial KOOL ad is an important first step, but when the findings of this research are presented you should be prepared with a recommendation as to the next steps that we should take in development and testing.

I would like to emphasize that, in my opinion, we must confine our campaign to the smoking and health issue and not be drawn into any other aspects such as the economic results, the legality, the unfairness, etc. If this campaign is effective, it will immediately draw fire, and we cannot bear to have in our ads or in our literature a single word that cannot be thoroughly documented. {2111.02, pp. 1–2}

Burgard then spells out the objectives for this campaign:

Objective No. 1: *To set aside in the minds of millions the false conviction that cigarette smoking causes lung cancer and other diseases;* a conviction based on fanatical assumptions, fallacious rumors, unsupported claims and the unscientific statements and conjectures of publicity-seeking opportunists.

Objective No. 2: *To lift the cigarette from the cancer identification as quickly as possible* and restore it to its proper place of dignity and acceptance in the minds of men and women in the marketplace of American free enterprise.

Objective No. 3: To expose the incredible, unprecedented and nefarious attack against the cigarette, constituting the greatest libel and slander ever perpetrated against any product in the history of free enterprise; a criminal libel of such major proportions and implications that one wonders how such a crusade of calumny can be reconciled under the Constitution can be so flouted and violated.

Objective No. 4: To unveil the insidious and developing pattern of attack against the American free enterprise system, a sinister formula that is slowly eroding American business with the cigarette obviously selected as one of the trial targets.

Objective No. 5: To prove that the cigarette has been brought to trial by lynch law, engineered and fostered by uninformed and irresponsible people and organizations in order to induce and incite fear.

Objective No. 6: *To establish—once and for all—that no scientific evidence has ever been produced, presented or submitted to prove conclusively that cigarette smoking causes cancer* [emphasis added]. {2111.02, pp. 3–4}

It is interesting to note how these goals, in particular "lift[ing] the cigarette from the cancer identification as quickly as possible," are completely at odds with the quest for a less dangerous cigarette, which had been a major research and development priority for years (see chapter 4). Burgard had direct line authority over research and development at B&W. Meanwhile, the company's parent, BAT (in its laboratories in England and in Germany), was working on technical approaches to reducing the toxicity of cigarettes while at the public level it, too, was pressing forward with disinformation campaigns questioning the health dangers of smoking.

The sequence numbers on the memo from Burgard to Pittman indicate that it was filed in conjunction with another document, titled "Smoking and Health Proposal," which contains the text of a presentation on "a proposal . . . for a B&W project to counter the anti-cigarette forces" {2111.01}. The proposal being discussed is the same one suggested in the Burgard memo. Although the document is undated, the context of the discussion places it around 1969, when the Burgard memo was written. The initials "JVB" (most likely those of J. V. Blalock, B&W's director of public relations) and "CM" (probably those of Corny Muije, position unknown, who is referred to in the document) appear in the margin on the first page. Evidently Blalock and Muije made a joint presentation to someone in the company. After summarizing the status of the anti-cigarette activities, the speaker notes that the anti-cigarette forces are better organized and more efficient than the tobacco industry:

I think the anti-cigarette forces can be characterized as dedicated opportunists. They are quick to act and seem to be totally unprincipled in the type of information they use to attack the industry.

The pro [tobacco] forces, on the other hand, and I'm speaking primarily of the Tobacco Institute, seem to be slow to act, mainly defensive, and rather narrow in the area of defense. The Tobacco Institute has probably done a good job for us in the area of politics and as an industry we also seem to have done very well in turning out scientific information to counter the anti-smoking claims. There is no question, though, that we have been inept in getting our side of the story, good though it may be, across to the news media and to the public. {2111.01, p. 2}

Following a discussion of the justification for the project, the speaker indicates that he views the problem as a marketing one. Thus, the project was designed to sell B&W's side of the smoking and health issue just as the company would sell a new brand of cigarettes. And, as the text of the document indicates, the project was clearly designed to confuse the general public about the scientific evidence on smoking and health.

In thinking over what we might do to improve the case for cigarettes, I have looked at the problem somewhat like the marketing of a new brand. Here is a chart where I have defined the basic marketing elements which I see in the smoking and health problem. Our consumer I have defined as the mass public, *our product as doubt, our message as truth—well stated, and our competition as the body of anti-cigarette fact that exists in the public mind* [emphasis added]. {2111.01, pp. 3, 4}

It seems rather curious that the speaker would suggest selling doubt with a message of truth, but he sheds some light on the rationale in the course of explaining why he has so defined the consumer, the product, and the message:

We have chosen the mass public as our consumer for several reasons:

This is where the misinformation about smoking and health has been focused.

The Congress and federal agencies are already being dealt with—and perhaps as effectively as possible—by the Tobacco Institute.

It is a group with little exposure to the positive side of smoking and health.

It is the prime force in influencing Congress and federal agencies—without public support little effort would be given to a crusade against cigarettes.

. . .

Doubt is our product since it is the best means of competing with the "body of fact" that exists in the mind of the general public. It is also the means of establishing a controversy. Within the business we recognize that a controversy exists. However, with the general public the consensus is that cigarettes are in some way harmful to the health. If we are successful in establishing a controversy at the public level, then there is an opportunity to put across the real facts about smoking and health. Doubt is also the limit of our "product." Unfortunately, *we cannot take a position directly opposing the anti-cigarette forces and say that cigarettes are a contributor to good health. No information that we have supports such a claim.*

Truth is our message because of its power to withstand a conflict and sustain a controversy. If in our pro-cigarette efforts we stick to <u>well documented fact</u>, we can dominate a controversy and operate with the confidence of justifiable self-interest [italic emphasis added]. {2111.01, pp. 4, 5}

Thus, this project was to be a classic example of the tobacco industry's attempts to instill in the public mind the notion that there is a controversy surrounding the scientific evidence about cigarettes and health so that further government regulation would be prevented. The speaker does not suggest that the industry has sufficient facts on its side to *refute* the evidence on the other side, nor does he believe that is necessary to accomplish B&W's main purpose. According to the speaker, B&W merely has to sell a sufficient amount of doubt about the scientific evidence to establish a controversy; it can then disseminate a sufficient amount of "truth" to *sustain* a controversy.

The speaker then discusses the potential for using brand advertisements to convey a political message:

We have seen research this morning which indicates that there is at least a potential for using our own ads to communicate the other side of the cigarette story. Before putting this type effort into practice, however, we would want to be absolutely certain that there is no damage to our advertising or to the consumer acceptance of our brands. So the first step for the immediate future would be research. We are recommending basic research to unearth specific problems in smoking and health that we can deal directly with. {2111.01, p. 5}

This effort was part of an organized campaign that was carefully researched and designed by Corny Muije, who describes the research that was needed:

What was shown today specifically demonstrates what happened when a certain type of information was supplied with the KOOL Adios II ad.

Indications are that the KOOL copy effectiveness was enhanced. We need more evidence that this is true. Furthermore, we need to establish whether this solely hinges on the Adios II ad and the specific body copy used.

Also, is this an effective approach when the information is supplied with ads for VICEROY, RALEIGH, and BELAIR? {2111.01, p. 6}

After noting that there will be two phases to the research program, Muije continues:

> *It is essential that we ascertain which type of anti-cigarette information has most affected the smoking public. What claimed health hazards are currently accepted by the general public.*
>
> A general survey with detailed questioning should establish this. During Phase II we should also investigate consumer reaction to at least three distinct anti-cigarette approaches. In addition, consumer reactions to maybe a dozen specific anti-cigarette claims could be probed.
>
> The purpose of Phase II is to establish which past information and which current anti-cigarette claims are most damaging. From this we should learn which information should be of greatest interest to the public. We could then tailor our efforts more precisely to achieve the greatest effect [emphasis added]. {2111.01, pp. 6–7}

This discussion suggests that B&W was not so much interested in the actual scientific evidence about smoking and health as it was in the public perception of the evidence. Once the company could ascertain what the public believed, it could then tailor its own public relations efforts to help smokers rationalize their behavior.

After estimating the costs of the second phase of the research, Muije introduces Phase III, test marketing:

> None of the research, up to this point, will have let us know the effect of sustained repeated exposure of B&W cigarette ads with body copy of different content.
>
> Prior to a nation-wide commitment, one or more test markets would be called for.
>
> At this point it is impossible to say whether one or more test markets would be desirable.
>
> Regardless, in each instance we recommend that a consumer survey be conducted prior to the start of the test market and another one at the end of the test market.
>
> A comparison of the pre and post surveys will enable us to evaluate the effect of the total campaign. {2111.01, pp. 7–8}

At this point another speaker, probably Blalock again, replaces Muije:

> We would like to have the Executive Committee's approval to initiate the research program that Corny has just explained and at the same time to start a task force study of the smoking and health question and develop a detailed plan of action for B&W.
>
> Such a plan would cover:
> Sources of information about smoking and health.
> The selection and clearance of information to be used by B&W.

The development of new information about smoking and health.

Means of anticipating and countering the release of misinformation.

Channels other than our own advertising for getting messages to the public.

Ways to use and perhaps focus industry efforts in support of our own program.

Agency participation in the program.

Internal administration and implementation of the program.

Thorough evaluation of potential advantages and disadvantages of public action on B&W and its brands. {2111.01, pp. 8–9}

It is not clear from the documents whether this program moved beyond the concept, design, and test market stages. However, it is clear B&W was actively researching why people believed that smoking is dangerous and was trying to develop specific counterstrategies to allay the fears of the general public. This activity came at a time when public health officials were calling for stronger warnings and a ban on television and radio advertising for tobacco; when anti-cigarette television ads, ordered by the Federal Communications Commission, were reducing cigarette consumption (16); and when discussions that would lead to modestly strengthened warnings on cigarette packages were under way (4).

RJR'S PROJECTS A AND B

In 1970 the tobacco industry was actively discussing various public relations strategies to undermine public awareness of the dangers of smoking. The instructions to the law firm hired to analyze the Brown and Williamson documents (see chapter 1), which describe the relationships among Project Truth (see above) and Projects A and B, provide the context for the following discussion:

PROJECT TRUTH / PROJECT A / PROJECT B: Documents relating to any of these public issue campaigns involving the tobacco companies and TI. "Project A," developed in 1970, consisted of three TV spots on smoking and health that would be substituted for some regular TV commercials for which time had already been contracted. The spots were rejected by the network. Ruder & Finn proposed "Project B," which called for TV and print advertising that might position tobacco beside liquor in terms of public tolerance. In the fall of 1970, TI distributed two public service TV spots, produced by Ted Bates, to counteract the anti-smoking spot announcements. This activity was called "Project Truth." {1001.01, p. 12}

On February 20, 1970, J. W. Burgard sent a memorandum to E. P. Finch, B&W's president and chairman of the board, summarizing and commenting on the recommendations of the Tobacco Institute's Communications Committee for 1970, which evidently included plans for certain advertising campaigns. After stressing the need to prepare and approve effective copy, Burgard discussed the possibility of using the material B&W had already been preparing for presentation to editors and others in connection with Project Truth. Burgard's comment makes it clear that the lawyers were heavily involved in that project:

> I suggest this because we are hopeful that we can have such a presentation approved before too long, and I am painfully aware of the fact that we have been working intensively on this for over six months, with the full and almost daily cooperation of not only our own Law Department but of outside counsel. {2112.01, p. 1}

Although Burgard notes that the committee's recommendations did not cover R. J. Reynolds's "Project A" proposal, he offers his opinion of the project:

> I still feel that this is quite worthwhile if, again, the copy submitted by Reynolds is approved. If we attempt to make any major changes in their proposal, I am afraid this also will bog down in the pursuit of effective approved copy. {2112.01, p. 2}

A separate document, which is untitled and is neither signed nor dated, but appears to be a summary of various proposed advertising strategies and B&W's analysis of them, has as its first item a discussion of "Project A"—an R. J. Reynolds television series:

> Full agreement of group. Esty [perhaps Gil Esterle, International and External Technical Services Dept.] would produce and supply, through Tobacco Institute, the special spots to the six companies for insertion in network prime-time schedules. The B&W-proposed share plan was adopted; i.e., each company would give one minute for every 10 minutes of present schedule. Copies of estimates are attached, showing an approximate dollar value for the series of $275,000 per week, or $14,508,000 on a 12-month basis. Except for production costs (on a market share basis), the companies would not be committed to spend any extra dollars for the series, since they would simply be substituting the spots for already purchased time on an allotted basis. Nor would any extra agency commissions be involved; each company's agencies would receive commissions on already contracted time.
>
> In developing the series, Esty would have the legal advice and counsel of some designated lawyer(s), not a committee of company counsels (it is understood that Dave Hardy would act for B&W and Philip Morris). Before the series is run, heads of the networks would be given a special presentation (of course the entire series has to be approved by the network continuity people). {2112.04, p. 1}

The other ideas discussed in this document include newspaper advertising to introduce the television series; a benchmark opinion survey to determine public attitudes toward the smoking controversy; media briefings; communications with physicians on research efforts and studies that cast doubt on the anti-smoking theory; television network specials; participation on educational television programs; and employment of a public relations agency by the Tobacco Institute {2112.04, pp. 1–3}.

As the instructions indicate, "Project B" called for television advertising, and the documents include two of the proposed ads, a one-minute spot and a thirty-second spot. They are worth setting out in full:

STAGE I—One-Minute TV Spot:

This is a message from the people who make cigarettes—and are proud of it. It is a plea for common sense. You've seen the anti-smoking commercials. Dramatic and frightening, they do not appeal to your reason, but rather to your emotions. The fact is, a clear and consistent picture does not emerge from research findings concerning smoking and health. Many statistical connections have been cited against smoking—but these figures work both ways. Some figures which are as questionable as any others, for instance, indicate that people who smoke moderately are actually healthier than non smokers. (PAUSE) Our common sense tells us that emotional charges and counter charges will not resolve this controversy. Such emotionalism may even discourage needed intensive research by dedicated scientists. In the field of tobacco and health research, we in this industry provide more money, without strings, than all the voluntary agencies in this country combined. We have great confidence that this impartial research will lead the way in providing fair and accurate information regarding cigarette smoking. Until the answers are in, we must count on your common sense and sense of fair play. And we do. {2112.02}

and

STAGE I—Thirty-Second TV Spot:

This is a plea for common sense. You've seen the anti-smoking commercials. Dramatic, frightening, they do not appeal to reason, but rather to emotion. The fact is, a clear and consistent picture does not emerge from research findings concerning smoking and health. (PAUSE) Emotional charges will not resolve this controversy. Intensive research by dedicated scientists will. We provide more money for this research than all the voluntary agencies combined, and more than any agency of the Federal Government. Until the dilemma is resolved, we must count on your common sense. And we do [emphasis in original]. {2112.03}

On March 3, 1970, J. V. Blalock wrote a scathing attack on Project B in a memorandum to Finch, Burgard, and Yeaman {2112.05}. In his memo Blalock notes that the project was presented as an alternative to

Project A, that it was presented in three stages, and that B&W had certain responses to each stage:

Stage I—"Person to person dialogue—reasonable and responsible."
Because words are spoken on television, a dialogue is not necessarily established with the viewers, particularly people who have been bombarded by anti-cigarette propaganda. The public doesn't feel it owes the tobacco industry anything. We must believe that people can be persuaded if presented a realistic argument or viewpoint; that is our task—what to say and how to say it. Certainly, we would be foolhearty indeed to put our trust in Ruder & Finn's reasoning by saying on television: "Until the dilemma is resolved, we must count on your common sense and sense of fair play." We have to do a great deal more than that, or go down with a faint smile of misguided trust!

Stage II—"Reassurance."
Ruder & Finn charges that Reynolds' "Project A" is "an angry attack" and "seems argumentative and accusative." Their suggested print ad (Page 14) calls the anti-cigarette propaganda "widely-distorted, semi-hysterical campaign of fear . . ." Nowhere in "Project A" is there such an extreme statement (we may believe the propaganda is just that, but to say so in those terms would immediately destroy credibility). Reynolds' "Project A" takes a position that appeals to reason: "You've been told (about lung cancer, heart disease, etc. as related to smoking) but why haven't the anti-smoking people told you (about the substantial number of scientists who doubt those statements?)" Of course, we should tell smokers about industry research efforts, but we can hardly give them any comfort by telling them that "Being alive today is a risky business" (Page 21). The whole argument made in these print ads smacks of fumbling and sweet dodging.

Stage III—"Risk-benefit."
At this point, we would be ill-advised to equate the amount of risk with the degree of benefit derived from smoking. Ruder & Finn are victims of a misconception when they say: "The broad intention envisioned . . . is to achieve for the Tobacco Industry a position similar to that currently held by the liquor and beer industries." Neither industry has ever unitedly spoken of moderation or used a "risk-benefit" argument. These are elements which Reynolds' "Project A" have left out, and I believe Ruder & Finn's "Project B" fails completely to advance a convincing argument for this or other phases of its alternative to "Project A."

*   *   *

There seems little advantage to go further into this proposal, because the basic premise by Ruder & Finn is not supported by their suggested television and newspaper advertisements. What they have done is to say what in their opinion is wrong with "Project A"; they have not proved that their "Project B" is a suitable alternative [emphasis in original]. {2112.05, pp. 1–2}

Blalock attaches comments by Burgard, with which he wholeheartedly agrees:

1.   Doubt that in public mind there is any real difference in feeling about the tobacco industry "sense" and their feeling about liquor.

2.   Suggestions make nice reading to us but fail as "advertising" to capture the interest of the always indifferent public—too long, too wordy, too involved. Any campaign that requires the viewer or reader to make a sequentially reasoned decision is doomed to failure if we can believe past advertising experience.

3.   An unsupported statement by the industry that what you have heard "is not true" is an unbelievable self-serving declaration. It lacks credibility and is so sweeping as to be fraught with danger.

4.   Project "B" fails to consider that the anti-cigarette attacks have been going on for years and we are late in the struggle. You don't talk "common sense" when some one is attacking you with a meat axe.

We can always test the Project A commercials to see what the reaction is [emphasis in original]. {2112.05, p. 3}

Although Blalock and Burgard totally rejected "common sense" as a means of warding off attacks on the industry, eight years later that tactic was to become the centerpiece of the industry's efforts to defeat an initiative measure in California that would have restricted smoking in public places and workplaces. Indeed, the campaign committee established by the industry was called "Californians for Common Sense" (see chapter 10).

KEEPING TRACK OF SCIENCE AND SCIENTISTS

In considering its public relations problems resulting from scientific evidence on smoking and health, BAT recognized that it must not only generate supportive reports in the scientific literature (see chapter 8) but also keep abreast of developing science in general, and of scientists and physicians who might be spreading anti-tobacco information. In a 1968 memorandum to attorney B. G. Pearson in the BAT Public Relations Department, A. D. McCormick, a senior person in BAT R&DE in Millbank, writes:

[Mr. Widdup, deputy chairman of the BAT Australian company] suggested that just as we list certain territories as "red territories" for the purpose of information about the Rothmans' group [one of BAT's competitors], we could designate certain territories "red territories" for smoking and health purposes. *Obvious candidates would be the U.S., Canada, Australia and, perhaps, South Africa. The idea would be to set up a system whereby we would keep companies in these territories informed of (a) industry policy or contemplated action; (b) a check-list of major scientific papers with industry comments;*

*(c) list of particularly favorable or unfavorable scientists and doctors, with a
warning system should they be travelling to any particular territory.*

The kind of situation with which he would like to be able to deal would
be—by way of example—when Dr. Keogh, the anti-smoking man from Vic-
toria, asked him what was the industry's answer to Harris's paper showing
he had caused some cancers in rats by getting them to inhale cigarette smoke.
As Widdup did not know of the paper he couldn't give a sensible reply. T.R.C.
had in fact known of the paper and discussed the industry's comments on it
some time previously. This would be a case where information should be
passed on to "red territory" companies ahead of time [emphasis added].
{2104.01}

The tobacco industry as a whole has adopted this practice and has formalized it through an organization known as INFOTAB, based in London, which keeps track of developments and individuals worldwide that
are perceived as threats to the tobacco industry.

The tobacco industry also sponsored reports and meetings to provide
citable sources for information that it needed for public policy and political purposes. For example, the lawyers took over control of work on
the economic costs of smoking.

INFOTAB, although retaining jurisdiction of the social costs issue, has passed
the ball for development of a position back to the U.S. Tim [Finnegan] believes, and understands that the INFOTAB members now agree, that George
Berman tends to use unacceptable arguments, perhaps as a result of his personal belief that causation is proven. Recently a SWOP held a workshop at
[the] Wharton [School of Business] which Berman conducted. Something like
10,000 invitations were issued and only 22 attended. This turned out to be
fortunate because the theme of Berman's presentations was that costs associated with smoking and health are not social costs but transfer payments. Tim's
objective is to take the lead of the social cost program away from Berman
and put U.S. lawyers in the forefront of preparing an industry position primarily through the development of witnesses who can present a position. I
told Tim you had written a superb memorandum describing the application
of various disciplines to the subject of social costs and I sent a copy to him
when you approved. {1825.01, p. 1}

The tobacco industry's use of economic symposia to advance its argument that tobacco is good for the economy is similar to its sponsorship
of workshops on secondhand smoke designed to counter scientific evidence that secondhand smoke is dangerous (17). Here again the industry used its lawyers to develop a response to a smoking-related health
problem when it decided that the scientists were using "unacceptable
arguments."

CONCLUSION

The tobacco industry's public relations efforts during the "safe" cigarette era consisted largely of an attempt to confuse the public about the scientific evidence on the dangers of smoking. Whether those efforts involved in-house handbooks, books and magazine articles written on behalf of the industry, or advertising campaigns, the thrust of the material was the same: create doubt in the public mind about what the scientific evidence really says and then attack the notion that the government should meddle in the tobacco industry's business without having definitive proof of harmful effects of smoking. To this end, the industry enlisted the support of powerful friends in the political world as well as in the media, and sometimes failed to disclose the fact that certain people expressing a viewpoint sympathetic to the industry had direct financial ties to the industry.

REFERENCES

1. Johnston J. *Testimony before the Subcommittee on Health and the Environment.* Committee on Energy and Commerce, US House of Representatives, 1994.
2. USDHEW. *Smoking and Health. Report of the Advisory Committee to the Surgeon General of the Public Health Service.* US Department of Health, Education and Welfare, 1964. Public Health Service Publication No. 1103.
3. Kitchin C. *You May Smoke.* New York: Award Books, 1966.
4. Wagner S. *Cigarette Country: Tobacco in American History and Politics.* New York: Praeger, 1971.
5. USEPA. *Respiratory Health Effects of Passive Smoking: Lung Cancer and Other Disorders.* Indoor Air Division, Office of Atmospheric and Indoor Programs, Office of Air and Radiation, US Environmental Protection Agency, 1992. EPA/600/6-90/006F.
6. Skolnick A. Burning mad tobacco firms turn up heat on major news media. *Science Writer* 1994 Summer:1–5.
7. Naureckas J. When journalists boost the tobacco industry, follow the money. *Extra!* 1994 September/October:18–19.
8. Jones C. Philip Morris aided periodical. *Richmond Times-Dispatch* 1994 June 30:B10.
9. Secondhand smoke: Is it a hazard? *Consumer Reports* 1995 January:27–33.
10. Wolinsky H, Brune T. *The Serpent on the Staff: The Unhealthy Politics of the American Medical Association.* New York: Putnam, 1994.
11. Slade J, Kopelowicz A. An analysis of "R. J. Reynolds' position paper on the health effects of smoking": I. The constitutional hypothesis. *Tobacco Products Litigation Reporter* 1986;1(8):5.97–5.105.
12. Eysenck H. Smoking and health. In: Tollison R, ed. *Smoking and Society: Toward a More Balanced Assessment* (pp. 17–88). Lexington, MA: Lexington Books, 1986.
13. Slade J, Nissenblatt M. An analysis of "R. J. Reynolds' position paper on the health effects of smoking": II. Lung cancer. *Tobacco Products Liability Reporter* 1986;1(9): 5.107–5.113.

14. Slade J, Hahn A. An analysis of "R. J. Reynolds' position paper on the health effects of smoking": III. Heart disease. *Tobacco Products Liability Reporter* 1986;1(9): 5.115–5.121.

15. Slade J, Kabis S, Vasen A. An analysis of "R. J. Reynolds' position paper on the health effects of smoking": IV. Chronic obstructive pulmonary disease. *Tobacco Products Litigation Reporter* 1987;2(2):5.11–5.21.

16. USDHHS. *Reducing the Health Consequences of Smoking: 25 Years of Progress.* US Department of Health and Human Services, Public Health Service, Centers for Disease Control, Center for Chronic Disease Prevention and Health Promotion, Office on Smoking and Health, 1989. DHHHS Publication No. (CDC) 89-8411.

17. Bero L, Galbraith A, Rennie D. Sponsored symposia on environmental tobacco smoke. *JAMA* 1994;271:612–617.

CHAPTER 6

Agricultural Chemicals and Cigarette Additives

If one applies a given material to tobacco, three things are important:

1. The characteristics of the material itself.
2. The characteristics of its pyrolysis products [i.e., products produced by burning].
3. The possible alterations in the chemistry of the plant material which may affect the biological activity.

> *Dr. R. B. Griffith, B&W director of research,*
> *April 1967 {1302.01, p. 2}*

INTRODUCTION

The documents include a number of discussions by B&W officials concerning the chemicals used in the growing and storage of tobacco (agricultural chemicals, such as sucker control agents, pesticides, and fumigants) and in cigarette manufacture (additives). Thirty years ago, B&W officials made genuine attempts to ensure that the agricultural chemicals and additives used in their products were nontoxic, and they expected the suppliers or makers of these materials to take responsibility for ensuring safety. Company officials in this era expressed specific concerns about the possibility that the combustion products of additives might themselves be toxic. More recent documents have a more defensive character, with officials frequently pointing out that a material in question has been declared "Generally Recognized as Safe" (GRAS) for use in food, either by the Food and Drug Administration (FDA) or by the Flavor and Extract Manufacturers' Association (FEMA). Additives on these lists, however, are declared safe in a product that is eaten, not in one that is burned to generate an inhaled smoke. As discussed later in this chapter, Dr. R. B. Griffith, B&W's director of research, recognized in 1967 that a material considered safe when eaten is not necessarily safe in other forms, particularly when it is burned and inhaled in smoke.

Unlike additives to foods, additives to tobacco products are not subject to government regulation in the United States. Since the mid-1980s the cigarette manufacturers have been required to submit a list of tobacco additives used in cigarettes to the Department of Health and Human Services (1), but the department is barred from publishing the list. Moreover, the manufacturers are not required to specify which brands of cigarettes use which particular additives. Quantitative information is similarly lacking. The tobacco companies are not required to disclose anything at all about additives to cigarette papers (such as fillers and adhesives) or to filters (such as plasticizers). In April 1994 public pressure forced the major cigarette makers to publish a version of this list (2), which included 599 materials that might, or might not, be added to any particular brand of cigarettes.

The first page of a file memo dated November 1, 1988 (probably from B&W's law firm in Louisville), provides the following nonexhaustive classification of nontobacco materials that might be found in cigarettes:

flavors
sugars
humectants
casings or sauce materials
insecticides
herbicides
fungicides
rodenticides
pesticides
water conditioners
manufacturing machine lubricants and other chemicals which come in contact with the tobacco and may leave residues on the tobacco {1324.01}

While this classification gives the reader some idea of the range of materials that find their way into cigarettes, the list does not include additives to papers or to filters.

The tobacco industry has used a wide range of additives in cigarettes for decades. Documents dating from as early as April 1965 show that BAT had an "Additives Guidance Panel" to discuss issues related to additive toxicity. In at least one instance B&W continued using an additive even when research suggested that it might pose a health risk to consumers and the panel advised against its use.

AGRICULTURAL CHEMICALS

SUCKER CONTROL AGENTS: MH-30 AND PENAR

To promote optimal leaf growth, farmers remove the terminal buds from tobacco plants about two months after transplantation from the seed bed into the field (3, 4). This procedure prevents flowering, which results in increased nicotine content in the leaves (4). Removing the terminal bud also controls the total number of leaves the plant will bear. In the absence of the terminal bud, new shoots arise from the axils of the leaves. These "suckers" must be removed by hand, or their growth must be inhibited by chemicals, to avoid sapping nourishment from (and lowering nicotine levels in) the developing leaf. Sucker control agents are chemicals that are sprayed on tobacco plants to slow the growth of suckers and thereby enhance crop yield. These agents—such as MH-30 (maleic hydrazide) and Penar (dimethyldodecylamine acetate)—eliminate the laborious task of removing suckers by hand and therefore lower the labor costs of growing tobacco.

In the mid-1960s the toxicology of sucker control agents was a matter of concern to the Sucker Control Committee, a committee composed of representatives from the tobacco industry and the US Department of Agriculture (USDA). Dr. R. B. Griffith wrote an extensive summary of an April 1967 meeting of this group, in which he had participated {1302.01}. At that time emerging data were suggesting that a commonly used sucker control agent, MH-30, was toxic. Experiments had exposed selected strains of mice to high doses of MH-30, and the significant toxicity that resulted called into question the safety of this agricultural chemical. In his memo Dr. Griffith notes that the USDA has very limited authority to act in such a situation:

> Although they [the USDA Pesticide Regulation Division] are greatly concerned, the law requires that others must demonstrate a potential effect on health which is irrefutable. However, they are prepared to act when such knowledge indicates that they should move. {1302.01, p. 1}

The committee members then compared the expected dose of MH-30 to human smokers with the dose administered to the mice; they concluded that the mice had been exposed to two million times the dose that a human smoker consuming two packs of cigarettes daily would ingest.

The committee discussion moved from MH-30 to a consideration of studies on Penar as a possible cause of chromosomal aberrations in plants:

At this point in the discussion, *I pointed out that the tobacco problem was unique*. If one applies a given material to tobacco, three things are important:

    1.   The characteristics of the material itself.

    2.   *The characteristics of its pyrolysis products* [i.e., products produced by burning].

    3.   The possible alterations in the chemistry of the plant material which may affect the biological activity.

I went on to point out that unusual chemical effects had been noted for each of the new sucker control materials now being considered and *that there was no way of predicting the effect that these chemical changes might have on the biological effects of the smoke produced by the treated tobacco*. I expressed the opinion that this was a very serious problem and that it was highly desirable for some way to be found to subject treated material to biological tests. In this connection mouse skin painting was not enough since it does not measure whole smoke. Present problems facing the industry certainly indicate the need for assurance that any material used will not result in any detrimental biological effects [emphasis added]. {1302.01, p. 2}

Dr. Griffith's comments reveal a concern with the toxicity of combustion products of additives and of the residues of agricultural chemicals. Although mouse skin painting is an important test for "biological effects" (i.e., carcinogenicity; see chapter 4), it might miss important effects because, as Dr. Griffith pointed out, it relies on painting smoke condensate, rather than whole smoke, onto the experimental animal. In other words, materials in the vapor phase, which are too volatile to be part of the "tar," are not tested in skin-painting experiments. Mouse skin might show no damage from a particular preparation of tobacco smoke condensate, but the smoke might still be highly carcinogenic.

A participant at the meeting indicated that a committee formed by British tobacco companies was "contemplating a series of biological tests" of the new sucker control agents, and that these tests could be replicated in the United States. The memo concludes:

Although everyone there [i.e., in Britain] seemed to recognize the magnitude of the problem, no one seemed to know what, if any, actions could be taken. *It was agreed that none of this information would be discussed with the chemical suppliers of any of the sucker control materials, and that no public discussions of this subject could take place until after . . . [the] papers* [describing the toxicity of MH-30 in mice] *have been published* [emphasis added]. {1302.01, p. 3}

A year later, Penar was the subject of correspondence between scientists at BAT and B&W. Dr. S. J. Green, a senior R&D scientist at BAT in London, transmitted a Tobacco Research Council (TRC) report on

Penar to Dr. Griffith in mid-April 1968. Griffith, in turn, sent copies to Addison Yeaman, B&W's general counsel, and Dr. R. A. Sanford, a fellow scientist at B&W {1303.01}. The report gave preliminary results suggesting that Penar is toxic. The authors recommended additional testing of Penar-treated tobacco, and they urged B&W to report the alarming initial results to regulatory authorities in the United States and Canada:

> The tests on [Penar-]*spiked tobacco have now been going for 31 weeks and results reported from Huntingdon* [Imperial Tobacco's laboratory in England] *at this stage are so disquieting that we consider that they should be reported to the U.S.D.A. and Canadian Department of Agriculture* [emphasis added]. {1303.02, p. 1}

We found no indication in the documents whether the data were, in fact, reported to the appropriate government authorities.

Shortly after this report was received in Louisville, on May 1, 1968, Dr. Griffith sent Yeaman a status report along with some background documents on the growing evidence of toxicity from sucker control agents {1317.09}. The report conveys a tone of urgency and helplessness. Griffith recognizes that, although Penar appears to be carcinogenic, he and the cigarette manufacturers have limited power to do anything about it, because Penar is produced by an independent company and is applied to tobacco in the field, months before the tobacco is bought by the cigarette makers.

> The tobacco manufacturer is completely at the mercy of the people who use various chemicals on tobacco. Of the chemicals used, MH-30 and Penar have probably been investigated most extensively, and there are certainly indications that these could have detrimental biological effects from smoke. *As you know, we have been sitting on the MH-30 "powder keg" for three years and no positive steps have been taken by the government agencies to provide any relief.* We now have, as a result of Dr. Green's letter of April 16 [{1303.01; 1303.02}], information which suggests that Penar could be even more of a problem than MH-30. In Dr. Smith's report of April 18, he pointed out that there is a possibility that as much as 25% of the crop in North Carolina will be produced using a combination of MH-30 and Penar. It would seem that something must be done, and since this is an industry problem, we must consider every possible avenue, including bringing this to the attention of the "Less Hazardous Cigarette" Committee [discussed in chapter 4].
>
> If you and your opposite numbers [i.e., attorneys at the other tobacco companies] can agree that this is an industry problem which must be handled on an industry basis, it might be helpful to solicit specific suggestions from the Industry Research Directors [emphasis added]. {1317.09}

Griffith's proposal to deal with the problem directly on an industry-wide basis is in line with the general policy of the R&D establishments

throughout BAT in the 1960s: they were earnestly seeking to lower toxicity in ways that did not fundamentally threaten the product itself (see
chapter 4). Thus, the B&W general counsel could be asked to confer
with his opposite numbers at competing companies about this "industry problem," because the problem was potentially soluble without
threatening B&W's core business. Government could regulate these agricultural chemicals if necessary, and tobacco production would go on.

J. E. Kennedy and R. P. Newton of B&W R&D wrote a "private and
confidential" file note in mid-1968 titled "The Relative Carcinogenicity
of Sucker Control Agents Maleic Hydrazide (MH) and Dimethyldodecylamine Acetate (Penar)" {1303.03}. It was circulated to Ed Finch,
B&W's CEO, Yeaman, and Griffith. The note analyzes two published
studies on maleic hydrazide and the unpublished Huntingdon study on
Penar. It emphasizes the relatively huge doses of both agents involved in
these experiments and describes the combustion behavior of the compounds. According to the report, maleic hydrazide was not changed at
high temperature and was therefore not expected to contribute other
compounds to cigarette smoke. Penar, on the other hand, decomposed
to dimethylamine, dodecaene, and acetic acid. Dimethylamine, in turn,
was expected to produce dimethylnitrosamine, which Kennedy and
Newton describe as "a strong carcinogen" {1303.03, p. 2}.

In August 1968 Imperial scientists shared their data on the carcinogenicity of Penar with Dr. T. C. Tso, a senior scientist at the US Department of Agriculture, while Dr. Tso was visiting England. This interchange
is discussed prominently in a September 13, 1968, file note by Dr. Griffith, which tells of his visits earlier in the month to USDA offices in
Beltsville, Maryland. He had meetings there with Dr. Tso and with Dr.
Leon Moore, who was in charge of the USDA's tobacco program
{1303.04}. After summarizing the data on Penar, Dr. Griffith notes:

> Dr. Tso and the people in England consider that these results indicate a very
> serious potential problem with Penar. This information is being given to the
> Penar manufacturers and a summary statement has been sent to Dr. T. W. Ed-
> minster, Deputy Administrator of ARS [Agricultural Research Service], with
> a request that he pass this information on through normal channels to the
> Pesticide Division of the USDA [emphasis added]. {1303.04, pp. 1–2}

Dr. Griffith had thought from a telephone conversation with Dr. Tso on
August 28 that Dr. Tso might want additional toxicology work to be
done on Penar, but "this impression is erroneous. He intends to accept
the English results as definitive for Penar" {1303.04, p. 2}. The additional work was to be done on other sucker control agents.

Dr. Tso is obviously impressed with the procedures being used in England and fully recognizes that valid work should not be repeated. On the other hand, the results obtained on Penar definitely indicate the need for such tests on other compounds used on tobacco. {1303.04, p. 2}

During this same September 1968 visit, Dr. Tso also talked with Dr. Griffith about the work of the Tobacco Working Group and the "Less Hazardous Cigarette Committee" in the United States. The discussion centered on cooperation and collaboration on the production of a standardized cigarette for testing.

The notes of Dr. Griffith's visit to Beltsville also summarize his meeting with Dr. Moore. Dr. Moore and Dr. Griffith agreed "that Penar was a very serious potential problem, but that this was only a specific example of a general problem" {1303.04, p. 3}. At the time, only MH-30 and Penar had been tested, and both had been found toxic. Griffith suggested that a general framework for approaching questions regarding agricultural chemicals should be developed to "prevent the feeling on the part of anyone that the USDA or Industry was attacking any individual company" {1303.04, p. 4}. The exchange indicates that Griffith was interested in developing a systematic approach to dealing with the potential toxicity of agricultural chemicals, and he clearly felt that government regulators had a major role to play. His view on pesticides sharply contrasts with B&W's position on cigarettes—that the government should play no role in regulating toxicity of cigarettes. Griffith endorsed government regulation of potentially toxic agricultural chemicals, but B&W has never wanted the government to regulate its manufactured tobacco products.

Griffith's file note concludes with his encouraging Dr. Moore to share the Penar results from England with other US tobacco product manufacturers. Griffith had known of the results because of the free exchange of research results between BAT and B&W. Other US manufacturers did not enjoy this access to the UK industry's joint research results. Moore indicated that his contact at Imperial Tobacco (John Campbell) had not given him permission to share the data. Griffith encouraged him to try to obtain that permission.

I expressed the opinion that if I were a company who did not have access to the information, I would be very disturbed. *The Penar situation could explode at any minute and a company without prior knowledge could be caught in a very embarrassing position.* Dr. Moore recognized this and promised to try and obtain permission from Mr. Campbell to pass this information on to the total American Tobacco Industry [emphasis added]. {1303.04, p. 4}

The carcinogenicity of Penar was later confirmed through long-term mouse skin–painting experiments conducted within the BAT system. A report two years later, dated May 18, 1970, from C. I. Ayres, a scientist in R&D at BAT in Southampton, describes the results of a 72-week-long experiment in which tobacco smoke condensates derived from tobaccos treated with two different concentrations of Penar were painted on the skins of mice {1308.01}. The report was sent to the R&D department at B&W as well as to BAT officials in Australia and Montreal. It seems to have originated at BAT's laboratory in Southampton. It refers to the experiment as the "remaining" Penar experiment, suggesting that its long-term results may have complemented short-term assays completed earlier. The experiment would have begun no later than sometime in 1968. In his report Dr. Ayres summarizes the experiments on 1,056 mice:

> I am enclosing the latest results (H 685) from the remaining PENAR experiment. *The position is unchanged, i.e., there is the indication that the addition of PENAR to cut tobacco leads to an increase in the tumorigenicity of the condensate* [emphasis added]. {1308.01, p. 1}

Thus, by 1970 BAT had demonstrated that an agricultural chemical could detectably increase the already high toxicity of tobacco.

Penar was finally reformulated at some time in the 1970s—years after the initial data which indicated that the original formula was carcinogenic had been developed.

Maleic hydrazide, another sucker control agent, was also reformulated. The diethanolamine salt was replaced with the potassium salt because of concerns that nitrosamines might be produced when tobacco treated with diethanolamine salt was burned (4, 5). Maleic hydrazide has continued in widespread use: in the mid-1970s about 3 million pounds were used on tobacco in the United States (4). The B&W Leaf Division reported that it was having difficulty meeting the standards set by the West German government for permissible levels of maleic hydrazide in tobacco in the 1971 tobacco crop {1317.07}. The report notes, "there is no systemic alternative to maleic hydrazide, but contact suckering formulations based on the long-chain alcohols octanol and decanol are coming into favour, especially in Canada" {1317.07}.

An April 12, 1984, memorandum from K. J. Brotzge, associate research biologist, to E. E. Kohnhorst, vice president for research, development, and engineering (RD&E) at B&W (with copies to Ivor Wallace Hughes, chairman and CEO; Thomas Sandefur, executive vice president; Ernest Pepples, senior vice president and general counsel; and others

{1003.01}), describes the "annual pesticide residue meetings" held at North Carolina State University the previous week {1318.01}. The meeting reviewed an ongoing monitoring program that analyzed levels of residues of agricultural chemicals in various brands of cigarettes. The work was supported by grants from the North Carolina Tobacco Foundation, American Tobacco, B&W, Liggett & Myers, Lorillard, Philip Morris, R. J. Reynolds, and the Tobacco Advisory Committee (UK). The program had supported a graduate student's master's degree work in toxicology. Maleic hydrazide, the sucker control agent, was still evident in cigarettes.

PESTICIDES

Pesticides have been of concern to tobacco industry scientists because of both the potential toxicity of their residues and the regulatory requirements of some governments. For example, a May 1958 memorandum from the B&W Research Department discusses the possibility of using an outside laboratory to conduct pesticide residue studies for the export department {1317.06}. The analyses may have been required for export of products to West Germany, which regulated levels of some additives and pesticide residues of tobacco products (see below).

A December 1968 letter from the Research Department at Imperial Tobacco in Bristol to the Tobacco Research Council in London documents the results of the department's analyses of DDT residues in samples of the 1967 US tobacco crop {1304.01}.

> In our view these figures indicate an unacceptably high contamination [with DDT residues] of the tobacco and we think that they should be brought to the attention of the U.S.D.A. with the request that action is taken to ensure that levels in future crops are lower. {1304.01}

An early meeting of a group called the Agricultural Chemicals Study Group was suggested to review the matter. There seemed to be some urgency to the deliberations:

> If there is support for our views it would then be possible for the matter to be raised with the U.S.D.A. in time for them to take some action in regard to the 1969 crop. {1304.01}

The *Congressional Record* for July 28, 1969, includes an eight-page exploration of the problem of pesticide residues in tobacco by Senator Gaylord Nelson (D-WI) {1307.01, pp. 2–3}. In this entry Nelson declares his support for a ban on DDT and notes that tobacco has been exempted from regulations limiting the levels of pesticides used on crops.

The first page of a progress report from the B&W Leaf Division's review of the 1971 crop mentions DDT residues in US tobacco {1317.07}. The report indicates that US leaf has levels of DDT residues that "continue to approach the level demanded by the West German legislation, but the levels of maleic hydrazide are still very high."

A June 1983 memorandum from R&D within B&W discusses the advantages of substituting an insecticide named Fican-Plus for Diazinon {1317.01}. The proposed substitute is described as "not as toxic to mammals" and therefore "a desirable replacement"; it also might render the pyrolysis products (the results of burning the chemicals in a cigarette) less toxic. Once again, the company's research scientists are intent on reducing the potential toxicity of a chemical used in tobacco production, as well as the potential toxicity of pyrolysis products of the chemical.

The report of B&W's delegate to the industry-wide "annual pesticide residue meetings" for 1984 (see above) includes a description of a smoke panel test that was to become part of the evaluation of new pesticides for tobacco {1318.01}. This test was to be used to determine whether new pesticides altered the actual smoking experience in any way. The smoke panel is described as follows:

> A toxicologist, Dr. Lamar Dale, was hired as an independent consultant. He is to review data packages from pesticide manufacturers when development of a pesticide for tobacco has progressed to the point that smoke flavor evaluations are needed. His evaluation will serve as a basis for judging the safety to tobacco company panelists who smoke experimental cigarettes treated with pesticides. {1318.01, p. 2}

Dr. Dale had been hired to do these evaluations for the entire US cigarette industry. Included in the specific information requested by Dr. Dale was "pyrolytic products at smoldering and ignition temperatures (acutely toxic products, i.e., HCN, CO, etc.)" {1813.02, Appendix III, p. 1}. The report noted that such information "will generally not be available. However, the safety to panelists can be judged through other available information requested" {1813.01, p. 2}. Thus, the committee representing the industry did not question the relevance to consumer safety of their consultant's requested information, but only its availability. The industry as a whole recognized that, in making the safety judgments about pesticide residues in cigarette tobacco, one must consider the toxicity of pyrolysis products (i.e., the results of burning them), not just the unheated form of the residue.

The fact that pyrolysis could increase the toxicity of additives had been recognized by Dr. Griffith in 1967, but the point seems to have been ignored by the industry in recent years. The additive list released by the cigarette companies in April 1994 indicated time and again that one material and another was GRAS or FEMA-approved (2), but nowhere in the listing is any consideration given to whether these additives are safe when inhaled.

ADDITIVES

Additives are used to make tobacco products more acceptable to consumers. They might prolong shelf life (humectants), make the smoke milder and easier to inhale (sugars and humectants), add flavor and aroma, improve the delivery of nicotine (ammonia compounds), and numb the throat (menthol and eugenol). For some time public health workers have pressed for disclosure of additives because some of them, or their combustion products, might be toxic (6). On at least one occasion the tobacco industry has considered additives to reduce the carcinogenicity of cigarette smoke. One such proposed additive, called Chemosol, is discussed in the documents.

By 1981 there was a tension between an increased need for additives in product design, because of pressures to lower tar and nicotine deliveries, and the increased likelihood of government regulation. BAT scientists at the Pichlarn, Austria, research conference in August 1981 concluded:

> While additives will assume increasing importance in product design, the freedom to use them could become increasingly restricted. {1178.01, p. 14}

The documents disclose several instances in which B&W was reluctant to abandon the use of additives that independent tests on animals had found toxic. Of course, the company was under no regulatory obligation to stop using these additives; however, it appears to have voluntarily discontinued use of some additives by 1994, probably because of the threat of public disclosure and government regulation.

CHEMOSOL: AN ADDITIVE TO REDUCE CANCER

In the late 1960s the American cigarette companies briefly joined forces to sponsor the study of a cigarette additive, Chemosol, which promised to greatly reduce the risk of smoking-induced cancer. The willingness of these companies to come together for such an extraordinary activity speaks eloquently to the seriousness with which the whole industry privately regarded the cancer risks of cigarettes. In addition, the Chemosol story illustrates the extent to which lawyers controlled critical pathways of scientific endeavor about sensitive subjects within the industry.

Chemosol, described in the documents as a "fuel additive," had been developed under the name "flowebin" by a physician named Max Bindig from Munich, Germany {1807.06}. When used as an additive in cigarettes, it was supposed to promote more complete combustion, which would reduce the levels of the carcinogen benzo(a)pyrene (or benzpyrene) in mainstream smoke. When the rights to flowebin were acquired by a US company, the Chemical Research and Development Corporation, the additive was renamed Chemosol and the company was renamed the American Chemosol Corporation.

During 1966 Dr. Perry Hudson, a biologist affiliated with Columbia University, who ran a research laboratory called the High Tor Foundation, conducted a mouse skin–painting experiment in which cigarettes treated with Chemosol were compared with cigarettes that had not been treated {1807.02}. In this experiment mice exposed to standard tobacco smoke condensate developed a high percentage of malignant tumors, whereas animals exposed to Chemosol-treated tobacco smoke condensate did not develop tumors. This result suggested that Chemosol reduced the carcinogenicity of tobacco smoke condensate.

In the spring of 1967, Joachim Schumacher, vice president of McDonnell & Company, agents for the owners of Chemosol, wrote Ed Finch, president of B&W, about the additive {1807.06}. The letter was a follow-up to a meeting between Schumacher and B&W general counsel, Addison Yeaman. While Schumacher was offering B&W an opportunity to obtain an exclusive license for Chemosol, B&W seems to have been committed from the beginning to bringing this potential additive to the attention of the industry as a whole {1807.07}. The file copy of a letter to the executive director of the Council for Tobacco Research, dated December 12, 1967, states:

> Some time ago Ed Finch was approached by representatives of Chemical Research and Development Corporation with an offer to negotiate with Brown & Williamson for an exclusive license to an undefined additive to tobacco called CHEMOSOL. It was claimed that CHEMOSOL 1) very significantly reduced the benzo-a-pyrene content of the mainstream smoke, and 2) that smoke condensate from tobacco treated with CHEMOSOL was virtually free of biologic activity. Finch replied that under no circumstance would Brown & Williamson consider such a proposal, but was willing to act as the conduit of information from the promoters of CHEMOSOL to the United States cigarette industry. {1807.07}

Dr. Griffith reviewed the data on Chemosol that Dr. Hudson had prepared and shared his thoughts in a July 19, 1967, memorandum to Addison Yeaman {1807.01}. Although he was impressed with the quality of the technical report and the soundness of the mouse skin–painting protocol that Dr. Hudson had used, he expressed considerable skepticism about Chemosol. He strongly recommended an attempt at replication of Dr. Hudson's study in another laboratory.

Plans for such a replication apparently were already under way when Dr. Griffith wrote this memo. By August 1, 1967, the Hazleton Laboratory in Falls Church, Virginia (a private laboratory), had submitted a draft protocol for testing Chemosol {1807.08}. Finch's initial decision to involve the entire industry in any development of Chemosol was maintained: nine companies (including B&W, Lorillard, R. J. Reynolds, Philip Morris, and American Tobacco) were sponsors of the 1967 protocol that Hazleton had developed (7). However, the experiment had still not been done by the time the matter was brought to the attention of a congressional committee in April 1969.

During the House hearings on cigarette package labeling in 1969, Dr. Hudson testified about his work on Chemosol. He said that it was capable of reducing the benzo(a)pyrene level in cigarette smoke by 34 percent. He described a mouse skin–painting experiment in which only 5 percent of the mice receiving the condensate from Chemosol-treated cigarettes, compared with 25 percent of those whose skin had been painted with the conventional condensate, developed cancer (7). Dr. Hudson also indicated that scientists in academic medicine and from the National Cancer Institute had reviewed the work done on Chemosol and had found it promising. His striking testimony was covered in the *New York Times* the following day (8), and by the end of August the tobacco industry was publicizing its agreement with Hazleton to proceed with the experiment (9). It appears that the glare of publicity got this project moving again.

On September 10, 1969, representatives of Hazleton met with the research directors of the major tobacco companies to discuss the protocol. Five days later, another meeting was held with representatives of Hazleton, three tobacco company representatives, and two lawyers from Covington and Burling (counsel for the Tobacco Institute) to discuss the fine points of the proposed protocol. The meeting is documented by a detailed set of notes written the following day by Allan J. Topol, one of the two lawyers present {1807.08}. Topol wrote these notes in the form of a memo to the other lawyer who was there, H. Thomas Austern. Austern was a prominent expert in food and drug law at the time. He had represented the Tobacco Institute before the Federal Trade Commission a few years earlier (10). The lawyers (purportedly on behalf of the research directors) sought to add defensive language to the protocol. According to Topol's memo,

> AJT [Topol] stated that the research directors had decided that the objective [statement in the protocol] should include a sentence stating that the relationship of skin painting to smoking and health had not been established. {1807.08, p. 1}

This embellishment was proposed despite the fact that mouse skin painting was being used to guide product development of less toxic cigarettes within the industry (see chapter 4). The Hazleton spokesman, a Mr. Gargus, disagreed with this change on the grounds that such a disclaimer belonged in the final report, not the protocol.

Although Austern was present as counsel for the consortium of tobacco companies sponsoring the research, he made a number of substantive scientific suggestions about the conduct and organization of the project. He asked whether a sufficient number of cigarettes would be available for the entire project, a question that led to agreement to raise the number to be made from 500,000 to 1 million. He offered the services of the Tobacco Institute Testing Laboratory to conduct preliminary quality control testing of the experimental cigarettes, and he suggested that organoleptic tests (human panel tests of subjective smoking qualities) be added to the protocol. He also suggested that the protocol specify the type of cigarette paper to be used in the manufacture of the experimental cigarettes.

Hazleton had planned to assay the smoke of experimental cigarettes for benzo(a)pyrene levels, but Austern objected

> in view of the claims made by Chemosol for benzo(a)pyrene reduction, and in view of the decision of the research directors at the meeting of September 10, 1969, that no decision would now be made as to the test for benzo(a)pyrene content, and that such a decision would be made at the termination of the biological tests. {1807.08, p. 3}

The tobacco company sponsors apparently did not want to consider collecting data that might validate Chemosol's claim for reducing benzo(a)pyrene levels unless the additive was first proven to protect mice from developing cancers. The report indicated that Hazleton's proposed assay of the condensate for benzo(a)pyrene would have been for routine quality control. It is interesting, then, to speculate as to why the attorney chose to object to the use of such a routine procedure. Our hypothesis is that if the experiment showed no protection, but benzo(a)pyrene levels were, in fact, lower, this result would suggest that other carcinogens in the smoke were responsible for cigarettes' carcinogenicity.

Austern also objected to the use of benzo(a)pyrene as the carcinogen to be employed for a positive control in the experiment. It was routine practice to include a positive control in these studies, and benzo(a)pyrene was the one that Hazleton had used in the past. (In fact, BAT later used benzo(a)pyrene—which it described as a "pure carcinogen"—as a positive control in precisely this way in its Janus mouse skin–painting experiments {1138.02, p. 4}; see chapter 4.)

> Mr. Gargus explained that benzo(a)pyrene had been employed because it was the best known carcinogenic agent and the one generally used in experiments of this type . . . HTA [Austern] *suggested that Hazleton employ some control other than benzo(a)pyrene in view of the repeated assertions made by Chemosol for benzo(a)pyrene reduction, and in view of the psychological implications of "benzo(a)pyrene" in the cigarette controversy.* Mr. Gargus rejected these suggestions, and Mr. Jessup [of Hazleton] stated that unless Mr. Gargus was satisfied on the scientific grounds, Hazleton would not enter into the contract [emphasis added]. {1807.08, p. 4}

Hazleton retained its preferred positive control, but Austern's attempt to get it changed is an example of how an attorney placed public relations concerns—not the lawyer's traditional concern with liability—ahead of scientific judgments.

Topol's account also describes a substantive discussion about the publication of the results of the experiment. Austern sought to establish control of the results by the tobacco companies (see chapter 8):

> With regard to publication of the results, Mr. Gargus suggested that Hazleton be authorized to publish the results of its study in a scientific journal even prior to submission of a report by Hazleton to the sponsors, and prior to Hazleton's submission of its final results to the sponsors. In this way, Mr. Gargus stated, Hazleton could secure its scientific reputation by making sure that Hazleton published its test results. Under this approach no-one would see the Hazleton results until they were published. HTA [Austern] disagreed with this suggestion, stating that the sponsors were paying for the work and should certainly see the results before they were published. In addition, publication is generally a matter of the sponsors' discretion. {1807.08, p. 5}

Austern prevailed. After discussion, Gargus agreed to submit a copy of the report to the nine sponsoring tobacco companies for review prior to publication. However, he insisted that there be an explicit clause in the contract relating to publication rights. This matter was to be decided later, after Austern had had an opportunity to discuss it fully with his clients.

The following suggestion was also made at this meeting:

> HTA [Austern] further suggested that AJT [Topol] should be present at any future technical discussions between Hazleton and industry representatives. {1807.08, p. 6}

In other words, a Covington and Burling lawyer was to participate in all scientific discussions about this experiment between Hazleton and the sponsors.

An interesting facet of the Chemosol story is Ed Finch's insistence that the additive be tested and developed as an industry-wide joint project. Finch may have felt this way for two reasons. In the United Kingdom BAT was part of an industry-wide consortium, the Tobacco Manufacturers' Standing Committee (TMSC), which was committed to the joint development of safe cigarette technology through its Harrogate research lab. Moreover, B&W may still have harbored memories of the reaction felt within the company when Lorillard had gone out on its own in 1962 and developed a filter that selectively removed phenols (see chapter 4). Eight other cigarette manufacturers agreed with B&W's position that Chemosol should be examined jointly, despite the fact that the joint development of a commercially important additive might have invited examination of this activity from an antitrust perspective (see chapter 7).

The documents provide no information on whether the Hazleton protocol was ever implemented or, if it was, what the results may have been. We are not aware that there was any further press coverage, either. There is no indication that Chemosol was ever used commercially.

What is certain is that nine cigarette manufacturers were willing to sponsor research on an additive that promised to reduce the risk of cancer from cigarette smoking; and this venture was coordinated by a lawyer who had worked for the Tobacco Institute. The record of the 1969 negotiation session about the protocol indicates that lawyers played a remarkably large role in discussions about the procedures for carrying out the scientific work. Moreover, there were plans for continued involvement by lawyers in the Chemosol studies at every significant step.

FREON

Tobacco used in cigarettes may be "puffed" or expanded by a variety of processes. Expansion decreases the mass per unit weight, which is one way to reduce "tar" delivery and total tobacco content of a cigarette. In the 1970s R. J. Reynolds developed a process called G-13, which used Freon-11 for expanding tobacco (11, 12). The process was used by RJR, Liggett & Myers, American Tobacco, and Lorillard. Only Philip Morris and B&W were not using this process as of mid-1977 {1309.01}. An undated and unsigned report, apparently reviewing toxicology studies conducted by RJR for B&W, indicates that in the 1970s RJR tested Freon-11 for its carcinogenicity in mouse skin–painting experiments and also attempted to determine whether Freon had any acute toxicity for the respiratory system {1309.04}. The report indicated that scientists at RJR found no evidence that Freon-11 was toxic under the conditions tested, but the report expressed reservations about these conclusions, since the data had not been evaluated by an independent, outside consultant.

A June 2, 1977, memorandum from Ernest Pepples, the general counsel at B&W, to Dr. I. W. Hughes, head of R&D, describes Pepples's objections to B&W's use of tobacco treated with the G-13 process {1309.01}. Environmental groups had filed petitions with the Consumer Product Safety Commission, and the Environmental Protection Agency was raising concerns that Freon could decompose into the poisonous gas phosgene (which had been used in World War I) when it was burned. The petitioners asked that Freon be banned from air conditioning systems because of this potential hazard. Pepples believed that the finding of phosgene in cigarette smoke might present an opportunity for a products liability claim {1309.01, p. 3}. Moreover, some scientists suspected that Freon could damage the ozone layer of the atmosphere. Pepples worried that the same thing was happening when the Freon residue on the tobacco was heated by the burning coal of a cigarette {1309.06}, although it was not then publicly known that Freon was widely used within the cigarette industry {1309.01, p. 2}:

> As we have previously discussed there are three problem areas in the use of the G-13 process:
>
> 1. The safety of the smoker particularly in light of the phosgene theory.
>
> 2. Safety of the workers at the site of the skid unit [where the freon treatment would be done].
>
> 3. The ozone theory which involves the safety of future generations of persons inhabiting the earth. {1309.01, p. 1}

Pepples also made a strong argument for environmental protection:

> There is another factor about which extensive comments are not needed. I refer to the morality of a step which would add 600 lbs. of F-11 [Freon-11] per day to the environment in the face of the already substantial scientific evidence that the chemical is actually harmful to the environment. {1309.01, p. 2}

Pepples recommended that other processes be developed.

A memorandum dated December 5, 1977, from Stanley L. Temko of Covington and Burling to the Committee of Counsel, a Tobacco Institute committee consisting of the chief counsels of the member companies, shared the news that the Consumer Product Safety Commission had denied the citizen petition "requesting a ban of 'Refrigerant 11' under the Consumer Product Safety Act" {1309.05}. With the threat of regulatory action against Freon diminished, Brown and Williamson began to utilize the G-13 process {1309.02}.

A May 1, 1978, memorandum from J. W. Webb, a research scientist at B&W, discusses the analysis of an expected shipment of expanded tobacco {1309.03}. Tests to be run included moisture content, glycerin content, residual Freon level, yield, percent fines, and fill value. These measures indicate that B&W was evaluating expanded tobacco made elsewhere for possible use. In June 1978 B&W signed a contract with Liggett Group to buy Liggett's excess capacity of G-13 processed tobacco {1309.02}.

CIGARETTES WITH "NOTHING ARTIFICIAL ADDED"

Cigarettes are more than shredded tobacco wrapped in paper. Additives are required for the tobacco, the papers, and the filter for a variety of purposes. The core need for some additives in modern cigarettes is revealed in a July 1977 memorandum summarizing a meeting at which B&W executives critically examined the claim "nothing artificial added" that RJR was then making about its new brand, Real {1311.01}. Real brand cigarettes had been launched by RJR in 1975, and a menthol version was marketed in 1977. Real contained glycerin (which could have been derived from natural sources) as a humectant; it also contained sugars (and possibly flavorings) for casing the tobacco used in the blend. The menthol version of Real might have contained natural menthol, but that was not yet clear to the B&W group.

B&W could match the RJR claim with a new brand if need be, and it could even use a claim of "all natural flavors." However, the use of "such artificial elements as cellulose acetate, plasticizers, freon, propylene glycol, humectants and some flavors" would preclude the assertion of a "pure organic" claim {1311.01, p. 1}. Propylene glycol, a manufactured chemical commonly used as a humectant by both B&W and RJR, could not be used in a cigarette claiming "nothing artificial added." Tobacco extracts were felt to be "nature identical" at best. Their use in a cigarette would preclude a claim of that brand's being "natural" {1311.01, p. 2}.

The observation that tobacco extracts are not "natural" runs counter to the impression sometimes given by tobacco companies that tobacco extracts are, simply, a form of tobacco. In 1988, when RJR explained its novel nicotine delivery device, Premier, to the scientific community, it described the tobacco extract used in the product as "spray dried tobacco" (13). This phrase was used to suggest that the extract was tobacco, just as certainly as tobacco leaf was. The contrary view expressed privately a decade earlier by B&W scientists in Louisville contradicts this contention.

EUGENOL

Eugenol, the active ingredient in cloves, is a local anesthetic agent. It is important for clove cigarettes (cigarettes made from a mixture of cloves and tobacco), which constitute an enormous share of the cigarette market in Indonesia, where BAT has long produced conventional, Western-style cigarettes in competition with clove brands. Traditional clove cigarettes have high tar and high nicotine yields and are made from dark tobaccos instead of the light or blond tobaccos used in Western-style brands. The dark tobaccos produce a harsher smoke, and it is thought that the cloves make it easier for a consumer to inhale the smoke because of the anesthetizing action of the eugenol (14).

B&W was using eugenol as an additive in its cigarettes in 1979 {1822.04}. Eugenol was approved as an additive in cigarettes by BAT's Additives Guidance Panel because of its successful performance in inhalation tests, Ames tests, and other tests from 1982 {1006.01}. The Additives Guidance Panel was an internal BAT group that met in London to review recommendations by its Research and Development Establishment on tobacco additives from various suppliers. Although the government in Jakarta forbade foreign companies from making clove cigarettes, Indonesian clove cigarette manufacturers had begun establishing markets for these products in Australia, Malaysia, and the United States by the early 1980s. This situation afforded BAT a potential market opportunity outside Indonesia for selling clove cigarettes. A summary of the toxicology of eugenol is contained in a 1982 report {1133.01}. This document may be the sort of report on which the Additives Guidance Panel based its decisions.

BAT's interest in eugenol was broader than the Indonesian market, however, and its conception of the pharmacological role of the compound was larger than the local anesthetic action. The BAT research conference held in Brazil in 1983 included a session devoted to eugenol

{1180.28, pp. BW-W2-03741–BW-W2-03742; 1180.07, p. 12}. The discussion centered on developing techniques for measuring eugenol so that its pharmacokinetics and pharmacology could be worked out. Of particular interest to the BAT scientists was its possible action as a central nervous system (CNS) depressant, one that was possibly synergistic with barbiturates and alcohol {1180.28}. The conference summary on eugenol states:

> Recognizing the potential for eugenol-flavoured cigarettes in countries outside Indonesia (eg Australia, Malaysia, USA), support was given for the proposed limited GR&DC [Group Research and Development Centre] programme to assess the pharmacology, biochemistry and toxicology of eugenol and its smoke products. *The study will include the possible interaction of nicotine as a stimulant with eugenol as a depressant.* Significant progress can be expected on this project within one year [emphasis added]. {1180.07, p. 12}

COCOA

Cocoa has long been an ingredient in American blend cigarettes. In the 1970s the National Cancer Institute's (NCI) cigarette testing program found that cocoa added to a tobacco blend increases the carcinogenicity of cigarette smoke condensate {1319.03}. While the results were not statistically significant, they prompted the British government to ban the use of cocoa in tobacco products. By 1983, however—after additional toxicological data were submitted to the British government's Independent Scientific Committee—the cocoa ban was lifted in the UK for additions of cocoa up to 5 percent of the tobacco weight {1319.03}

An article about cocoa came to the attention of senior executives at B&W in June 1984. The article itself is not in the documents, and it is not clear how it came to B&W's attention. General Counsel Ernest Pepples shared the article with B&W executive vice president Thomas Sandefur, who in turn passed it on to E. E. Kohnhorst, vice president of R&D {1319.02}. Kohnhorst asked Gil Esterle, B&W manager of smoking and health affairs, and Jim Rosene, a B&W research scientist, to analyze it {1319.01}. Esterle and Rosene gave their report to Kohnhorst by early July {1319.03}.

Esterle and Rosene's report confirms that cocoa is used extensively by the industry as an additive and summarizes the NCI findings that cocoa increases the carcinogenicity of tobacco smoke condensate. In B&W products, the report indicates, cocoa levels in cigarettes are about 0.5 percent and up to 5 percent in pipe tobaccos; Philip Morris and R. J. Reynolds use about the same amounts of cocoa, but Lorillard has replaced cocoa with a proprietary substitute. Lorillard's substitution of something else for cocoa had been verified by the absence of theobromine (an alkaloid in cocoa) from Lorillard brand cigarettes. The document continues:

> In the recent past, we attempted with only very limited success to delete cocoa from our cigarettes. Cocoa is incorporated in most of our new products. To eliminate cocoa from all our brands would be a multi-year, costly program, with all indications of minimal success as measured against competitors [sic] products that use cocoa. Consequently, *we recommend not actively pursuing a cocoa deletion/replacement program at this time. Rather the industry should defend the use of cocoa* [emphasis added]. {1319.03, pp. 2–3}

A handwritten summary of this report indicates that Kohnhorst shared the main points with Sandefur {1319.01}. So, even though Lorillard had successfully stopped using cocoa in its cigarettes, B&W decided not to do so itself because of economic concerns. The data indicating that cocoa increases the carcinogenicity of cigarette smoke did not seem overwhelming to B&W at the time, and there was no governmental pressure for it to make the change.

COUMARIN (DEER TONGUE)

Coumarin, which imparts a vanilla-like flavor and is a flavor fixative, was used as a food and tobacco additive for many decades. It was especially valued by tobacco product designers as a flavor booster in low-tar brands. Most commercial use was abandoned when it was discovered that coumarin caused liver damage in both rats and dogs and was suspected of being carcinogenic.

Some background on the B&W attitude toward coumarin is reflected in the January 1978 minutes of an internal BAT Additives Guidance Panel meeting on November 15, 1977 {1310.02}. The minutes indicate that numerous additives were approved for use, and that coumarin received special consideration:

> The Hunter Committee [an independent committee in the UK which advised the government on smoking and health] have now considered the Final Report from BIBRA [British Industry Biological Research Association, a report apparently sponsored by BAT (see below)] but were unable to approve levels as high as those recommended by the panel at their last meeting. The reason for this was that the Hunter Committee took into account not only the intake of coumarin from tobacco smoking but also that likely to be ingested from foods in normal diets having a content of natural coumarin. Accordingly,

for the United Kingdom: THE PANEL RECOMMENDS THAT WHERE COUMARIN
IS USED AS A TOBACCO ADDITIVE THE RATES OF APPLICATION SHOULD NOT
EXCEED

    (i)   525PPM FOR CIGARETTE TOBACCOS

    (ii)   1023PPM FOR PIPE TOBACCO.

While the limits by the Hunter Committee must be observed in the U.K. the
Panel saw no reason to modify their general recommendation of revised limits (740ppm for cigarette tobacco and 1500ppm for pipe tobacco) for other
countries, where no legal restriction is imposed. {1310.02, pp. 1–2}

In other words, BAT would observe the UK's prescribed limit on coumarin
for products sold in the United Kingdom but not for products sold
elsewhere.

On June 6, 1984, E. E. Kohnhorst, sent Thomas Sandefur a memo on
coumarin in response to an inquiry from Sandefur {1320.02}. In this
memo Kohnhorst indicates that R. J. Reynolds's Now and Vantage cigarettes had coumarin in them in 1982 and 1983, respectively, but the
1984 products no longer did, and efforts were under way to remove
coumarin from the "RALEIGH/FIESTA flavor package."

> Coumarin is specifically rejected by FDA for use on foods. This rejection
> was based on very questionable animal studies; but, the FDA has not lifted
> the ban.
>
> BAT sponsored a study by British Industry Biological Research Associa-
> tion [BIBRA] on coumarin. The BIBRA study, which is published, showed
> that coumarin is of no health risk in long-term feeding to baboons.
>
> Presented with the BIBRA results, the UK Independent Committee on
> Smoking and Health (Hunter, Frogget) lifted this past refusal to allow use of
> coumarin on tobacco products. This was published in the London Gazette.
> So, coumarin can be used in the UK and other areas under English influence.
> BAT (Germany) presented the BIBRA finding to their government decision-
> makers and were subsequently granted limited approval to use coumarin. This
> was with low delivery cigarettes (need flavor to induce good smoking qual-
> ity). There was the requirement to repeat the early studies on coumarin to
> show they were in error. This accounts for cautious, limited use.
>
> The BAT Additives Guidance Panel (AGP), since the BIBRA findings, has
> opened [opined?] that coumarin can be used.
>
> BARCLAY originally had coumarin (12 ppm), but it was removed from
> the flavor formula in November, 1982. Export cigarettes produced by B&W
> have not contained coumarin since June, 1983. We do not sell licensees/
> associates coumarin or coumarin-containing botanicals [emphasis in origi-
> nal]. {1320.02, pp. 1–2}

Two weeks later, C. J. Rosene wrote General Counsel Ernest Pepples
(with a copy to Kohnhorst) about coumarin substitutes {1320.01}:

There are no compounds or formulated flavors available to us that can accurately replace coumarin as a flavor on tobacco. Coumarin itself and natural substances containing coumarin are prohibited from direct addition to food as cited under 21 CFR [*Code of Federal Regulations*] 189.130.

Two homologs, 6-methylcoumarin and dihydrocoumarin, exhibit coumarin-like qualities on tobacco but neither can be used as a direct replacement. Both compounds are FEMA-GRAS but are not listed as approved direct food additives by FDA.

We currently use an IFF [International Flavorings and Fragrances, Inc.]-formulated coumarin substitute on BARCLAY. It does not match coumarin very well either.

Attached is a list of domestic brands containing vanillin, mace oil, and glycerin, added either as pure compounds or as part of proprietary flavors. {1320.01}

While FEMA regarded the listed coumarin substitutes as "Generally Recognized as Safe," the FDA did not.

The following month, on July 19, Dr. Sam R. Evelyn from BAT's research laboratory in Southampton sent Kohnhorst a packet of material from his files on coumarin. The material includes reports and site visits to labs conducting animal studies on coumarin as well as a letter from a pathologist at the FDA who had re-reviewed slides from a supposedly positive animal study of carcinogenesis; he had not confirmed the initial report of cancer but had confirmed that coumarin caused liver damage. While the background material Evelyn provided his colleague at B&W is generally negative or noncommittal, his letter indicates that current work with coumarin-feeding experiments was showing some instances of metastatic cancer in the animals. He speculated that such results would likely lead some countries to ban coumarin from tobacco products {1323.02}. Even though the United States had not eliminated coumarin from tobacco as of 1994, it did not appear on a list of cigarette additives released by the six major cigarette manufacturers (2).

DIETHYLENE GLYCOL (DEG)

Humectants, or moisturizing agents, are used in cigarette tobacco blends to assist with aerosol formation and thus make cigarette smoke "milder." The more that nicotine can be dissolved in the tar droplets, the less irritating the smoke is to the consumer's throat and the easier it is to inhale. Diethylene glycol, more familiar to most readers as an automotive antifreeze, was introduced as a humectant in cigarettes in the 1930s by Philip Morris.

Humectants were reviewed by BAT's internal Additives Guidance Panel in April 1965 {1310.01}. The minutes of the April 9 meeting make the following observations about humectants:

> Di-ethylene glycol After some discussion, the Panel members present agreed that because a) there is a known cumulative effect of small doses of this material in the kidneys, and b) there are some other doubtful aspects, it would advise against its use.
>
> Glycerol as a tobacco additive The Panel took the view that, although there was no known reason at present to suppose that this material should not be used on tobacco products, it should, in view of the observations (not supported by references) made on page 62 of the U.S. Surgeon General's Report "Smoking and Health" [the 1964 report] and because of its wide use in the Group, be investigated by R.&D.E. [Research and Development Establishment] both biologically and chemically.
>
> Propylene glycol as a tobacco additive The Panel agreed that this material should also be investigated by R.&D.E. both biologically and chemically. {1310.01, pp. 1–2}

The 1964 Surgeon General's report stated (15, p. 62):

> Cigarette manufacture in the United States includes use of additives such as sugars, humectants, synthetic flavors, licorice, menthol, vanillin, and rum. Glycerol and methylglycerol are looked on with disfavor as humectants because on pyrolysis [burning] they yield the irritants acrolein and methylglyoxal. Additives have not been used in the manufacture of domestic British cigarettes since the Customs and Excise Act of 1952, Clause 176, and probably longer, inasmuch as Section 5 of the Tobacco Act of 1842 imposed a widespread prohibition on the use of additives in tobacco manufacture.

Despite the recommendation from the Additives Guidance Panel, B&W was still using DEG twenty years later. In June 1984 R. H. Sachs, deputy general counsel for B&W, wrote to Ernest Pepples, J. G. Esterle, and C. J. Rosene about recent discussions between B&W and Union Carbide, the company that was selling diethylene glycol to B&W {1322.02}. In the course of the discussions, a Union Carbide sales representative said that the company had not known that B&W was using DEG in smoking products and that it would not sell DEG to B&W for this purpose. According to Sachs,

> Scientific references were cited to us as the bases for their action. Our scientists read the references, but could not see what Union Carbide was so upset about.
>
> We received a letter from the Union Carbide sales representative stating that DEG could not continue to be used on smoking tobacco because of health concerns, that Union Carbide would be glad to supply a substitute, and that Union Carbide only recently found out about our use of DEG on smoking tobacco.

I contacted the Union Carbide General Counsel to discuss the matter. After an investigation, a lawyer in his office called me to say:

1.   Union Carbide had absolutely no problem with our use of DEG on smoking tobacco or cigarettes.

2.   Union Carbide had mistakenly thought that we were using the product in <u>chewing tobacco</u>. They are of the opinion that the use of DEG in chewing tobacco would be a health hazard because it would be "ingested".

3.   The sales representative was in error in writing the letter. Union Carbide would draft a follow-up letter that we can review before it is sent. They are willing to cooperate in any way they can to rectify this situation.

While Union Carbide is satisfied that our continued use of DEG in smoking tobacco does not pose a health hazard, we should not let the matter rest there. If the "ingestion" of DEG applied to chewing tobacco is a problem (as Union Carbide seems to indicate it is), then how is it that they are so sure that its inclusion in smoking tobacco poses no problem?

We will look into this matter further [emphasis in original]. {1322.02, pp. 1–2}

The memo includes handwritten notations indicating that Earl (Kohnhorst) asked Gil Esterle whether the effort to eliminate DEG was continuing. Esterle replied that it was. He noted that DEG was not "Generally Recognized as Safe" by either the FDA or FEMA, and that it was not used in foods.

[I]f we need to someday release to government we will need to vigorously defend and public reaction would be negative (I don't trust confidential disclosures to government). We should replace but with a good match. {1322.02, p. 1}

The list of additives released by the tobacco industry in April 1994 does not include DEG (2).

Public relations seems to have become the guiding force for managing potentially toxic additives such as DEG, as it finally became for dictating how to handle matters related to the toxicity of tobacco (see chapter 4). The operative approach was that ingredients for cigarettes must be proven dangerous, and an acceptable substitute be available, before changes would be made. The usual expectation for consumer products, however, is that safety should be established *before* a product is used.

DISCLOSURE OF ADDITIVES

Since 1981 or even earlier, public health workers had been calling for legislation requiring that manufacturers specify the additives used in tobacco products. In 1984 they received a phantom of what they had sought. Section 7 of the Comprehensive Smoking Education Act (Pub. L. 98-474), passed in 1984, included the requirement they had been seeking—namely, that manufacturers must disclose the additives to the Department of Health and Human Services—but added conditions that rendered the "disclosure" virtually worthless: the additives were to be shared only as an aggregate list, quantitative information was not required, and the information was to be treated as a "trade secret" and not disclosed to any unauthorized person. The veil of secrecy that this useless provision imposed was partially torn down in April 1994, when the cigarette manufacturers, under public pressure, voluntarily released an additives list. The B&W documents provide some background on the industry's attitude toward additives and their disclosure.

LAWYER CONCERNS OVER ADDITIVES

From a legal standpoint, the tobacco industry has had good reason to be concerned about the potential hazards of additives. While it is one thing, in terms of products liability, to provide an essentially "natural" product to a consumer, it is quite another thing to alter that product by adding dangerous chemicals to it. For example, one might compare the difference between cigarettes without additives and those with additives to the difference between an apple that naturally contains arsenic in the core and an apple that has also been sprayed with DDT. The industry has generally defended products liability suits on an "assumption of risk" theory; that is, the smoker knew that cigarettes might be dangerous and assumed that risk in deciding to smoke. With the advent of the cigarette warning labels in 1965, this defense became even more formidable, because juries (who were unaware of the addictive nature of cigarettes) refused to believe that smokers did not know the risks they were encountering. However, those juries might have taken a different view if they had been told that the cigarettes smoked by the plaintiff were not merely made of cut, blended tobacco, but, in fact, contained numerous harmful additives that presented health dangers in and of themselves. There is also, when one considers potential health risks, a difference between an additive in its original state and an additive when burned in a cigarette. An additive that might be totally benign from a human health standpoint when in its original state might, nevertheless, be a serious health hazard when burned in a cigarette in combination with hundreds of other chemicals. Thus, even if the manufacturer of an additive had conducted sufficient testing to ensure its safety, a tobacco company using the additive in its cigarettes was still faced with the problem of determining the safety of the additive when burned in a cigarette.

Attorneys at B&W actively worked to keep abreast of the latest research dealing with cigarette additives. On December 26, 1978, Ernest Pepples sent a memo {1822.01} to Dr. J. G. Esterle, referring to an attached report (not in the documents) by the National Cancer Institute (NCI) on its bioassay of dl-Menthol for possible carcinogenicity and an attached list (also not in the documents) of chemicals being tested for carcinogenicity in the NCI program. Pepples asked, "When you have had a chance to look over the list please give me a call." Whether or not Esterle phoned Pepples, he did send him a reply memo on January 8, 1979, enclosing "a listing of chemicals which are included in the list of chemicals being tested for carcinogenicity in the NCI program and which are known or we consider likely to be present in cigarette additives" {1822.03}. Two days later, Pepples sent a letter to Fred Panzer at the Tobacco Institute asking him to "track" progress NCI had made in testing the very list of chemicals that Esterle had sent along to him {1822.02}. The list consisted of:

<u>Chemicals Which Are Currently Used</u>
    Benzyl acetate
    Cinnamaldehyde
    Eugenol
    D Limonene
    Safrole (mace)
    Titanium dioxide (filter tow, paper)
<u>Chemicals Which May Be Present in Current Additives</u>
    Allyl isovalerate
    Benzyl alcohol
    2,6 di t Butyl p cresol
    Cinnamyl Anthranilate
    Furfuryl alcohol
    Geranyl acetate
    Gums
    Isophorone
    α Methyl benzyl alcohol
    Propyl gallate
    Pyridine {1822.04}

Among the chemicals listed as being currently used, only cinnamaldehyde was named by the cigarette industry as an additive to tobacco in 1994 (2). Titanium dioxide is still used as a whitening agent for cellulose acetate filter tow, but it is not added to tobacco.

B&W'S POLICY ON TESTING ADDITIVES

In 1967 Dr. R. B. Griffith, director of research at B&W, informed a group of USDA scientists and other officials that they must test combustion products of residues in tobacco to be assured of their safety {1302.01, p. 2}. By the 1980s this sensibility is no longer evident in the documents. Rather, concern about the toxicology of combustion products is termed "unscientific" and is projected onto critics and potential regulators.

Dr. J. G. Esterle, manager of smoking and health affairs at B&W, wrote a memo to Dr. R. A. Sanford, vice president for R&D, on September 11, 1981, about a "suggested program for testing biological activity of our cigarette additives" {1314.01}. The proposed program first takes note of B&W's additive policy and a criticism this policy has received.

> B&W's policy on cigarette casing and flavoring ingredients is:
> "To be used as a casing or flavoring in any of our cigarette products, an ingredient added to tobacco shall meet one of the following criteria:
>> 1.   The ingredient has been used historically in cigarettes for many years.
>> 2.   The ingredient appears on an approved list such as the GRAS list (Generally Recognized as Safe) or the FEMA list (Flavor and Extract Manufacturers' Association).
>> 3.   The ingredient is a substance found in tobacco or tobacco smoke."
> Adherence to this policy provides B&W with a very favorable position in defense of our usage of flavors and casings. *Yet, the regulatory and anti-smoking agencies have identified, at least from a PR standpoint, a weakness. This is that the additives are potentially altered during smoking which may provide a new health risk to the smoker.* However unscientific this attack may be, we should be prepared to respond. The program, described here, is designed to provide that response [emphasis added]. {1314.02, p. 1}

These criteria permitted B&W to use any current additive, since only *one* of the criteria need be met and the first one essentially grandfathered all existing additives regardless of possible dangers. Moreover, the concerns expressed in the 1960s by a company scientist about the need to examine the combustion products of pesticides for toxicity are now instead attributed to outside, anti-tobacco critics.

The proposed solution was to conduct Ames testing of cigarette smoke from cigarettes, with the test additives added at ten to twenty times the normal level {1314.02}. The Ames test is a test of mutagenicity which has been used as a screening test to predict carcinogenicity. Other screening tests were considered but discarded as inappropriate. The concern seems to have been focused exclusively on the possible carcinogenicity of pyrolysis products of additives. Esterle suggests that each flavor formula for each brand be systematically tested. The initial wave of testing was to be completed by July 1982. The tone of this proposal is purely defensive. The impression one gets is that the purpose of the test is not to determine whether there might be real problems but simply to obtain data that might be used if the company were forced to describe the toxicology of its additives in connection with a lawsuit or if the federal government were able to require the disclosure of additives.

INTERNAL DEBATE OVER DISCLOSURE OF ADDITIVES

Two weeks after Esterle had formulated the defensive strategy for testing additives, J. K. Wells III, B&W's corporate counsel, wrote Pepples a "thinkpiece on the additives issue" {1316.01}. In his memo Wells summarizes discussions at a Committee of Counsel meeting held two days earlier. Representatives of B&W and five other companies attended the meeting and presented their views about disclosure of additives in the face of increasing pressure from the Department of Health and Human Services (HHS) and Congress. Wells describes the positions of the other five companies as follows:

RJR:	Continue meetings with HHS at the industry's initiation and two or three meetings from now submit to HHS a list of commonly used casings and flavorings which would include about thirty items.
PM:	Submit a list of about fifty items soon.
AMERICAN:	Submit a list of the most heavily used casings and flavorings at any time.
LORILLARD:	Stall any disclosure by industry as long as possible; industry should immediately appoint an independent panel of reputable toxicologists to review a list of as yet undetermined items.
L&M:	Stall disclosure and industry should immediately appoint one independent toxicologist to review a list. {1316.01, p. 1}

Horace Kornegay of the Tobacco Institute indicated that the pressure from Congress was based on the industry's failure to disclose. Stanley Tempko, a lawyer at Covington and Burling, indicated that an industry-sponsored review panel would lack credibility.

The memo lists a series of pros and cons regarding disclosure. In favor of disclosure was the argument that there are no known toxicological problems, only "uncertainty," and that disclosure would solve the problem and reduce congressional criticism. Against disclosure was the argument that this is part of a long-term attack, that "anti-industry activists" would use such a list to their advantage, and that adverse scientific opinion would form around the list.

The pros and cons of an independent panel are also enumerated in the memo. The approach avoids legislation and mandatory disclosure while improving the public image of the companies. On the other hand, "products liability litigation risk is increased because of the possibility that the industry appointed panel might conclude that certain additives have problems," and the panel is "unnecessary because the problem will go away if the industry simply discloses some number of its additives" {1316.01, p. 3}.

Bob Northrip, an attorney from Shook, Hardy, and Bacon, proposed that each company do a critical review of its own additives and discard those with problems:

> If company testing began to show adverse results pertaining to a particular additive, the *company control would enable the company to terminate the research, remove the additive, and destroy the data.* Hopefully, the company testing would be done prior to adoption of an additive, but if tests were made of an additive in current use the additive would be discontinued and eliminated from the C&B [Covington and Burling] list before HHS had the opportunity to make adverse comment [emphasis added]. {1316.01, p. 3}

Such a company-by-company sanitized list could then be channeled through Covington and Burling, the Tobacco Institute's counsel, to HHS.

Wells then puts forth the B&W position:

> Key factors in assessing the industry position on additives will probably be:
>
> (1)   The importance and possibility of improving the image of the industry's products through HHS sanction of industry self-policing.
>
> (2)   The assessment of the legislative and public affairs environment over the next five years.
>
> (3)   The assessment of the products liability risk.
>
> We cannot argue that there is no increased products liability risk inherent in the B&W position. However, the increased risk must be judged against alternatives forecast for the future. If, following disclosure, adverse scientific comment about currently used additives and the claimed failure of the industry to perform adequate testing prior to usage become major public affairs issues, the result would also be an increase in products liability risk. Is

it feasible to expect each of the companies to do review and testing of its additives and remove problematical additives from usage and from the list? If so, then the risk of adverse finding by industry toxicologists is substantially reduced. If not, then the Northrip scheme to prevent adversity subsequent to disclosure is not available.

There appears to be some confusion that the recommendation of an independent industry panel of toxicologists is primarily for the purpose of developing information about our additives. Of course, this is not the case. The industry panel is a formal mechanism for self-policing as part of an industry strategy to gain HHS sanction. The panel is not intended as a substitute for each company's own review and testing of its additives.

The best pitch for B&W's position on additives might be as follows:

The industry can improve public acceptance of its products through HHS approval of industry self-policing of additives. Self-policing will involve research at some point in the future when the research can be satisfactorily set up; immediately the formal mechanism for self-policing would involve only literature review and opinion. It is assumed that the companies will have done their own private review and research of additives and eliminated any which cannot be defended. {1316.01, p. 4}

One of the interesting aspects of the Wells memo is the weight assigned by Wells to public relations and marketing ("public acceptance of [industry] products"). Indeed, the tenor of the memo is that such considerations were deemed of greater importance than the products liability and regulatory concerns that were the lawyer's professional responsibility. Also striking is the suggestion that a panel might serve as a mechanism for self-policing, without having as a primary purpose the development of information about additives, and would instead limit itself to literature review. The industry panel seems proposed primarily as a means of maintaining the privacy—secrecy—of the past use of additives that "cannot be defended." The lawyers seemed to assume that such additives existed. (Indeed, the memo states that Bob Northrip assumed that four or five additives would have problems, not as his own assumption but "because it had been stated as a probability at the table" {1316.01, p. 3}.) If such additives were eliminated from any list given to HHS, then their past use—and the research on health effects—need not be disclosed. Indeed, the suggestion was that past use of toxic additives be affirmatively concealed by destroying adverse data.

The speculation in 1981 that disclosure would blunt criticism was validated in 1994. Following a crescendo of criticism in Congress and in the press about the "secret" additive list, the cigarette manufacturers released a general, overall list in the spring (2). A few days' worth of press stories followed, but little else came of the disclosure.

In the midst of congressional consideration of the bill that required disclosure of additives to HHS, B&W hired outside consultants to test its additives. The Additives Guidance Panel within BAT was to be excluded completely from the project. It is not at all clear that they would even be informed of the project. A note in the documents summarizes a conversation among E. E. Kornhorst; Dr. I. W. Hughes, a B&W scientist; Ernest Pepples, general counsel; and T. Sandefur, who would soon become president. The note, written by Kornhorst on June 8, 1984, reads as follows:

> We are going outside to obtain the best expert in toxicology/biological testing. The purpose of this effort will be:
>
> A.   To gain an understanding to develop protection for existing nontobacco additives in products.
>
> B.   To develop clearance for any new additives in new products or product improvements.
>
> Ernie Pepples and myself will be the only B&W contacts. Once an initial protocol is developed by outside consultants, we will review the same with BAT, given their high involvement with biological and [toxicological] testing. In addition to standard toxicology, the reaction product of combustion might also be considered.
>
> The current Additives Guidance Panel will not be involved in any way in this activity. {1321.01}

The documents contain no information about this program of toxicological testing, nor does the note indicate what exactly prompted this course of action, although the pending congressional action, as well as the revival of products liability suits at about the same time (e.g., the *Cipollone* case, discussed in chapter 7), may be more than coincidental.

CONCLUSION

A large number of chemicals are used in the growing, processing, and manufacture of tobacco. Residues of agricultural chemicals and chemicals added during manufacture contribute to the final product. Additives enhance the finished product in numerous ways.

From the late 1960s through the early 1980s, BAT's Additives Guidance Panel systematically reviewed additives. In the 1960s a B&W scientist expressed concern about the toxicology of combustion products of residues in tobacco. By the 1980s this perspective was characterized internally by some at B&W as "unscientific" and was regarded as a tactic by industry opponents in public health. Throughout the period, from the

1960s through the 1980s, legal, public relations, and regulatory concerns about agricultural chemicals and additives are evident in the documents.

The cooperative industry work on Chemosol demonstrates that the US cigarette companies could come together to investigate an additive that promised to reduce the cancer risk posed by smoking. It also demonstrates the central role industry lawyers had in guiding scientific research. The discussions about eugenol at the Brazil research conference in 1983 reinforce the evidence that BAT was interested in the pharmacological effects of smoking on its consumers.

The overall approach to agricultural chemicals and to additives reflected in the documents parallels that taken with nicotine and with health concerns about smoking. In the 1960s the companies honestly grappled with difficult technical issues, and the goal of a safe cigarette seemed within reach. By the 1980s, the documents were filled with defensiveness and concerns about potential regulations, public relations, and products liability.

REFERENCES

1. USDHHS. *Reducing the Health Consequences of Smoking: 25 Years of Progress.* US Department of Health and Human Services, Public Health Service, Centers for Disease Control, Center for Chronic Disease Prevention and Health Promotion, Office on Smoking and Health, 1989. DHHS Publication No. (CDC) 89-8411.
2. Tobacco Institute. *Ingredients Added to Cigarettes* Washington DC: Tobacco Institute, 1994.
3. Tilley N. *The Bright-Tobacco Industry, 1860–1929.* Chapel Hill: University of North Carolina Press, 1948.
4. Tso TC. *Production, Physiology, and Biochemistry of Tobacco Plant.* Beltsville, MD: IDEALS, Inc., 1990.
5. Spears A, Jones S. Chemical and physical criteria for tobacco leaf of modern day cigarettes. *Recent Adv Tobacco Sci* 1981;7:19–39.
6. American Health Foundation. *Comments on Tobacco Additives.* Valhalla, NY: American Health Foundation, 1990.
7. House Commerce Committee. *Cigarette Labeling and Advertising—1969.* US House of Representatives, Committee on Interstate and Foreign Commerce, 1969. Serial No. 91 (12–12A).
8. A safer cigarette reported possible. *New York Times* 1969 April 30:48.
9. Tobacco industry will aid tests on chemical said to cut cancer. *New York Times* 1969 August 31:43.
10. Wagner S. *Cigarette Country: Tobacco in American History and Politics.* New York: Praeger, 1971.
11. Voges E. *Tobacco Encyclopedia.* Mainz, Germany: Tobacco Journal International, 1984.
12. Hoffmann D, Hoffmann I. On the reduction of nicotine in cigarette smoke. In: Wald N, Froggatt P, eds. *Nicotine, Smoking and the Low Tar Programme* (pp. 200–211). Oxford, England: Oxford University Press, 1989.

13. R. J. Reynolds Tobacco Co. *Chemical and Biological Studies on New Cigarette Pro-
    totypes That Heat Instead of Burn Tobacco.* Winston-Salem, NC: R. J. Reynolds To-
    bacco Co., 1988.
14. Slade J. Nicotine delivery devices. In: Orleans C, Slade, J. eds. *Nicotine Addiction:
    Principles and Management*, pp. 3–23. New York: Oxford University Pres, 1993.
15. USDHEW. *Smoking and Health. Report of the Advisory Committee to the Surgeon
    General of the Public Health Service.* US Department of Health, Education and Wel-
    fare, 1964. Public Health Service Publication No. 1103.

CHAPTER 7

Legal Concerns Facing the Industry

I suggested that Earl [Kohnhorst] have the documents indicated on my list pulled, put into boxes and stored in the large basement storage area. I said that we would consider shipping the documents to BAT [outside the US] when we had completed segregating them. I suggested that Earl tell his people that this was part of an effort to remove deadwood from the files and that neither he nor anyone else in the department should make any notes, memos or lists.

J. K. Wells, B&W corporate counsel
{1835.01, p. 2}

INTRODUCTION

By the early 1970s the evidence of the health dangers of smoking had accumulated to the point of causing serious legal problems for the tobacco industry. The industry was being attacked on many fronts and faced increasing government efforts to regulate it in various ways. By the mid-1980s the industry also had to contend with a new wave of products liability lawsuits, filed by plaintiffs who were encouraged by the new significance attached to products liability law regarding toxic substances. If any one lawsuit could be won by a showing that the tobacco industry was responsible for the death or disease of a smoker, the eventual liability of the industry might bankrupt it. With this threat in mind, the industry's lawyers were working hard to protect against potential lawsuits.

PROTECTING DOCUMENTS FROM DISCOVERY AND ADMISSION AS EVIDENCE

The documents include a great deal of material written by attorneys for B&W and BAT. These documents—consisting of letters, memoranda, and working papers—indicate that the attorneys for the two companies, particularly those at B&W, took a very strong interest, and played an unusually active role, in the details of scientific research being conducted over the years into the health dangers of cigarettes. In the normal corporate environment, company scientists are responsible for conducting research dealing with a company's products; company attorneys confine their work to legal matters. Although attorneys are kept abreast of research results, they usually learn, after the fact, what the scientists have discovered. However, as the documents demonstrate, B&W's attorneys were thoroughly involved in planning, and in many cases directing, scientific research projects. Attorney control over company research apparently was deemed necessary to assert control over evidence produced within the company so that it could not be used to prove that the company's products were dangerous, even though the evidence developed by the company scientists clearly contradicted this view. The attorneys appeared particularly interested in preventing potentially damaging research results from being disclosed in litigation against the company, to the point of avoiding knowing the results at B&W of certain projects conducted by BAT {1132.01; 1824.03}.

The attorney documents raise a question of immense importance in litigation involving Brown and Williamson and the other tobacco companies: whether some of these documents, or similar documents not yet made public, might be protected under the "work product rule" or the attorney-client privilege from discovery or admission as evidence in lawsuits against the companies for fraudulently concealing the health dangers of tobacco from the public. (Discovery is the process by which a party to a lawsuit obtains information from the opposing party prior to trial in order to prepare for trial. It is generally permitted with respect to any matter that is relevant to the pending suit, but the court may refuse to allow discovery if, for instance, a document is protected under the work product rule or the attorney-client privilege.)

In at least three pending lawsuits against the major tobacco companies [*Butler v Philip Morris*, Civil Action No. 94-5-53, Cir. Ct., Jones County, Mississippi; *Castano v American Tobacco Co.*, No. 94-1044, United States District Court, Eastern District of Louisiana; and *State of Florida v American Tobacco Company*, Cir. Ct of 15th Judicial District for Palm Beach County, Florida, No. CL95-1466AO] in which the plaintiffs have sought to use the Brown and Williamson documents in evidence, the tobacco companies have claimed a right to exclude certain of the documents from evidence under the work product rule and the attorney-client privilege.

WORK PRODUCT RULE

In 1947 the United States Supreme Court established the "work product rule" to protect the work of an attorney in preparing for litigation. Under this rule, when a court orders discovery of documents that have been prepared in anticipation of litigation or for trial by or for another party, the court is required to protect against disclosure the mental impressions, conclusions, opinions, or legal theories of an attorney of the party concerning the litigation [*Hickman v Taylor* 329 U.S. 495 (1947)]. The rule is codified in the Federal Rules of Civil Procedure, Rule 26(b)(3), and is followed in most, if not all, states.

However, the documents might be discoverable, and therefore admissible as evidence, under at least two theories, despite the work product rule. First, a "fraud exception" to the rule has been recognized in a number of cases. This exception provides that an attorney's mental impressions, conclusions, opinions, or legal theories may be discoverable if there is evidence indicating that the attorney was involved in, or had assisted a client in perpetrating, fraudulent or criminal activity ["Fraud Exception to Work Product Privilege in Federal Courts," 64 A.L.R. Fed. (*American Law Reports Federal*) 470, § 2]. Thus, a document otherwise protected by the work product rule would be discoverable if, in the court's opinion, the document shows that the attorney who prepared the document was engaged in fraud or criminal conduct or was assisting a client in such conduct.

A strong case can be made that B&W concealed the health dangers of tobacco products from the company's customers and the general public. The documents clearly show that the attorneys and the company were well aware of many of the dangers of cigarettes, including addiction, at least thirty years ago, even though the company, to this day, continues to deny that cigarettes are either dangerous or addictive. As previously noted, the documents also demonstrate that the attorneys were thoroughly involved in planning, and in some cases directed, company scientific research projects. Apparently this was done to allow them to claim an attorney-client privilege covering the results of the research and shield the results from disclosure. Furthermore, as the documents reveal, on different occasions B&W attorneys specifically planned to have scientific research papers from BAT routed to the attorneys (ostensibly for use in potential litigation), in order to protect them from discovery. The documents also show that Corporate Counsel for B&W reviewed "behavioral and biological studies" to identify scientific documents that were "deadwood," with instructions to ship the "deadwood" out of the country without leaving any documentary record of the process {1835.01, p. 2}.

In addition, the work product rule protects documents prepared in anticipation of litigation, but its application requires a more immediate showing than the remote possibility of litigation. The probability that some particular litigation will occur must be substantial before a document may be deemed to be in anticipation of litigation, and the mere fact that a particular event has a likelihood of bringing about litigation at some time in the future is not a sufficient showing. The probability must be substantial, and the commencement of litigation must be contemplated at the time the document is prepared. Thus, advising a client about matters that may or even likely will ultimately come to litigation does not satisfy the "in anticipation of" standard; the threat of litigation must be more real and imminent than that. In order for the work product rule to apply, a specific claim must have arisen to make the prospect of litigation identifiable [23 Am. Jur. 2d, *Depositions and Discovery* § 53, and cases cited therein]. Although, even at the time of the earliest attorney documents, there was litigation against some of the tobacco companies with respect to the health dangers of cigarettes, nothing in any of the attorney documents marked "Work Product" indicates that the attorneys were contemplating a particular lawsuit against B&W, as opposed to the possibility of litigation against the industry generally in the future.

ATTORNEY-CLIENT PRIVILEGE

While the work product rule bars the disclosure of certain work of an attorney in preparation for litigation, the attorney-client privilege bars the disclosure of documents that contain confidential communications between an attorney and his or her client, and neither the attorney nor the client can be compelled to disclose them. Of particular importance with respect to the documents involving B&W's own attorneys is the fact that a corporation can claim the attorney-client privilege and prevent the discovery of communications made to house counsel as well as to outside counsel [23 Am. Jur. 2d, *Depositions and Discovery* § 30].

Just as the fraud exception may prevent application of the work product rule, the existence of an unlawful purpose prevents the attorney-client privilege from applying. The privilege does not generally exist where the representation is sought to further or conceal criminal or fraudulent conduct, whether past, present, or future. Thus, a confidence received by an attorney in order to advance a criminal or fraudulent purpose is beyond the scope of the privilege [81 Am. Jur. 2d, *Witnesses* § 393]. For example, communications between attorney and client having to do with the client's contemplated criminal acts, or in aid or furtherance of such acts, are not covered by the attorney-client privilege [§ 395]. This rule is equally applicable to communications as to tortious acts [§ 398], and, generally, where an attorney is consulted for the purpose of obtaining advice to assist in the perpetration of a fraud, or in the continuation of an ongoing fraud, the communications are not protected by the privilege [§ 399]. As explained earlier, the fraud exception to the work product rule might apply to the attorney documents; that exception might be applicable to communications for which the attorney-client privilege is claimed. For example, if it could be shown that a "Privileged" communication from a B&W attorney to a B&W executive were in furtherance of a fraudulent attempt to conceal the dangerous nature of the company's tobacco products, that communication would not be protected by the attorney-client privilege. In fact, as discussed below, that is precisely what a federal district court has held in a recent case against the tobacco industry.

FEDERAL COURT RULINGS

In at least two federal court cases, documents similar to those we discuss were ruled not protected from disclosure by the attorney-client privilege.

As discussed in chapter 1, B&W obtained subpoenas from the Superior Court for the District of Columbia, ordering two congressmen who serve on the House Subcommittee for Health and the Environment to appear in court and to produce the B&W documents in their possession. When the matter was removed to the United States District Court for the District of Columbia, Judge Harold H. Greene quashed the subpoenas. As discussed, he rejected B&W's contention that the subpoenas should be granted because the documents had been stolen by the individual who supplied them to the subcommittee. In addition, he rejected B&W's argument that the subpoenas should be granted because the documents had been obtained by the individual in violation of an attorney-client privilege [*Maddox v Williams* 855 F. Supp. 406, at 414, 415 (D.D.C. 1994)].

Whereas Judge Greene's rejection of the attorney-client privilege was based largely on public policy grounds—the right of the public to know the truth about the health dangers of tobacco products supersedes B&W's

rights with respect to the documents—the decision in the other case was based squarely on the fraud exception to the attorney-client privilege.

In 1983 a wrongful death action was brought against the Tobacco Institute and several tobacco companies. The plaintiff sought to discover various documents pertaining to the "Special Projects" program of the Tobacco Industry Research Council (TIRC), later known as the Council for Tobacco Research (CTR), and asserted the fraud exception to the attorney-client privilege. (For general discussion of TIRC and CTR, see chapter 2; for discussion of the "Special Projects," see chapter 8.) The plaintiff's general theory of fraud in the case was that the defendants knew of the dangers of cigarette smoking, concealed information that demonstrated the dangers of smoking, and affirmatively misled the public about the risks of smoking. As part of that theory, the plaintiff maintained that the tobacco industry had perpetrated a public relations hoax by advertising CTR as an entirely independent and objective scientific research body that would investigate the supposed hazards of cigarette smoking and report the results of those cigarette studies to the public. The plaintiff contended that, in fact, no meaningful research was conducted and that it was never the industry's intention to discover or publish the truth about the risks of smoking. In contrast to the defendants' promotion of CTR's "independence and objectivity," the plaintiff alleged that the defendants guided CTR to sponsor research tending to prove that other causes existed for the illnesses attributed to smoking, in an effort to perpetuate doubts about links between smoking and disease rather than to uncover the truth. In 1992 a federal district court ruled on the discovery issue and determined that the plaintiff had presented sufficient prima facie evidence of fraud by the defendants to warrant invoking the fraud exception to the attorney-client privilege [*Haines v Liggett Group, Inc.,* 140 F.R.D. 681 (D.N.J. 1992)].

Although this decision was later vacated by the United States Court of Appeals because of a procedural error [*Haines v Liggett Group, Inc.,* 975 F.2d 81 (3d Cir. 1992)], the district court's opinion by Judge H. Lee Sarokin includes this general observation:

> All too often in the choice between the physical health of consumers and the financial well-being of business, concealment is chosen over disclosure, sales over safety, and money over morality. Who are these persons who knowingly and secretly decide to put the buying public at risk solely for the purpose of making profits and who believe that illness and death of consumers is an appropriate cost of their own prosperity!
>
> As the following facts disclose, despite some rising pretenders, the tobacco industry may be the king of concealment and disinformation. [140 F.R.D. at 683]

Our analysis of the Brown and Williamson documents yields the same conclusions.

SPECIFIC STRATEGIES TO AVOID DISCOVERY

The attorneys at B&W and BAT routinely labeled their documents "Work Product" or "Privileged," to prevent them from being subject to discovery by an opposing party in litigation or from being admitted as evidence in a trial. The attorneys at B&W also devised two other methods to avoid discovery of sensitive information. One method was to develop special procedures for handling documents sent to B&W from BAT and affiliated companies, so that they would become privileged. The second was particularly ingenious: it was simply to remove certain documents and all traces of their existence from the premises.

SPECIAL PROCEDURES FOR HANDLING DOCUMENTS SENT TO B&W

To maintain the company's unwavering public position that there was no scientific evidence of any health dangers (and the implication from its silence that the company had certainly not discovered any in its own exhaustive research), the attorneys developed special procedures for the handling of internal scientific documents. These procedures were designed to allow the company to claim that the documents came within the attorney-client privilege. This use of the attorney-client privilege appears to have been very broadly applied to sweep up work that would normally have been conducted for scientific rather than litigation purposes. As such, the adoption of these private procedures to maintain secrecy seems completely inconsistent with the public claims made by the tobacco companies that they were spending millions of dollars on research for the scientific purpose of evaluating the safety of tobacco consumption.

The purpose of these procedures is explicitly spelled out in the memorandum that established them: a June 15, 1979, memo, marked "Restricted," from J. K. Wells, the corporate counsel, to Ernest Pepples. After describing the current procedures under which scientific materials from BAT are received at B&W, Wells states that he has not come up with any better ideas for handling the materials than Pepples had previously outlined:

> The [scientific] material should come to you under a policy statement between you and [BAT's laboratory in] Southampton which describes the purpose of

developing the documents for B&W and sending them to you as use for defense of potential litigation. It is possible that a system can be devised which would exempt the Engineering reports [which Wells has previously stated are almost never concerned with smoking and health] because it might be difficult to maintain a privilege for covering such reports under the potential litigation theory.

Continued Law Department control is essential for the best argument for privilege. At the same time, control should be exercised with flexibility to allow access of the R&D staff to the documents. The general policy should be clearly stated that access to the documents and storage of the documents is under control of the Law Department and access is granted only upon approval of request. A secured storage area of the documents should be arranged, perhaps in the R&D library [as opposed to the law library] and the policy statement would designate the same terms and conditions of storage for the documents as were spelled out for the literature retrieval service files [emphasis added]. {1824.02, pp. 1–2}

After suggesting that the documents might be divided into different categories according to how sensitive the documents are, the memo continues:

The abstracts of the documents should be circulated only for the less sensitive categories and then only to a list given prior approval by the Law Department.

The policy should explicitly make Dr. Sanford [director of research and development] the agent of the Law Department with regard to these procedures. {1824.02, p. 2}

These procedures would have put the Law Department in control of the dissemination of internal scientific reports.

Five months later, on November 9, 1979, Wells sent another "Privileged" memo to Pepples on the same subject. Evidently, the proposal in the June memo had not been adopted, because this memo discusses the problem as if it had just arisen:

I have discussed with Gil Esterle [International and External Technical Services Department] various alternatives for handling BAT scientific reports which come to B&W in a way that would afford some degree of protection against discovery. . . . One alternative discussed was that all BAT scientific reports would be sent to you [emphasis added]. {1824.01, p. 1}

Wells notes that this procedure would be cumbersome because the vast majority of the documents are routine—that is, not sensitive—and then states:

The cost sharing agreement between B&W and BAT, under which B&W pays for BAT scientific research and receives reports, is an obstacle because as presently written it would probably contradict the position that you were acquiring the reports for purposes of litigation. . . .

I recommend a second alternative, which would be that all BAT scientific reports be shipped directly to Dr. Esterle under a formal arrangement that Dr.

Esterle was assigned to be your agent for the acquisition of scientific materials in anticipation of litigation. Dr. Esterle would separate the reports which were relevant to smoking and health, or otherwise sensitive, for special handling as described below and place the routine reports into regular R&D circulation [emphasis added]. {1824.01, p. 1}

After explaining that this procedure would provide work product coverage for sensitive documents under federal and Kentucky law, Wells continues:

There would still be the matter of the cost sharing agreement. Regardless of the initial recipient of the documents, *in order to be covered by the rules of civil procedure they must be "prepared in anticipation of litigation."* Appropriate paper work should be established with BAT, including any amendments to the cost sharing agreement to establish that documents of a certain nature are prepared for B&W in anticipation of litigation. *I have in mind paper work which would make the statement as a policy between the parent and sibling, but that in the operational context BAT would send documents without attempting to distinguish which were and were not litigation documents* [emphasis added]. {1824.01, pp. 1–2}

These cost- and risk-pooling agreements are discussed later in this chapter.

More than six years later, on February 17, 1986, Wells sent another memo to Pepples, this time dealing with the question of whether B&W should receive certain scientific reports from affiliated companies generally, and how B&W can receive such reports without receiving information that would be useful to a plaintiff. The memo includes references to specific projects and notations as to whether B&W is interested in them. Wells summarizes his discussion with Esterle and David Gordon, controller in the B&W R&D administration, on this subject:

[W]e should approach these projects on the basis of whether the reports are limited to the information from good science and whether the information is useful in the United States market. *Our market is a "tar" and nicotine market, and information pertaining to other constituent delivery levels and biological effects will not be helpful.*

B&W will receive concise reports, estimated to be about one-half page in length, twice each year for each project it wishes to follow. While the brevity of the reports will reduce the potential for receipt by B&W of information useful to a plaintiff, disadvantageous information could be included and the reports could serve as road maps for a plaintiff's lawyer.

I have advised that we can receive reports from some of these projects notwithstanding the risk. The reason is that we cannot shut out the flow of information: the BAT will find ways to get information into B&W from the scientific projects it is running in its laboratories worldwide. The only way BAT can avoid having information useful to plaintiff found at B&W is to obtain good legal counsel and cease producing information in Canada, Germany, Brazil and other places that is helpful to plaintiffs [emphasis added]. {1824.03, p. 1}

The memo goes on to summarize the discussions among Wells, Esterle, and Gordon about eight specific projects, selected from a longer list (see table 7.1), in which the scientific staff had expressed initial interest. The list below includes the title of each research project, as described in the B&W database, followed by Well's comments:

> No. 430. [New/novel products: filter: aerosol testing (special cigarette developments).] Among things of interest, the project apparently intends to investigate the retention of smoke particles in the respiratory tract. *Such data could be used by the plaintiff. I have taken under advisement the question whether B&W should receive reports from this project. I propose to suggest to RD&E* [Research, Development, and Engineering] *that we ask for more information before we decide. The work will occur in Germany, and the German scientist who designed the program should seek counsel before providing the additional information. Hopefully, the problem area will disappear.*

TABLE 7.1   EXCLUDED PROJECTS, 1986

Country	Accession Number	Project Title
Brazil	39	Nicotine, Nitrate & Nitrosamine
	49	Va. & Bur. Blend Nitrosamine
Canada	313	Nicotine & Smoking Behavior
	331	Additives Biological
	324	Mainstream Biological
	329	Smokeless Products Biological
	305	Sidestream Irritation
	605	Ambient Smoke
Germany	430	Aerosol Testing
	440	Cuts Per Inch (CPI)
	453	Nicotine Within the Smoker
	441	Core Blends
	448	Smoke Indices
	469	Low Sidestream
	471	Degradable Filter
UK	493	Chemical Filtration
	514	Product Development & Innovation
	494	Nitrosamines
	495	Free Radicals
	500	Biology: Leaf Studies
	501	Biology: Ames
	487	Sidestream Visibility
	485	Ambient Smoke Nitrosamines
	496	Other Smoke Components

%Total effort excluded: 21% {1824.03, p. 3}.

No. 514. [Product development & innovation: smoking pleasure & satis-faction.] RD&E is interested because apparently the project includes work on better quality low delivery cigarettes. However, the description contains a statement that the low delivery is intended to "satisfy another identified con-sumer need for personal reassurance." The project will be done in the U.K. David [Gordon] will ask for more information about the work to be included in the project before requesting reports.

No. 487. [Smoke control: sidestream reduction: visibility.] *RD&E is in-terested in work dealing with sidestream smoke reduction, but is not inter-ested in the biological testing of products produced. David [Gordon] will ex-plain this to Allen Herd and ask whether projects could be run without biological testing.*

No. 496. [Smoke control: chemical reaction mechanisms: other smoke components.] *After discussion, RD&E is not interested.*

No. 313. [Investigation of the effects of nicotine enhancement on human smoking behaviour.] RD&E is interested in information which relates the "tar"/nicotine ratio to subjective smoke quality. *However, this project could produce data pertaining to nicotine such as pharmacological information which would be helpful to plaintiffs. RD&E will begin receiving this infor-mation, but will not be interested unless the work deals predominantly with subjective smoke quality.*

No. 331. [The influence of additives on the mutagenicity of smoke con-densate.] *After discussion, RD&E decided it is not interested.*

No. 305. [Sidestream smoke and irritation.] RD&E will receive these reports.

No. 453. [Smoker reaction/behavior: product testing: the influence of nico-tine within the smoker.] RD&E is interested in information pertaining to the role of nicotine in the smoker's subjective perception of smoke quality. *If the reports stick to research data, the reports would be interesting. However, if the reports include discussions of pharmacological effects of nicotine, the in-formation will not be interesting and would be helpful to the plaintiff. RD&E will begin receiving reports from this activity and be prepared to inform BAT to cease sending the data to B&W if the science is not interesting* [emphasis added]. {1824.03, pp. 1–2}

Wells ends his memo to Pepples with the following plea:

> I recommend you discuss the problems involved in the projects with counsel for the BAT companies involved. {1824.03, p. 2}

Apparently, the projects deemed not "interesting" to the B&W re-search and development staff were those whose results might be useful to plaintiffs in products liability cases against the company. Thus, research results from elsewhere in BAT aimed at cosmetic improvements (less visible sidestream smoke), reduced irritation (which makes smoking easier), and customer satisfaction were of interest to B&W, but results that might delineate the toxicities of tobacco smoke or the pharmacological properties of nicotine were to be avoided. (See chapter 3 for a discussion of the research at BAT that indicated the addictive nature of nicotine and chapter 4 for a discussion of the research that, in the process of BAT's attempt to produce a "safe" cigarette, confirmed the toxic nature of tobacco smoke.)

REMOVING "DEADWOOD" DOCUMENTS

At one point, Wells decided that certain documents should simply be declared "deadwood," removed from the company's files, and shipped offshore. (This plan to protect problematic scientific information from discovery by simply removing it is not unique. As discussed in chapter 6, in 1981 industry lawyers discussed a plan to protect from discovery scientific evidence that additives were dangerous by simply destroying it {1316.01, p. 3}.)

> I explained I had marked certain of the document references with an X. The X designated documents which I suggested were deadwood [were] in the behavioral and biological studies area. I said that the "B" series are "Janus" series studies [mouse skin–painting studies demonstrating that tobacco tar is carcinogenic; see chapter 4] and should also be considered as deadwood.
> I said in the course of my review of scientific documents stored by RD&E, a great deal of deadwood had appeared, such as studies of the chemical composition of Canadian tobacco leaf in 1966. {1835.01, p. 1}

Perhaps aware of the incongruity presented by the picture of a highly placed company lawyer volunteering to weed out "deadwood" documents from company files, Wells somewhat self-consciously states that his suggestions were in the context of moving RD&E to a new building and of building a reference set for smoking and health materials.

> I suggested that Earl [Kohnhorst] have the documents indicated on my list pulled, put into boxes and stored in the large basement storage area. I said that we would consider shipping the documents to BAT when we had completed segregating them. *I suggested that Earl tell his people that this was part of an effort to remove deadwood from the files and that neither he nor anyone else in the department should make any notes, memos or lists.*
> I mentioned that Carol Lincoln [a B&W librarian] had said that offshore research and engineering studies sent to B&W in care of Earl and Bob Sanford [vice president, R&D] during roughly last one year period had not been

sent to her for logging in and that most of those documents may be in the offices of Earl and Bob and would not be reflected on the list which I had reviewed. Earl said he would send all of the studies in his possession to Carol, who would make a list of the documents and send it to me for review. Earl suggested that I should ask Bob Sanford to do the same [emphasis added]. {1835.01, pp. 2–3}

There is no clear indication in the documents of the purpose of the lawyer's supervision of the "deadwood" removal. There is no indication in the documents that the file purge was in contemplation of any particular litigation or proceeding. The circumstances outlined in the memorandum suggest that this was not a routine disposal of useless documents. In addition to the personal participation of an attorney from the office of general counsel and the specific instruction that no records be kept of what was removed, it seems unlikely that B&W would pay to ship garbage to England.

RISING FEAR OF GOVERNMENT REGULATION

In the early 1970s, even as the tobacco industry was continuing its efforts to develop a safe cigarette (see chapter 4), it was feeling increasingly threatened by possible government regulation. As the ensuing discussion indicates, there were many areas of regulatory activity and the industry adopted various measures to forestall further regulation or at least to counter its effects.

A February 14, 1973, memo, marked "Confidential," from Ernest Pepples, assistant general counsel at B&W, to J. V. Blalock, director of public relations, asks for news clippings relating to "salient problems now facing the cigarette industry" {1814.01}.

The first concern is "Cancer." More specifically, the author sees three threats posed by the activities of the National Cancer Institute and the American Cancer Society.

1.   Increased anti-smoking activities by government officials

2.   Possible legislative action to establish more stringent limits on the tar and nicotine content of cigarettes, and

3.   *Increased educational programs to prevent young, non-smokers taking up the practice of smoking* [emphasis added]. {1814.01, p. 2}

Second on the list is "The Attack on Heart and Lung Diseases":

This newly authorized program, associated with the Heart and Lung Foundation . . . contains the same seeds of difficulty for the tobacco industry. The same forces and considerations for quick and easy solutions are at work in this area. The new law setting up this program also provides for an assistant director for health information who could easily seize upon an anti-smoking campaign to establish an activist record. {1814.01, p. 2}

The third salient problem listed is "Jurisdiction over Tobacco":

Renewed efforts will be made to include tobacco in the list of products coming under control of the Food and Drug Administration, the new Product Safety Commission, or the proposed Consumer Protection Agency. Should any of these efforts succeed, the industry would be seriously harmed since tobacco would fall under the same category as cyclamates. {1814.01, p. 2}

Cyclamates, artificial sweeteners that were regulated as food additives, were a then-current example of a material that had been banned from foods by the FDA because of animal evidence of carcinogenicity at high doses. The statement in the memo probably indicates concern that even though, according to the industry, the poisons in tobacco smoke were dangerous only in high doses, tobacco would suffer the same fate as cyclamates. Saccharine, another artificial sweetener, had similar, but less compelling, evidence against it, but it has been permitted to remain in the food supply with a warning label.

Fourth on the list is "Passive Smoking":

The anti-smoking lobby is using the issue of the alleged health effect of smoking on the non-smoker to generate media publicity. This trend has been growing since 1970. It received prestigious support when the [Supreme Court] Chief Justice [Warren Burger] made a public display of his annoyance with tobacco smoke on a passenger train. Similarly, the current issue before the CAB [Civil Aeronautics Board] regarding smoking on airliners is also part of the same campaign. There is no medical evidence concerning the health effects of passive smoking. The real purpose [of the anti-smoking lobby] is symbolic to make smoking socially unacceptable and by limiting the public areas where it is permitted. {1814.01, p. 2}

By the early 1970s, then—when the first systematic studies on the respiratory effects of passive smoking on children were just beginning to appear and nearly a decade before the first papers implicating passive smoking as a cause of lung cancer were published—B&W had identified passive smoking as an important issue. (See chapter 10 for a full discussion of passive smoking.)

The fifth item is headed "Implications of Biological Research." Here the author expresses concern about the publication of a study by W. Dontenwill and co-workers (1) funded by the German tobacco industry. The study demonstrated that inhaled smoke produced laryngeal cancer in Syrian golden hamsters:

> There is the likelihood that the Dontenwill work will be published in the U.S.A., and implied in this work are directions for product modification. This approach has some support by anti-smoking scientists in the U.S.A. and is likely to lead to political pressure of the industry to change products. Actions by foreign manufacturers will have effect in the U.S.A. {1814.01 pp. 2–3}

"Addiction" is also a problem:

> Some emphasis is now being placed on the habit-forming capacities of cigarette smoke. *To some extent the argument revolving around "free choice" is being negated on the grounds of addiction. The threat is that this argument will increase significantly and lead to further restrictions on product specifications and greater danger in litigation* [emphasis added]. {1814.01, p. 3}

Finally, "Excise Taxation" is listed as a concern because:

> It appears that the anti-smoking groups may find that one of the most successful methods of reducing the use of tobacco products will be the enactment of a high rate taxation on such products, since by this method tobacco products can be priced at a level so as to place the product beyond the financial reach of many consumers. {1814.01, p. 3}

That "many consumers" may be a euphemism for young people is illustrated by the following excerpt from the instructions for the document review project conducted by the law firm of Wyatt, Tarrant & Coombs for B&W (see chapter 1):

> If a document discusses or contains testimony of an industry representative speaking at a proceeding, it will receive a significance of "1" underline the issues being discussed are not related to smoking and health (e.g., fire-safe cigarettes). (Excise taxes are related to smoking and health, because taxes influence the price of cigarettes. *The price affects the ability of young people to buy cigarettes*) [italic emphasis added]. {1000.01, p. 28}

There is also a second concern relating to excise taxation:

> A second basis for attack appears to be the introduction of legislation providing for a tax level graduated on the basis of tar and nicotine content. {1814.01, p. 3}

Indeed, New York City had enacted such a tax in 1971, and just a few months after this memo was written, a New York County trial court upheld the validity of the tax and the accompanying administrative regulation requiring that cigarette prices reflect the amounts of tax attributable to the tar and nicotine content of cigarettes sold [*Long Island Tobacco Co., Inc. v Lindsay* 343 N.Y.S.2d 759 (N.Y. Sup. Ct. 1973)]. The court stated that the regulation was "clearly designed to preclude the seller from absorbing the tax and to discourage through higher prices the consumer's use of cigarettes with relatively higher levels of tar and nicotine" [at 763]. This case was subsequently affirmed without opinion by New York State's highest court, the Court of Appeals [*Long Island Tobacco Co., Inc. v Lindsay,* 313 N.E.2d 794 (N.Y. 1974)]. In 1976 a bill was introduced in Congress to tax cigarettes on the basis of tar and nicotine content.

Clearly, the author of this list of concerns (probably Pepples) was quite accurate about most of the items, and twenty years after the list was compiled, much of it is still relevant. While the scientific issues surrounding cancer and heart and lung diseases have long since been settled, and the industry barely makes a pretense of contesting the existence of these health problems, the addiction issue (in part because of the exposure of the documents discussed in this book) has become the new battleground. Whereas, in all the intervening time, jurisdiction over the industry by the listed federal agencies never materialized, it has now become a distinct possibility because of the addiction issue. (The FDA, however, had started to raise questions about nicotine addiction several months before these and related documents began to surface in the press in mid-1994.) The author of the list of concerns correctly forecast the problems to the industry from the passive smoking issue and the increase in excise taxes, but it is doubtful that, in his wildest dreams, he actually foresaw the enormous cost to the industry from the emerging nonsmokers' rights movement, both in actual dollars and as an influence on the public perception of smoking. It should also be noted that, while the industry has always fought even minimal increases in tobacco excise taxes, it has consistently raised the prices of tobacco products, often well beyond the rate of inflation.

Ten years later, three areas of regulatory concern—smoking in the workplace, the treatment of grass-roots lobbying, and fire-safe cigarettes—were the subject of a memorandum by R. H. Sachs, reporting on a meeting held on December 8, 1983, by the Committee of Counsel (a Tobacco Institute committee consisting of the chief counsels of the member tobacco companies).

Smoking in the Workplace—We discussed the draft of a model ordinance prepared by C&B [the law firm of Covington and Burling]. [Stanley] Temko [an attorney at Covington and Burling] lamented that suggestion to add language for some sort of "equal accommodation" for smokers was difficult. [Roger

L.] Mozingo [Tobacco Institute vice president] does not need the model ordinance at present. {2220.01, p. 2}

This memorandum was written just one month after the tobacco industry had suffered a major defeat by the passage of Proposition P in San Francisco, a referendum that ratified a city ordinance requiring that nonsmokers be protected from secondhand smoke in office workplaces (2). Numerous cities throughout the country were asking for copies of the ordinance so that they could replicate it, and the "model ordinance" referred to in the memorandum was undoubtedly being drafted by the industry as a countermeasure. The industry typically presents its own sham versions of nonsmokers' rights laws when faced with the possible enactment of meaningful legislation.

The memorandum also discusses the possible use of scientific studies on this subject:

Shook, Hardy [and Bacon, an industry law firm] reported on a Swedish case wherein descendants of a lung cancer victim were awarded compensation because of prolonged exposure to tobacco smoke at work. (I talked to Morini about this case. He was aware of it, and is presently checking it out.)

A settlement agreement is near in the Lee case (Mass.) [an action by a state employee seeking a smoke-free workplace, that was settled favorably for the employee] and an accommodation has been worked out in the Orange County (Cal.) case [reference unclear].

There was a deep split of opinion with respect to commissioning scientific studies, using Battelle, with respect to smoking in the workplace. B&W and Lorillard are in favor of proceeding. ATCo. [American Tobacco Company] is strongly against it. RJR [R. J. Reynolds] and PM [Philip Morris] both expressed grave reservations but were not in a position to give a final answer. It looks like it's dead. {2220.01, p. 2}

This discussion appears to relate to work that Battelle (a contract research organization) was conducting on secondhand-smoke levels in workplaces. Battelle had been funded to do this work through CTR Special Account 4 (discussed in chapter 8) during 1981–83, so the work appears to have been halted (the memorandum is from December 1983). Since Special Account 4 was administered by the law firm of Jacob, Medinger, and Finnegan, perhaps expenditures could have been made even if not all the tobacco companies agreed on a given project.

The tobacco industry's evolving grass-roots lobbying effort also commanded comment in the same memorandum:

Tax Treatment of Grass Roots Lobbying—Temko reported that the Treasury is still reviewing this issue and that it is conceivable that new regulations could be issued in the Spring. C&B will keep an eye on it. {2220.01, p. 2}

The tobacco industry has responded to the growing (and genuine) non-smokers' rights movement (discussed in chapter 10) by conducting its own grass-roots lobbying through so-called "smokers' rights" organizations (3–5). The tobacco industry's serious interest in this issue is yet another indication of how important and large an effort the industry was anticipating.

Another item in the list of concerns related to fires caused by cigarettes when they were inadvertently left to burn on a combustible surface, such as bedding or other furniture. Although a few cigarette brands have been found to be relatively fire-safe (including a B&W brand, Capri), in that they will either self-extinguish before igniting furniture or will not burn hotly enough to ignite an adjoining surface, most brands are not fire-safe. As a result, cigarette-caused fires are the leading cause of fire deaths in the United States. There have been various attempts at both the state and federal levels to legislate a requirement that cigarettes be fire-safe, but none has succeeded. In 1984 Congress passed a bill sponsored by Congressman Joseph Moakley (D-MA) that established a three-year research committee, the Technical Study Group, to determine whether a fire-safe cigarette was technically and economically feasible. In 1987 the committee submitted its unanimous conclusion that such a cigarette was feasible. Then, in 1990, another bill by Congressman Moakley established a new committee, the Technical Advisory Group, to oversee the development of a test method for determining whether or not a cigarette is fire-safe. In August 1993, on an 11-to-4 vote (the four tobacco company representatives being in the minority), the committee reported to Congress that it had developed a sufficient test. Thus, the requirement that cigarettes be made fire-safe awaits only congressional regulatory action. It is in this context that the discussion of this issue in the memorandum should be read:

Fire Safe Cigarettes—John Rupp (from Covington & Burling) reported that we are gaining some support from within the International Association of Fire Chiefs. In the past they have supported Congressman Moakley's bill [to require "fire-safe" cigarettes]. This year, after hearing a presentation from the tobacco industry, led by Dr. [Alexander] Spears from Lorillard, IAFC set up a committee to reconsider their position. The efforts we have put behind building a relationship with the organization may be paying off.

The companies agreed to proceed with an industry examination of ignition propensity in order to develop a model for a testing methodology. Scientists from each company will meet to discuss this. Covington & Burling will provide counsel at these meetings for the purpose of antitrust oversight.

Rupp reported on efforts to get a meeting with Moakley to see if there is any way to reconcile our position. There are two troublesome areas: federal preemption and trade secret confidentiality. On the first issue, our position has been to push for "perpetual" preemption. Rupp and others think this is unrealistic. Moakley has accepted the idea of some federal preemption and Rupp would like to see us accept 18 months after publication of the study. He is also seeking more flexibility on the trade secrets issue. He mentioned allowing information to be turned over to permanent Congressional committees "with some safeguards". Rupp would like to hear from each of the companies on this by the middle of next week. {2220.01, p. 1}

Whereas one might think that an association of fire chiefs would be the least likely organization to inhibit fire safety legislation, there is evidence to the contrary. The "efforts" expended to build a relationship between the industry and the fire chiefs consisted of the payment of money to provide services for the organization. Indeed, during the 1980s the tobacco industry provided millions of dollars in grants, equipment, and public relations services to the fire chiefs' association, other firefighter organizations, and numerous individual fire departments around the country, to enlist their support in opposing meaningful legislation regarding fire-safe cigarettes (6).

The legislation surrounding fire-safe cigarettes is another example of how the tobacco industry uses preemption as a general political strategy to limit its political exposure and liability. Preemption at a federal or state level protects the tobacco industry broadly from local activities, over which they have less control. Moreover, obtaining preemption only requires action by a relatively few powerful members of Congress or a state legislature, as opposed to dealing with a plethora of local jurisdictions. Indeed, as discussed later in this chapter, by the late 1960s the tobacco industry had accepted mild federal warning labels on tobacco packages, and, later, bans on radio and television advertising, in order to preempt possible state action with respect to consumer warnings and limits on tobacco advertising (7). The tobacco industry still uses preemption as a major strategy today, particularly in the effort to stop passage of local laws requiring smoke-free workplaces and public places.

STRATEGIES TO DEFEAT GOVERNMENT REGULATION

As the threat of government regulation of tobacco increased on several fronts, the tobacco industry developed several strategies for counteracting government action. The principal strategy was simply to create as much controversy as possible over the link between smoking and disease (see chapter 8). Beyond this, the industry also developed specific methods for minimizing the impact of legislation aimed at smoking itself (such as the requirements for warning labels and the disclosure of the tar and nicotine content of cigarettes) and legislation aimed at limiting smoking in public places and the workplace.

In 1976 Ernest Pepples, B&W's vice president and general counsel, composed a long, thoughtful analysis of the smoking and health controversy, entitled "Industry Response to the Cigarette/Health Controversy." Pepples begins by noting the means by which the industry has coped with the smoking and health controversy:

> *The tobacco industry has reacted to the challenge of the smoking and health controversy in the following ways:*
>
> (1)   *Produce more filter brands with lower tar delivery.*
>
> (2)   *Support scientific research to refute unfavorable findings or at a minimum to keep the scientific question open.*
>
> (3)   Conduct information campaigns against claims by the anti-smoking lobby.
>
> (4)   Voluntarily meet some of the demands of the anti-smoking lobby, such as agreeing to publish the FTC ratings on tar and nicotine in cigarette advertising.
>
> (5)   Corporate diversification to minimize the potential adverse financial consequences of the controversy on cigarette sales [emphasis added]. {2205.01, p. 1}

The fact that Pepples regarded filters and low tar as responses to the "smoking and health controversy" (item 1) contrasts with the industry's public stance that these innovations were made in response to "consumer demand" and had nothing to do with health. This memo is an explicit acknowledgment that these things *did* have everything to do with health. Tying the two together leads to the conclusion that filters and low tar have to do with health concerns of consumers, and to the extent that the innovations allayed concern without providing protection, they are public relations devices for a public health problem.

Pepples then spells out the role of the Tobacco Institute, the industry's trade organization, and the Council for Tobacco Research (CTR), the entity established by the industry purportedly to do independent scientific research on the health effects of smoking (see chapter 2):

> The Tobacco Institute, founded in 1958, has been the focal point for criticism of research that indicates a connection between smoking and health. The Institute has attempted to keep the opposition honest. It has carefully scrutinized the sampling difficulties and statistical deficiencies in the studies which allegedly indicate correlations between smoking and disease. The Institute

also has vigorously opposed governmental control of the marketing of cigarettes. This rearguard action has bought time in which the companies could
adapt to the challenge, i.e. change themselves (through diversification) and
change their products.

The Council for Tobacco Research (CTR) has dispersed over $26 million
through 1973. During the past 20 years the industry has committed more
than $50 million to scientific research related to tobacco and health. In De-
cember 1972, five cigarette companies including Brown & Williamson gave
a $2.8 million grant to the Harvard Medical School for a 5-year investiga-
tion of any specific effects cigarette smoke may have in the development of
lung and heart diseases. In 1967, over $12 million was spent in the United
States on smoking and health research. In 1968, the figure increased to over
$15 million.

*The significant expenditures on the question of smoking and health have
allowed the industry to take a respectable stand along the following lines—*

*"After millions of dollars and over twenty years of research, the ques-
tion about smoking and health is still open"* [emphasis added]. {2205.01,
pp. 1–2}

Pepples viewed CTR as a means of keeping the "controversy" alive, although the industry maintained publicly that CTR was an independent
organization whose purpose was to determine whether smoking is
causally linked to disease. In essence, therefore, the industry was spending millions of dollars on research so that it could make the single statement that "the question about smoking and health is still open."

The Tobacco Institute also was used for the purpose of prolonging the
"controversy." The instructions for B&W's document review project
show that the lawyers were sensitive to this issue:

Documents discussing or containing public statements made by TI [the Tobacco Institute] in its role as spokesman for the tobacco industry. *Pay special
attention to documents suggesting that TI was used as a vehicle for the industry's alleged conspiracy to promote cigarettes through the "open controversy" PR program; that industry-sponsored smoking and health research
was used for PR;* or that the industry monitored governmental expenditures
on research to make certain the industry outspent the government on research
[emphasis added]. (1001.01, p. 32}

In "Industry Response to the Cigarette/Health Controversy," Pepples
also discusses the strategy of preemption.

The tobacco industry wanted to prevent the chaos of nonuniform state and
local regulation such as affects the alcohol industry. *To gain one crucial cost-
saving objective, uniform regulation, the industry compromised by adding a
health warning to the cigarette package. Another critic noted that "the label
might even be a boon of sorts, providing a new defense for the industry"* when

new health suits were brought by persons claiming to have been injured by cigarette smoking.

The broadcast ban which was enacted by Congress in 1969 called for the elimination of all TV and radio cigarette advertising after January 1, 1971 as well as strengthening the cautionary statement. The bill extended the preemption of state and/or local health regulation until June 1971. *The tobacco industry did not oppose the 1969 or the 1965 enactments* [requiring warning labels on cigarettes] *which were in some ways victories* [emphasis added]. {2205.01, p. 6}

Indeed, the tobacco industry testified in favor of the federal broadcast ban on cigarette advertising in July 1969.

Pepples concludes his 1976 analysis with a discussion of the implications for the tobacco industry of the disjointed nature of the federal government's regulatory authorities:

Some Conclusions and Observations

The foregoing discussion illustrates that the federated nature of the U.S. political system and the fragmentation of governmental authority and administrative responsibility are important in determining the type of governmental response.

The Congress is not staffed adequately nor is it properly structured to deal on a comprehensive basis with the medical aspects of the smoking controversy.

The independent regulatory bodies in the United States have been established to accomplish government regulation in technical areas. The FTC [Federal Trade Commission], FCC [Federal Communications Commission] and FCPSC [Federal Consumer Product Safety Commission] have been on very doubtful statutory ground in treating the smoking/health issue. They have been slowed by the limits in the procedures found in their statutory charter. As a result broad consideration of the smoking/health problem has been made difficult. Compared with public agencies in other countries they have been relatively free, however, to respond to the problem.

The FTC and FCC actions in this area have been unexpected and precedent-setting. They have mainly stemmed from the efforts of individual personalities. While the agencies have taken a high profile attitude, they have not had the power to act on issues of this type which lie outside their expertise and outside their legislative mandates. *Congress has not extended their mandates to deal with the smoking/health problem and in fact has expressly prevented proposed agency actions from taking effect.* In addition to the FTC, FCC and FCPSC the Departments of Agriculture, Treasury and Health, Education and Welfare have all dealt with portions of the total picture. A disjointed nature of governmental response has been augmented by the multiplicity of possible places where the action could occur [emphasis added]. {2205.01, pp. 6–7}

Pepples is saying, in effect, that Congress should not play a major role in tobacco control but should leave it up to an agency that is properly structured. When discussing potential regulatory agencies, he does not mention the FDA.

Pepples continues:

> Each agency is affected by interest group pressures that oppose compromise and cooperation with its opponents. For example, U.S. tobacco price supports and export subsidies are two programs (the latter begun after the Surgeon General's Report) that have been criticized as being in direct conflict with the government's smoking and health program. Also in Britain the Exchequer has been notably reluctant to give up tobacco taxes from cigarette smokers.
>
> The oversight by Congress of its departments is not effective in resolving differences between departments. Each pressure group struggles to define the issue in its own terms so that the goals and actions of government will be congruent with its desires. The Treasury has sought to collect revenues, Agriculture has sought to maintain and increase employment, income and productivity of farmers while the health interests have sought to reduce disease. The antismoking forces were able to gain a foothold in the FAA [Federal Aviation Administration], FCC and FTC and in the Department of Health, Education and Welfare. *The fact that one hand of the government does one thing and another hand does something quite different reflects the division of authority and responsibility which has made each agency vulnerable to the narrow interests of particular pressure groups* [emphasis added]. {2205.01, p. 7}

There is a certain irony in Pepples's complaint about the multitude of government agencies involved in regulating tobacco and their disjointed efforts. Had a single federal agency been given the power to regulate tobacco in a comprehensive manner, its coordinated approach might well have resulted in much stricter control of tobacco. Had regulation been consistent, we would not have had federal price supports for tobacco growers, and tobacco exports would not have been subsidized under the Food for Peace program along with programs to discourage smoking.

Pepples continues,

> Smoking and health as a political issue has been unpopular with all but a few politicians regardless of political party persuasions or country. Not only have strong economic interest groups opposed government action but a substantial portion of adult population indulge in the habit and derive significant pleasure from the use of the product. While it is reasonable to assume that the public desires good health, it is not reasonable to assume that the public at large and especially the cigarette smoking public is favorable toward antismoking measures that entail giving up the pleasures of smoking. {2205.01, p. 7}

These views were supported by decades of experience. However, not long after this paper was written, some politicians, particularly at the local level, began to take up the cause of nonsmokers' rights and to react favorably to the idea of restrictions on public smoking.

Pepples, moreover, miscalculated the reaction of smokers to restrictions on public smoking. Polls over the past twenty years have consistently shown majority support among smokers for such restrictions. Many smokers view limitations on smoking as a way to help them quit, or at least reduce their consumption, and many also understand the need to control tobacco smoke pollution for the sake of others.

Pepples next discusses the impact of the efforts to regulate cigarette advertising on cigarette consumption:

> So far government efforts to regulate cigarette advertising have constituted the main thrust of government concern and the aggressive antismoking lobby is highly dissatisfied with the impact such efforts have had on total consumption. (The following page [not in the documents] shows in chart form the general upward trend in cigarette sales but suggests a significant loss of volume due to political factors.) *The reduction in cigarette advertising seems to have made the industry stronger economically. Profits have increased. The ban on television and other broadcast advertising does not seem to have reduced consumption. The concomitant reduction in the number of anti-cigarette commercials is considered to be a severe loss in the effort to keep public concern and awareness of the controversy at a fever pitch* [emphasis added]. {2205.01, p. 8}

Pepples then specifies the legitimate government role in regulating tobacco as a public health problem.

> *Like the meat industry* [because of muckrakers who demanded USDA regulation early in the century] *and recently the automobile industry* [because of Ralph Nader], *tobacco products are now coming under close scrutiny and governments are attempting to establish control over the products, as opposed to merely the advertising, to protect the public.*
>
> The warnings, the tar and nicotine ratings and the anti-cigarette commercials were all part of the effort to educate children and cigarette consumers not to smoke. Implicit in the policy of education is the idea that the consumers should make the basic decision and will make the "right" decision, provided they are given "more knowledge." In short, inform the public, and rely on an informed public to change the pattern of consumption. The government has not yet intervened directly to change the content of the product or limit its use. *The protection of nonsmokers also has become an important and growing focus of the antismoking lobby with the announced purpose of making cigarette smoking an unacceptable social custom which they compare to spitting.* At least 26 bills have been added to some 70 antismoking proposals in state legislatures for action in 1976, involving 26 states. Characteristically these measures would restrict the places where smoking may lawfully occur.
>
> It is clear, however, that many anti-cigarette zealots and some public officials believe that the responsibility of the government does not end with merely warning the public of the hazards. They advocate direct intervention. Senators [Edward] Kennedy (D-MA) and [Gary] Hart [D-CO] recently [in

1976] proposed a health research bill to be financed by a tax related to the tar and nicotine content of cigarettes. At about the same time, the British Minister of Health announced on national television that he intended to lay an order before Parliament bringing additives and substitutes under the Medicines Act, which order must be approved by resolution of each House.

The tobacco industry, of course, would prefer no regulation at all. *If there must be regulation, the industry is probably better off to have it at the federal level than be forced to fight off a multitude of nonuniform regulatory efforts at the state, county and town levels.* Even expanded regulatory efforts may be shaped by the industry to enhance stability in the market or by individual manufacturers to bolster market positions—for example, by capitalizing on official tar and nicotine ratings in cigarette advertising.

The manufacturers' marketing strategy has been to overcome and even to make marketing use of the smoking/health connection. Individual tobacco companies have benefited from government actions. Thus the "tar derby" in the United States resulted from industry efforts to cater to the public's concern and to attract consumers to the new filtered brands. The heavy use of television in the introduction of WINCHESTER [a cigarette-like little cigar made by R. J. Reynolds] represented a bald exploitation of the little cigar loophole in the broadcast ban law. The current duel between TRUE and VANTAGE and between CARLTON and NOW are other examples of competitive efforts to capitalize on the smoking/health controversy.

Market conditions are important in determining company response. In a rapidly changing cigarette market, it is difficult to obtain industry cooperation because cooperation tends to affect individual firms unevenly [emphasis added]. {2205.01, pp. 8–9}

In effect, preemption allowed the industry to accept certain defeats, while at the same time limiting the damage. Indeed, as Pepples noted, the radio and television advertising ban, which might have appeared at first to be a crippling blow to the industry, actually turned into an unforeseen advantage. As important as preemption was to the industry with respect to the issues discussed by Pepples in 1976, it was to become an even more crucial tactic for the industry in its battle against legislation regulating environmental tobacco smoke. In that battle the industry has focused on passing weak laws at the state level (where the industry has great political clout) that preempt stronger ordinances passed by cities and counties (where industry influence is relatively weak).

LEGAL CHALLENGES TO REGULATION

On August 14, 1978, Ernest Pepples sent a "Privileged" memorandum to several high executives at the company regarding a paper entitled "Up from the Bombshelter," which was written by Charles Morgan, a noted

civil rights attorney in the 1960s, who later represented the tobacco industry. Although the documents include only a tiny fragment of the paper, we know from those fragments and from Pepples's memo that Morgan believed the industry should adopt aggressive legal measures to
challenge government regulation of tobacco. For example, at one point,
Morgan states:

> We recommend the initiation of litigation to strike down legislation which
> forbids private property owners to allow free and unrestricted assembly by
> smokers in their businesses, restaurants, hotels, bars, stores, and similar fa-
> cilities. {2211.01, p. 57}

Pepples explained that the paper had been reviewed and discussed by the
Committee of Counsel, a Tobacco Institute committee consisting of the
chief counsel of the tobacco companies, and by Horace Kornegay, then
president of the institute, and that the memo dealt "with the main cur-
rents of the deliberations arising from [the] paper" {2210.01}.

In his analysis of Morgan's paper, Pepples notes:

> Although some of the specific recommendations in Morgan's paper seem im-
> practical, there is already wide agreement with one of his underlying ideas;
> namely, that now it has become timely for the industry to adopt a more ag-
> gressive stance in objection to some of the anti-industry measures being pro-
> posed. {2210.01}

Pepples then explains that challenging the Federal Trade Commission's
attempts to impose further restrictions on cigarette advertising is a
worthwhile endeavor because the industry has a reasonable chance of
prevailing and there is "genuine value to be gained by winning":

> The hard part is to find the right thing to stand and fight about and the right
> time and place to do so. The FTC wants to do something more about ciga-
> rette advertising because the display of the health warning in advertising has
> not been sufficiently "effective." By effective the FTC means a reduction in
> sales of cigarettes. The Commission attack will be founded on the now fa-
> miliar premise that cigarette advertising tends to overcome the effect of the
> Surgeon General's warning and in so doing the advertising amounts to an un-
> fair practice within the meaning of Section 5 of the FTC Act.
>
> We can fight on that battlefield. We have a good argument and we will
> not be alone. The First Amendment issue is raised by the attempts to regulate
> the commercial expression on the vague ground of "unfairness." Here the
> FTC goes far beyond the familiar notions of falsity, deceit and misrepresen-
> tation. There is no lie or deceit present in cigarette advertising, whether you
> view the words alone or as a whole with the imagery. The FTC has to make
> its case in the mushy area of "unfairness." While "unfairness" under the Act
> may prove a flexible tool in regulating conduct, such as bait-and-switch

practices, the attempts to use it for the expansive regulation of the substance of expression contained in advertising runs right up against First Amendment considerations.

Another important legal issue concerns the res judicata effect to be given to the 1972 Consent Order under which the Surgeon General's warning is required in cigarette advertising. The Consent Order was based on a broad-ranging complaint that covers almost all of what the Commission is likely to come up with the next time around. Whatever legal validity and strength the FTC contentions in that complaint may have had, they should be taken as settled and not be open for relitigation time and time again [emphasis in original]. {2210.01, pp. 1–2}

Res judicata is a legal term meaning, literally, a thing that is definitely settled by judicial decision. When that is the case, the issue—in this instance the effect of the Surgeon General's warning—may not be opened up again by the same court or another court. Thus, Pepples is saying that the 1972 Consent Order settled all the issues relevant to the order and that the FTC contentions surrounding the order should receive no further hearing.

These are "good" legal issues, there is a reasonable chance of prevailing, and there is a great deal of genuine value to be gained by winning. Moreover the issues are sufficiently basic and of broad applicability that the industry will not necessarily be standing out there alone. For example, as to the First Amendment issue the makers of sugared cereals are already locked in battle, and the beer industry may soon be, on some of the same grounds as those that will be of concern to the cigarette industry. {2210.01, p. 2}

However, there were two important areas of concern that the attorneys did not believe were worth pursuing, despite Morgan's recommendations. The first of these was the ban on broadcast advertising on cigarettes, which the attorneys believed could not be challenged successfully on constitutional grounds and, in any event, was not worth fighting about:

He [Morgan] also says that the time is right for attacking the broadcast ban on cigarette advertising, again resting his arguments in the federal constitution.

With respect to Morgan's ideas about the broadcast ban, the First Amendment issues are theoretically interesting. The ban is a clear restriction of expression. *The Court has recently affirmed that commercial forms of expression are protected by the First Amendment. But we are the wrong industry and this is the wrong issue on which to try to enlarge on this new-found constitutional protection for advertising.* The Court has left many questions about the protection of commercial speech unanswered and this might be a very bad case to bring on early, before the Court has developed the rule more fully. *The Court has already hinted that mere product advertising may enjoy the lowest degree of protection. Add to the foregoing factors that the case involves issues of the public health and the protection of children and one can see that a negatively-inclined Court would have plenty of ammunition to use against the First Amendment argument.*

Judges are only people and people are not favorably inclined toward this industry. On crucial points in the debate, the public opinion percentage scores against the industry read like a thermometer in July. Over 90 do not believe anything we say. Over 90 think cigarettes are dangerous. Even among smokers we lose. People say they want to quit. In an unaided poll a strong majority said that public smoking should be banned. *About half of the people believe that ambient smoke is hazardous. With these kinds of attitudes floating around, Courts will likely be very negative toward cigarette advertising and any First Amendment argument which is advanced to get cigarettes back on TV* [emphasis added]. {2210.01 pp. 2–3}

This frank assessment of the unpopularity of the tobacco industry and the extent to which the public was aware of the dangers of smoking for both smokers and nonsmokers indicates that the industry was far ahead of most politicians of the day in these realizations. In 1978 it was still only a rare politician who understood the industry's credibility problems and was willing to stand up to it. Pepples continues:

We have some discouraging history in this regard too. When the industry tried to impose the Fairness Doctrine in reverse—giving tobacco companies a right to reply to free anti-cigarette ads—Lewis Powell [an attorney at the time, who later became a justice of the Supreme Court] was hired and brought the case in the friendly 4th Circuit [of the US Court of Appeals]. Although it should have been won, the case was lost. It's bad law but there it is.

Even if the broadcast ban now were struck down, the pressures from government and non-government sources for counterads would be tremendous. The Fairness Doctrine may no longer require stations to carry anti-ads, as Morgan notes, but it certainly doesn't forbid stations to do so. The resumption of advertising on television would almost certainly be accompanied by the return in force of anti-smoking announcements [emphasis added]. {2210.01, p. 3}

Since the television and radio advertising ban was upheld in court, Pepples was undoubtedly correct in his assessment that it was not worth challenging. More recently, however, the advertising issue has shifted dramatically: there has been serious discussion of banning cigarette advertising altogether or of severely restricting its content. In August 1995 the FDA proposed a moderate set of restrictions designed to reduce the appeal of cigarettes and smokeless tobacco products to children and adolescents (8). The industry, of course, does not view such restrictions in the same way it did the broadcast ban. After the broadcast ban it merely shifted its advertising to another medium, and it vigorously opposes any across-the-board restrictions or prohibitions.

In addition, Pepples rejects the notion that restrictions on public smoking are unconstitutional:

> Similarly the recommendation for a wave of industry sponsored litigation attacking the constitutionality of public smoking ordinances is not convincing. A basic fallacy in Morgan's arguments is the assumption that the case involves an issue concerning the right of assembly and association. None of the anti-smoking ordinances in fact restricts a smoker's right of association or assembly. None of them exclude smokers from any place or infringe the rights of smokers to associate with whom they choose and assemble where they please. Instead they regulate activity or conduct. The ordinances do invoke the police power to restrict the activity of smoking in certain places.
>
> A second major fallacy is the failure to recognize this police power aspect. *The states have extensive authority to regulate the use of privately owned commercial property especially where questions of public health and safety are concerned.*
>
> With respect to the litigation recommended, the chances for success are relatively slight and with a small chance of winning, the prizes to be won would be practically valueless. If an anti-smoking ordinance is knocked down the most likely result would be the environmental protection "No Smoking" signs would be taken down and Fire Marshall's "No Smoking" signs would be put back up. No doubt the anti-smoking ordinances cover a somewhat broader group of public places than the Fire Marshall's have traditionally covered, but the Fire Marshall's authority is broad and could be more widely exercised in the future. One has to conclude, therefore, that the practical effort of a victory over the anti-smoking ordinances would be something less than sweeping [emphasis added]. {2210.01, pp. 3–4}

This analysis is particularly interesting for two reasons. First, it provides further evidence that the industry recognized nonsmokers' rights and clean indoor air as crucial issues in 1978, long before the mainstream health establishment did. Second, it indicates that the industry's chief lawyers agreed that they could not challenge a clean indoor air law on constitutional grounds; thus, they clearly conceded that public smoking is not a constitutionally protected right. Pepples's recognition that public smoking laws regulate conduct and do not interfere with constitutional freedoms is in sharp contrast with the position the tobacco industry has consistently taken when opposing the passage of such laws. In fact, the industry always frames the issues in terms of the effect of a proposed law on the "rights" of smokers (chapter 10).

PRODUCTS LIABILITY CONCERNS

Under products liability law, the manufacturer of a product, as well as other entities in "the stream of commerce" linking the manufacturer to the consumer, may be held liable for injuries sustained by the consumer as a result of some defect in the product caused by negligent manufacture or design. Under the doctrine of strict products liability, the manufacturer may be held liable even in the absence of negligence, as long as the product was defective and the defect caused the injury. The tobacco manufacturers were not concerned with products liability until the link between smoking and disease could be established, but when that link was finally forged, products liability litigation threatened the very existence of the industry.

Prior to the products liability litigation that began in the 1990s, there had been two waves of litigation against the tobacco industry (9). The first wave began in the mid-1950s, after the evidence of a relationship between smoking and lung cancer was published, and it lasted for about a decade. The second wave began in the mid-1980s, when public concern over health and the environment had reached a new peak and products liability law regarding toxic substances had taken on a new significance.

Many of the cases in the first wave were abandoned by the plaintiffs, who simply ran out of money after being worn down by the tobacco industry's use of procedural tactics to cause endless delays and obstacles. Of the cases that did proceed to trial, most were decided in favor of the defendant tobacco companies on grounds that they could not foresee any risks associated with the use of their product. In one major case, however, following rulings by an appellate court that favored the plaintiff and forced a new trial, the defendant won at the second trial by convincing the jury that the plaintiff had assumed the risk of contracting lung cancer.

In the second wave, the industry continued its successful procedural tactics. One of those tactics was to resist all discovery of tobacco industry documents and then to obtain confidentiality orders on materials finally produced, so as to prevent the information from being shared with other plaintiffs. The second wave of cases failed to produce a clearcut victory for a plaintiff. They foundered on a variety of legal theories, including preemption of state tort law by the federal Cigarette Labeling and Advertising Act of 1965, which required warning labels to be placed on all cigarette packages, and the lack of proof that cigarette smoking was the cause of the plaintiff's disease. But playing the most important role was the defense of freedom of choice or assumption of risk. Even when juries determined that the tobacco companies were at fault to some degree, they found that the plaintiffs were aware of the risks associated with smoking and nonetheless continued the activity over a long period of time. And those findings have persisted despite attempts to portray tobacco as addictive. One further legal theory proved to be damaging to the plaintiffs. This was the proposition that "good" tobacco—that is, tobacco that has not been in some way adulterated by the manufacturer— is not defective, and therefore cannot give rise to liability based on the production of a defective product. In fact, legislation in a number of states, most notably California, has created a defense in products liability litigation that prevents recovery where the product involved, such as tobacco, is inherently unsafe.

In any event, the assumption of risk defense, which was so important to the industry during the second wave of litigation, may eventually be overcome. For example, a plaintiff may be able to prove that the industry fraudulently withheld crucial information about the health dangers of smoking from the public, so that smokers, in fact, could have believed that the risks of smoking were still unproven or, at least, could not have known the degree of those risks. A key component of such proof would be that the industry fraudulently withheld its knowledge of the addictive nature of tobacco, thereby preventing people from realizing the difficulty they might have in stopping to smoke once they started.

INVOLVEMENT OF LAWYERS IN SCIENTIFIC RESEARCH

On May 29 and 30, 1984, attorneys from B&W and BAT held a conference on US products liability litigation. This conference took place less than a year after the famous *Cippolone* case was filed [*Cippolone v Liggett Group, Inc.*, 593 F. Supp. 1146 (D.N.J. 1984)]. That case, which would wind its way through the courts for several years, is the only products liability case in which the tobacco industry has ever been held liable for damages caused by tobacco (an award to the husband of the plaintiff, who had died during the litigation), although even that award was subsequently overturned on appeal. The conference is summarized in a June 12, 1984, memo to the file by J. K. Wells, B&W's corporate counsel. Wells first discusses the attribution problem (see below) and then "Project Rio, Project Ship and other biological testing programs." Project Rio, a version of the safe cigarette project in the early 1980s, was extremely sensitive:

Within the limited time available, we were able to hold significant discussions about implications for U.S. products liability litigation only regarding Project Rio. BAT Legal acknowledged the needs for lawyer involvement in the project and for possible restructuring, but there was not enough time to plot a course of action. Alec [Morini, of BAT] said that he had not been aware of Project Rio until about two weeks prior to the meeting when he heard it mentioned briefly in a description of Southampton work. {1830.01, p. 2}

Wells then summarizes the status of the discussions, and it becomes clear that there are differences between the two companies on the degree to which the lawyers should be involved in scientific work:

[I]t is fair to say that BAT Legal are informed about the danger of the admissibility of BAT statements on smoking and health in U.S. products liability litigation. BAT Legal will offer counsel to BAT activities which pertain to smoking and health but no specific steps and no specific projects (other than Project Rio) were identified. Alec is concerned about the BAT senior management position [yet to be formulated] on the involvement of BAT Legal in R&D programs. {1830.01, p. 2}

After noting the success of the discussions, Wells proposes some follow-up activities:

[W]e should arrange a meeting in London with BAT Legal . . . to delineate more specific counsel to the BAT, including proposals for the structure and organization of BAT programs and statements which would hold to the minimum feasible level their potential impact upon U.S. products liability litigation. Topics would include proposals for organizing programs already on the table and general procedural guides for lawyer counseling of ongoing and future programs. For example, if Project Rio must continue, *restructuring probably will be required to control the risk of generating adverse evidence admissible in U.S. lawsuits. . . . Direct lawyer involvement is needed in all BAT activities pertaining to smoking and health from conception through every step of the activity.*

The problem posed by BAT scientists and frequently used consultants who believe cause is proven is difficult. A sound recommendation must be based upon consideration of several factors, including the basis upon which senior management relies in concluding that the opinion of the scientist is incorrect; the overall reliance of senior management on opinions of the scientist; the responsibilities assigned to the scientist; and the company's duty to encourage scientific inquiry [emphasis added]. {1830.01, p. 2}

Wells also expresses concern as to whether BAT senior management will go along with the lawyers' recommendations with respect to their involvement in R&D programs. He ends with a reference to the question of whether BAT or BATUS (the US-based holding company of BAT, owner of B&W and other major assets) could be held as a party in a US products liability lawsuit based on consumption of B&W products by the plaintiff {1830.01}

In effect, this document tells us that the B&W attorneys saw the need for themselves and the BAT attorneys to become totally involved in the research process in order to prevent potentially damaging research information from becoming known. The problem was that the attorneys in England, where products liability law was not as well developed as it was in the United States, were reluctant to become so intimately involved in scientific work. The B&W attorneys also recognized that at least some BAT scientists and consultants were convinced that the cause-and-effect relationship between smoking and disease had been proven. This was all the more reason to keep BAT scientific information away from the United States. However, in a July 8, 1985, memo to David A. Schechter, general counsel at BATUS, Sidney S. Rosdeitcher, an attorney at Paul, Weis, Rifkind, Wharton & Garrison in Washington, DC, concludes that documents in the possession of BAT Industries or BATCo would be discoverable by a plaintiff in a US lawsuit. Specifically, Rosdeitcher states:

> You should not assume that discovery would be prevented by British law or a British government blocking order.
> Neither Brown & Williamson nor B.A.T. could solicit the issuance of a blocking order without risking sanctions by the U.S. courts.
> Even if the British government issued a blocking order, a U.S. court would require Brown & Williamson to make a good-faith, affirmative effort to convince the U.K. government to waive the blocking order.
> If the U.S. court did not believe that such an effort had been made, or if it believed that Brown & Williamson or B.A.T. had solicited the blocking order, it could impose severe sanctions against Brown & Williamson, such as adverse factual findings (i.e., finding facts favorable to the plaintiff on matters in dispute), fines, and a default judgment.
> You should act on the assumption that discovery of the documents would be available.
> In the Appleton case, B.A.T. did not resist document demands from the FTC; B.A.T. negotiated certain modifications in the scope of those demands, and then agreed to produce documents located in the U.K. {1836.02}

"CARELESS" STATEMENTS BY COMPANY SCIENTISTS

As discussed in chapter 4, during the 1960s and early 1970s the tobacco industry believed it could create a "safe" cigarette, and it directed much of its research toward that goal. The scientists who conducted this research naturally had many discussions about the existing or suspected health dangers of cigarettes and how they might be eliminated. These discussions, in turn, were troublesome to industry lawyers, since statements by those scientists, if discovered by a plaintiff's attorney, might be used against the industry in products liability lawsuits.

Toward the end of the first wave of litigation, one of the tobacco industry's principal outside counsel, David R. Hardy (of Shook, Hardy, Ottman, Mitchell, and Bacon), wrote a lengthy letter to DeBaun Bryant, general counsel at B&W, giving his observations and opinion about BAT's possible involvement in US smoking and health litigation. (The same subject arose fifteen years later; see the discussion above on lawyers' involvement in scientific research.) In this letter, written on August 20, 1970, and marked "CONFIDENTIAL, FOR LEGAL COUNSEL ONLY," Hardy notes that "BAT may well be involved in future cases either as a defendant or through deposition of its employees or discovery of its records in cases where Brown and Williamson (B&W) is a defendant" {1840.01, p. 1}. But the real emphasis of the letter is on the "effect of statements made by employees of either BAT or B&W."

> It would, no doubt, be virtually impossible to determine to what extent statements have been made which would be damaging to defendant's position in a smoking and health case, but *I have seen sufficient documentation from you to conclude that the dangers I describe in this letter have a very real foundation.* For example, the minutes of a conference at Kronberg, Germany, held from June 2 to June 6, 1969[{1169.01}] and attended by research personnel of both BAT and B&W, reflect statements such as the following:
>
> (i)   ". . . a mouse-skin safer cigarette is a worthwhile objective . . . ",
>
> (ii)   ". . . it was necessary to set up some hypothetical model of *how smoke aerosol could cause cancer in the basal cells of the human lung epithelium*",
>
> (iii)   ". . . there is a possibility that the experiments taking place at R. & D.E. [Research and Development Establishment], Southampton, with the membrane of the chicken embryo *might be showing genuine carcinogenic effects in days*" and
>
> (iv)   "*The conclusion of the Conference was that at the present time the Industry had to recognize the possibility of distinct adverse health reactions to smoke aerosol: (a) Lung Cancer (b) Emphysema and bronchitis* . . ." [emphasis added]. {1840.01, p. 2}

Hardy then refers to an interesting example of industry doublespeak. Despite the industry's relentless efforts through its public relations apparatus to make the public believe there is no medical proof of the dangers of smoking, Hardy notes the following "admission," undoubtedly crafted by an attorney, made at a BAT research conference:

At the St. Ives Conference, May 8 to 12, 1970, an opening statement was made which included an acknowledgment that tobacco manufacturers are not competent to give authoritative medical opinions and stating that "causation" is still an open question. {1840.01, p. 2}

Hardy complains:

> In the minutes of this Conference, however, we note a number of statements or expressions which could be most damaging notwithstanding the disclaimer in the opening statement. For example: (i) reference is made on page 6 to the fact that research "will continue in the search for a safer product"; (ii) on page 14 a product is characterized as "attractive" because less biologically active; (iii) on page 15 the phrase "biologically attractive" is used; and (iv) on page 18 reference is made to a "healthy cigarette". {1840.01, pp. 2–3}

Hardy explains why the types of statements quoted from the two conferences are worrisome:

> *It is our opinion that statements such as the above constitute a real threat to the continued success in the defense of smoking and health litigation. Of course, we would make every effort to "explain" such statements if we were confronted with them during a trial, but I seriously doubt that the average juror would follow or accept the subtle distinctions and explanations we would be forced to urge* [emphasis added]. {1840.01, p. 3}

Such statements, Hardy point out, if admitted into court, could tip the scales in the battle to convince a jury as to where the balance of the scientific evidence lies:

> As you know, with the testimony of independent and well-informed doctors and scientists, it has been repeatedly demonstrated in court to the satisfaction of impartial jurors that cigarette smoking has not been scientifically proved to cause disease. This is certainly one very good reason that the industry has attained a one hundred percent record of victories in its health litigation. Jurors are, however, aware that a substantial segment of the medical and scientific community has accepted smoking as a cause of disease notwithstanding the deficiencies in the proof. This group includes many well-intentioned but inadequately informed doctors and scientists who operate on a philosophy that if smoking <u>may</u> be hazardous to health no further inquiry is necessary. In other words, they are willing to settle for suspicion in lieu of proof in condemning cigarettes. We have been able to show this to be the case when such suspicion has been claimed by our known enemies to be established fact. Obviously our problem becomes entirely different and far more serious when agents and employees of the defendant cigarette company or its parent become the spokesmen against us.
> *Fundamental to my concern is the advantage which would accrue to a plaintiff able to offer damaging statements or admissions by persons*

employed by or whose work was done in whole or in part on behalf of the company defending the action. A plaintiff would be greatly benefited by evidence which tended to establish actual knowledge on the part of the defendant that smoking is generally dangerous to health, that certain ingredients are dangerous and should be removed, or that smoking causes a particular disease. This would not only be evidence that would substantially prove a case against the defendant company for compensatory damages, but could be considered as evidence of willfulness or recklessness sufficient to support a claim for punitive damages. The psychological effect on judge and jury would undoubtedly be devastating to the defendant. To be more specific:

(1)   *It would certainly be difficult for a defendant to effectively contest or question the work of some particular "anti-cigarette" scientists if such work had been labeled as "valid" by defendant's own people.* How, for example, would our position that "mouse-skin painting" does not provide data which can be extrapolated to humans stand up if the reference to mouse-skin painting "as the ultimate court of appeal on carcinogenic effects" from page 5 of the Kronberg minutes was offered in evidence by a plaintiff?

(2)   The testimony of outstanding and independent doctors and scientists of the type who have enabled us to win a number of cancer cases on the causation issue would be nullified or weakened by our own people's statements. Furthermore, after one experience of being disputed by statements of our own employees, it is doubtful that such independent experts would agree to testify again.

(3)   If a plaintiff's contention as to causation of a disease by cigarettes seems to be supported by statements and opinions of our own specific employees, this important issue on which we have prevailed in the past would undoubtedly be decided against us, despite our best efforts to explain them [italic emphasis added]. {1840.01, pp. 3–4}

Hardy concludes his letter with the following:

In conclusion, I would like to emphasize that, in our opinion, the effect of testimony by employees or documentary evidence from the files of either BAT or B&W which seems to acknowledge or tacitly admit that cigarettes cause cancer or other disease would likely be fatal to the defense of either or both companies in a smoking and health case. I am afraid that any attempted explanation to a jury that such statements were made only in the context of a "working hypothesis" for the further development of our products would fall on deaf ears. Clearly, the admission of such evidence would cause a plaintiff's case to attain a posture of strength and danger never before approached in cigarette litigation. It could even be the basis for an assessment of punitive damages if it were deemed to indicate a reckless disregard for the health of the smoker. Certainly such evidence would make B&W the most vulnerable cigarette manufacturer in the United States to smoking and health suits.

We, of course, know that the position of BAT, as well as B&W, is that disease causation by smoking is still very much an open question. Cigarettes have not been proved to cause any human disease. Thus, any statement by responsible and informed employees subject to a contrary interpretation could only result from carelessness. *Therefore, employees in both companies should be informed of the possible consequences of careless statements on this subject* [emphasis added]. {1840.01, p. 7}

Hardy obviously chose his words carefully. Even in such a confidential letter to a fellow attorney, he maintains the fiction that a statement by a corporate scientist subject to an interpretation that smoking causes disease could only occur through "carelessness."

In a letter written on November 5, 1970, Bryant passes along Hardy's concerns to E. G. Langford, an attorney at BAT:

> As you know, we have for some time been concerned over the possibility that the BAT might in the future be involved in smoking and health litigation in the USA. This involvement might be through the deposition of BAT employees or the discovery of BAT records in cases in which B&W is a defendant. We asked Dave Hardy to prepare an opinion for us on this subject, which he has done and I am enclosing a copy for your consideration. {1840.03, p. 1}

Langford acknowledges receipt of the letter in return correspondence on November 11, 1970, and makes some suggestions:

> I think the problem centers mainly on the R&D and to a lesser extent P.R. Departments and I know that both Departments are conscious of it, particularly since Pat Kelly's visit here last May. Nevertheless, in the light of Dave Hardy's Opinion the matter ought to be looked at again. It happens that Tony McCormick will be visiting you later this month, following a R&D Conference in Canada, and since he is responsible for both of the Departments I have mentioned above, I suggest that you discuss the matter with him. If you have any specific proposals to make we will certainly co-operate in every way we can. {1840.04, p. 1}

(For an example of how B&W's corporate counsel rewrote a scientific paper in 1984 to avoid having certain scientific statements linked to the company, see chapter 9, "The Blackman Paper: Rewriting Scientific Documents.")

ESTABLISHING LIMITS FOR SHARING OF INFORMATION

Among the many concerns of the attorneys at B&W was the extent to which information should be exchanged, both within and outside the associated companies. The documents indicate that this concern was a long-standing one, preceding the second wave of litigation by many years. A November 27, 1968, letter from Addison Yeaman, B&W vice president and general counsel, to G. C. Hargrove at BAT—marked "Private and Confidential"—states:

> Ed Finch [president of B&W] told me of his talk with you and in particular we discussed Tony McCormick's [a senior executive in the Research and Development Establishment at BAT] memorandum of 27th June to B. G. Pearson which had to do with exchange of pertinent information in the area of smoking and health. The approach is an interesting one and I should like to give it further thought and discuss its implementation with my opposite numbers [in a letter of December 11, 1968, Finch explains that this is a reference to the lawyers of the other tobacco companies in the U.S. who are members of the Tobacco Research Council {1809.03}] before trying to set up anything definitive. You will, of course, hear further from me on this. {1809.01}

The documents never specify the "information" to which they refer. A response from Hargrove to Yeaman, dated December 4, 1968, and marked "Private and Confidential," states:

> You will by now have received the documents with reference numbers F.1193 and F.1224 which I left with Ed Finch. Having consulted Mr. Dobson, I confirm that the information in these documents can be made known in confidence to the rest of your Group in the U.S. Industry, if you so wish. We would not, however, wish the source of this information to be disclosed—although admittedly it would not be very difficult for others in your Group to guess this. {1809.02}

The Finch letter, which was written to R. P. Dobson at BAT, discusses the difficulties in exchanging information between individual BAT companies, and the problems that might arise from such exchanges.

> *I am in complete agreement with your statement that the subject of the exchange of information* [on smoking and health] *between individual companies within B.A.T. is full of difficulty.* As you know, I have been and still am concerned about the problems that might arise as a result of individual companies corresponding with each other on this matter. . . . From this information, it seems to me you would know best how the information should be used and whether or not it should be transmitted to other companies. In addition, I also agree with your thought that there should be *personal visits* between the major companies to discuss the health matters whenever possible [emphasis added]. {1809.03}

Also of concern to B&W was the extent to which BAT might be sharing information with British government officials. A memo dated October 20, 1971, from Dr. I. W. Hughes, director of R&D at B&W, to his superior, J. W. Burgard, and to the general counsel, Addison Yeaman, is on the subject of smoking and health research at Imperial Tobacco Group

(ITG) in the United Kingdom {1121.01}. Dr. Hughes had just read a report about this research (possibly document {1120.01}). Although, he notes, much of the report is concerned with the technical program,

> there are a number of points mentioned which give an impression of the way I.T.G. may be planning its policy in terms of the Smoking and Health area.
>
> 1. Intention to make available to the Dawkins Committee some of the bio-systems developed at Huntingdon.
>
> 2. Visitation to Huntingdon by Sir Derrick Dunlop (Chairman of the Medicines Committee). Dr. Frank Fairweather (Member of the Cohen Committee and cited by the Committee as an authority on biological tests) may also be invited; the thought is that he might be influenced by such an unofficial channel as Huntingdon.
>
> 3. Visitation by Members of Parliament, senior officials of Dept. of Health to Huntingdon. {1121.01}

It is not clear what the Dawkins, Medicines, and Cohen Committees are, but in context they may be committees of the Royal College of Physicians or of another independent group interested in the toxicity of tobacco.

Dr. Hughes evidently wanted to draw the attention of senior management to these moves by ITG so that Mr. Finch might discuss them with a Mr. Carter, who was to be visiting soon. Dr. Hughes also suggests that Finch should not let it be known that B&W received information on ITG's plans through BAT:

> During Mr. Carter's visit to Mr. Finch, it might be useful to Mr. Finch to obtain from Mr. Carter an overview of the policy in the health area. If this is considered worthwhile, it might be preferable not to mention that we receive through BAT broad reports of the I.T.G./Huntingdon situation. {1121.01}

ATTRIBUTION OF STATEMENTS BY SUBSIDIARIES

When the health dangers of smoking became a serious issue, one of the problems facing BAT was the possible attribution to its tobacco companies of statements made or decisions taken by its other subsidiaries. This problem was the topic of several memos between corporate attorneys. In one memo, titled "Legal Considerations on Smoking and Health Policy" {1828.01}, which was unsigned and undated but apparently written by an attorney, the author summarizes the policy of BAT Industries Group in relation to smoking and health issues. The author then warns that BAT's nontobacco companies must be made aware of the group's stance, because the spread of "no-fault" liability may result in the future attribution to the group's tobacco companies of statements made or

decisions taken by other subsidiaries. The following excerpts demonstrate the industry's classic three-pronged stance with regard to the health
dangers of smoking: (1) a genuine scientific controversy exists; (2) individuals have a right to choose whether or not to smoke; and (3) further
research is needed:

> For this reason [the spread of no-fault liability] it is essential that statements
> about cigarette smoking or the smoking and health issue generally must be
> factually and scientifically correct. The issue is controversial and there is no
> case for either condemning or encouraging smoking. It *may* be responsible for
> the alleged smoking related diseases or it may not. No conclusive scientific ev-
> idence has been advanced and the statistical association does not amount to
> proof of cause and effect. Thus a genuine scientific controversy exists.
>
> The Group's position is that causation has not been proved and that we
> do not ourselves make health claims for tobacco products. *Consequently
> the Group cannot participate in any campaigns stressing the benefits of a
> moderate level of cigarette consumption, of cigarettes with low tar and/or
> nicotine deliveries or any other positive aspects of smoking except those
> concerned with the dissemination of objective information and the right of
> individuals to choose whether or not they smoke.* However, the Group en-
> courages constructive dialogue with the authorities, the dissemination of in-
> formation about the smoking and health controversy and research and new
> product development.
>
> Non-tobacco companies in the Group must particularly beware of any
> commercial activities or conduct which could be construed as discrimination
> against tobacco manufacturers (whether or not involving companies within
> the Group), since this could adversely affect the position of Brown &
> Williamson in current US product liability litigation in the US. If in doubt,
> companies should not hesitate to consult their inhouse consel, or BAT In-
> dustries Legal Department, who have up-to-date information on the legal sit-
> uation affecting the tobacco companies [emphasis added]. {1828.01}

The recommendation against participating in the promotion of health
claims for low-tar cigarettes is in sharp contrast to the industry's active
promotion of such cigarettes during the "tar derby" of the late 1950s
(discussed in chapter 2). However, the principal point being made here
is that the companies in the BAT group were not to engage in *any* dialogue concerning the health aspects of smoking and were to adhere
strictly to the three-pronged position on that issue, as outlined above.

The seriousness with which this policy was taken can be seen by what
happened to one unfortunate employee at US Tobacco, manufacturer of
moist tobacco products, who made an inappropriate statement regarding the health benefits of smokeless tobacco. This episode is recounted
in a 1977 confidential memo from Ernest Pepples, B&W vice president
for law, to J. E. Edens; C. I. McCarty, the company's chairman and chief

operating officer; and R. A. Pittman, the senior vice president for public relations:

> US Tobacco's General Counsel, Jim Chapin, sent me the attached article from the New York Post for March 16. It reports a most unfortunate interview with an over-enthusiastic employee of US Tobacco who is quoted as saying about so-called smokeless tobacco:
>
> > [F]rom what we understand, it presents the least possible danger of all. It's when you light tobacco that you start doing damage.
>
> Chapin says the statements quoted were unauthorized and do not represent his company's views. He has asked me to extend US Tobacco's apology to each of the cigarette companies and advised me that the individual quoted in the article is no longer employed at US Tobacco. Chapin says US Tobacco has instituted smoking and health seminars throughout the company. {1500.01}

On May 29 and 30, 1984, attorneys from both B&W and BAT held a conference on US products liability litigation. (For further discussion of this conference, see above section on involvement of lawyers in scientific research.) This conference is summarized in a June 12, 1984, memo to file by J. K. Wells, B&W's corporate counsel. The conference placed particular emphasis on the problem of the attribution to the tobacco companies of statements and actions by affiliated companies:

> Trial counsel described evidence rulings in United States courts pertinent to the admissibility of statements (used herein to include written and oral statements and actions whether internal or published) of an affiliate of B&W. A prudent lawyer in a U.S. products liability action must assume that any damaging statement will be admitted into the evidence and will be discussed by the plaintiff. It is likely that statements by a tobacco affiliate of B&W would be admitted and smoking and health research done in-house or by contract by any company owned by the BAT certainly would be admissible. Statements by a non-tobacco affiliate would be admissible where control or close functional relationship, either on a general line of business or a specific project basis, was shown. {1830.01, p. 1}

A February 4, 1985, letter from R. G. Baker, a senior scientist at BAT's Southampton laboratory, to D. A. Schechter, an attorney at BATUS, Inc., in Louisville, labeled as an "Attorney Work Product," discusses the need to set up guidelines for affiliated companies outside the United States to follow when making public statements. The letter suggests six questions to be considered:

> (1)   Does this particular statement amount to an admission [of anything that could be compromising in a lawsuit]?
>
> (2)   Does this particular statement amount to product assurance which can be attributed to an affiliated US defendant?

(3)   Is this statement admissible in cross examination of defendants' witnesses?

(4)   Are statements of this type by non-US affiliates discoverable?

(5)   What are the risks of overseas companies becoming parties of US cases? Is their public posture relevant to this question?

(6)   Given the range of company activities in the Group, what are the risks associated with expert status being attributed to employees of certain companies in the Group? {1829.01, pp. 1–2}

Included with the letter is a two-page legal analysis of the attribution issue put together by Baker. An introduction to this analysis states: "A substantial discussion took place about the risks of statements and positions of affiliates of Brown & Williamson being attributed to it. The intention is, so far as possible, to conduct matters so that no connection can be shown" {1829.02, p. 1}.

STRATEGY OF NO SETTLEMENTS

By the mid-1980s there was no doubt among tobacco industry executives about the seriousness of the products liability issue. A July 22, 1985, restricted briefing document titled "B&W's Public Issues Environment" outlines the potential importance of products liability actions against Brown and Williamson and the principal strategy to be followed: no settlement payments are to be made.

> B&W will continue the strategy of intensive litigation of each case with the objective of exploiting each case's favorable factors and a policy of no payments to plaintiffs in settlement of cases. In the event manufacturers experience losses in the smoking and health cases, the selection of contingency strategy would depend upon the scope of the losses. During the planning period the most attractive strategy probably will be to continue intensive litigation of the cases with no settlement payments and the acceptance of losses as charges against income. The current insurance coverage of $1,000,000 would quickly be absorbed and the adoption now of internal financial structures to fund losses could be a negative influence on juries. Such structures should be re-evaluated if losses occur. A possible contingent strategy of settlement also should be reassessed on an opportunistic basis. Pressure will develop in the Congress for superfund legislation [pursuant to which corporations that produce hazardous substances are taxed, and the resulting fund is used to pay for the costs associated with the release of hazardous substances] applicable to smoking and health lawsuits if large scale plaintiff victories occur; such a fund would be financed by contributions from cigarette manufacturers amounting to a large percentage of profits. {2228.02, pp. 1–2}

The strategy of refusing to settle with any plaintiff was one that the industry had devised when the first products liability actions were filed in the mid-1950s, and the industry has religiously observed it to this day. The tobacco companies decided that they would defend every suit, regardless of cost, and would do so regardless of how many appeals were taken. As part of this strategy, the industry also decided that it would spend whatever it must to exhaust the plaintiff's resources in each case. Thus, the litigation in this area became a war of attrition in which the richest party, rather than the one with the best legal case, would win (9).

MAINTAINING LEGAL DISTANCE BETWEEN B&W AND BAT

The briefing paper discussed above also notes the importance of maintaining some legal distance between Brown and Williamson and BAT, to protect the larger organization from involvement in a US lawsuit:

> *The BAT group must preserve the independent corporate status of B&W.* A smoking and health plaintiff could bring B&W's parent or parents into a case if the parent exercised such control over B&W as would support a plaintiff's argument that B&W was not an independent business entity. B&W's net assets should not be reduced below a level commensurate with B&W's operations as an independent entity. *Similarly any substantial reduction or dilution of pension plan assets, or dividend up or pledge of assets, would invite a court to pierce the B&W corporate entity and hold BATUS or even BAT responsible for B&W's liabilities.* Also, BATUS' or BAT's detailed direction of B&W's marketing plans could lead a court to the same result [emphasis added]. {2228.02, p. 2}

While there was concern that BAT might be dragged into US lawsuits because of its ties to B&W, the attorneys at B&W worried that the company might receive scientific information from BAT that would be useful to a plaintiff in litigation, and as described earlier in this chapter, they tried to devise methods for preventing the discovery of such information by a plaintiff. One might say that these two closely linked corporations were giving new meaning to the expression "hands across the sea."

B&W PARTICIPATION IN BAT RESEARCH

While B&W attorneys were busy trying to conceal the fact that the company was aware of certain information obtained from research conducted by BAT, the documents themselves tell us that B&W was actually an active partner in much of the BAT Group research and, therefore, must have known of most of the important information obtained from it. All the information in the documents about BAT research activities around the world is from the files of Brown and Williamson. While some research activities, such as work on smoker compensation and biological testing, were never conducted in the United States, there is abundant evidence that B&W actively participated in planning and funding at least some of this work and that the company benefited from receiving the results of these studies.

ACTIVE PARTICIPATION BY B&W PERSONNEL

B&W had at least one delegate at each of the seventeen research conferences held between 1962 and 1985 (see table 7.2). BAT representatives from the United Kingdom, Canada, and Germany also attended each research conference. Brazil was regularly represented by the mid-1970s while Australia was represented only occasionally. In addition, as described below, B&W scientists attended other BAT R&D meetings and conferences, including meetings on the direction of the biological testing programs, such as Project Janus.

B&W contributed experiments to Project Janus (see chapter 4) {1164.03; 1112.04}. A B&W scientist was a member of the Biological Testing Committee. Moreover, B&W scientists made site visits to BAT research labs in the United Kingdom. Dr. R. B. Griffith visited Southampton in the summer of 1965 {1105.01}, and Dr. Robert R. Johnson made an extensive visit in mid-1967 {1109.01}.

B&W scientists sometimes made comments on proposed agendas of research conferences and edited drafts of minutes that resulted from these meetings. For example, Dr. Robert Sanford of B&W made detailed suggestions to Dr. S. J. Green of BAT for revising draft minutes of the 1968 Hilton Head research conference (discussed in chapter 4) {1112.02}. The B&W general counsel, Addison Yeaman, received a copy of this letter. Dr. Alan Heard of BAT Southampton sent Dr. R. A. Sanford a questionnaire about the draft agenda for the 1980 Sea Island research conference. As described in chapters 3 and 4, Dr. Sanford responded with a number of comments about areas of research, such as inhalation, that should not be further pursued {1132.01}. In July 1983 the director of R&D at Millbank, Dr. L. C. F. Blackman, sent Earl Kohnhorst of R&D at B&W the proposed agenda for the 1983 research conference in Rio and asked him to comment on it {1180.05}. Similarly, draft minutes of the 1983 Rio meeting were sent to B&W for comment and feedback. Edits appearing in handwriting in the draft from B&W's files {1180.09} were incorporated into the final set of minutes {1180.07}. These editorial changes in-

TABLE 7.2 PARTICIPATION IN
BAT GROUP RESEARCH CONFERENCES
BY SCIENTISTS FROM B&W

Date	Location	No. Attendees	No. Countries	B&W Personnel Present
7/62	Southampton, England	10	6	J. G. Esterle
				R. B. Griffith
				A. Upfield
				T. M. Wade, Jr.
10/67	Montreal	9	4	R. B. Griffith
				R. A. Sanford
9/68	Hilton Head, SC	12	4	J. G. Esterle
				R. B. Griffith
				R. A. Sanford
9/69	Kronberg, Germany	10	4	R. B. Griffith
				R. A. Sanford
11/70	St. Adele, Quebec	16	4	R. A. Sanford
10/72	Chelwood, England	11	4	R. A. Sanford
1/74	Duck Key, FL	12	5	R. A. Sanford
				J. G. Esterle
4/75	Merano, Italy	11	6	R. A. Sanford
3/78	Sydney, Australia	15	6	R. A. Sanford
				J. G. Esterle
2/79	Chewton Glen[?]	16	6	R. A. Sanford
				M. L. Reynolds
11/79	London	10	5	R. A. Sanford
9/80	Sea Island, GA	8	5	R. A. Sanford
8/81	Pichlarn, Austria	10	5	R. A. Sanford
8/82	Montebello, Canada	10	6	R. A. Sanford
8/83	Rio de Janeiro	12	6	R. A. Sanford
				E. E. Kohnhorst
9/84	Southampton, England	26	6	E. E. Kohnhorst
				R. A. Sanford
				E. Parrack
9/85	Wallingford, England	8	4	E. E. Kohnhorst

NOTE: R. J. Pritchard attended the 1979 London meeting and the 1980 Sea Island meeting. Mr. Pritchard was with R&D of BATCO at the time of these conferences, but he later became the CEO of B&W.

SOURCES: {1102.01; 1165.01; 1168.01; 1169.01; 1170.01; 1171.02; 1172.01; 1173.01; 1174.01; 1175.01; 1176.02; 1177.01; 1178.01; 1179.01; 1180.08; 1181.01; 1182.01}.

cluded the excision of a phrase referring to a filter developed at B&W. Thus, under a discussion of research at the German affiliate, the draft minutes contain the following paragraph about filter variants:

A description was given of a number of filter designs capable of directing smoke to specific areas of the mouth. This technology, which is an extension of the B&W Actron concept, has led to patent applications. Results with other novel filters which make use of the principles of 'smoke elasticity' were given. {1180.09, p. 14}

The phrase "which is an extension of the B&W Actron concept" is lined out in the draft, and the final version of the minutes reflects this edit {1180.09, p. 14}.

The minutes of the Rio conference also discuss an information exchange system called Interbat {1180.07}. The minutes indicate that there were mechanisms within Interbat's structure to control the flow of "sensitive reports or information."

> With the growing interest and use of INTERBAT, CAC Companies should be reminded that facilities are available to limit or block access to sensitive reports or information. {1180.07, p. 16}

The CAC Companies were the members of the Chairman's Advisory Conference, BAT affiliates in the United States, Canada, Brazil, Australia, and Germany, the places outside the United Kingdom where BAT maintained research facilities. The draft minutes circulated at B&W include a marginal note stating, "We own 1/3 share" {1180.09, p. 15}, which indicates that B&W was a participant in the Interbat system. The documents do not indicate exactly what information was shared on the Interbat system, but it might be the information retrieval and sharing system recommended for BAT's R&D by a consultant in 1979 {1175.03, p. 7}. Southampton, Louisville, and Hamburg were each to have input into the design of the system, and this might explain the reason B&W bore a third of the costs.

Furthermore, the minutes of the Rio conference include a list of the dozen technical meetings that had been held over the past year (including a "smoking behaviour" conference in the United States in March 1983) and conclude,

> It was agreed that the meetings had been a highly effective means of exchanging technology throughout the Group, and that a similar level should be maintained in the future. {1180.07, p. 16}

These conferences covered a wide range of issues in research and development. The full list of immediate past and future BAT technical exchange meetings for 1982–1985, as it appeared in the Rio conference documents {1181.14}, is shown in table 7.3. The comment from the conference minutes suggests that participants at each conference included individuals from various BAT companies. These frequent exchanges (nine or ten a year) clearly permitted companies not doing the actual research

TABLE 7.3   SCHEDULE OF R&D CONFERENCES,
BAT, 1982–1984, AND CONFERENCES PLANNED
FOR 1985

Meeting Topic	Location	Date	
Tobacco Processing Seminar	USA	January	1982
Research Conference	Canada	August	1982
Production Conference	UK	November	1982
Combustion—Fundamental Mechanisms	UK	December	1982
Environmental Smoke	UK	March	1983
INTERBAT/Telecommunications	UK	March	1983
Smoker Behavior	USA	April	1983
Tobacco Processing Seminar	Germany	May	1983
Biological Studies	UK	May	1983
GRD&C Programme Review	UK	May	1983
Computer Modelling	UK	July	1983
Research Conference	Brazil	August	1983
Production Conference	Kenya	November	1983
Flavourists' Workshop	USA	November	1983
Near Infra-Red Workshop	UK	March	1984
Biological Studies	UK	April	1984
Nicotine	UK	June	1984
GR&DC Programme Review	UK	June	1984
Structured Creativity Conference	UK	June	1984
Smoking Behaviour/Marketing	Canada	July	1984
Research Conference	UK	September	1984
Swirl Conference	USA	October	1984
Production Conference	Malaysaia	November	1984

Proposed 1985 Conferences

Chemometrics
Biological
Research/Marketing (theme to be determined)
Flavourists' Workshop, or Flavour Applications
GR&DC Programme Review

SOURCE: {1181.14}.

work or receiving formal reports to benefit from the results of the work being done throughout the group. It may be that, after lawyers at B&W became more concerned about what was discoverable in its files in the late 1970s and early 1980s, these conferences were scheduled more often so that not as much paper would have to change hands.

B&W scientists also attended meetings other than the annual research conferences. For example, Dr. Sanford was one of eight participants from four operating companies who attended the R&D Policy Conference held at Chewton Glen and Torquay in February 1979 {1175.03}; and Earl Kohnhorst attended a Chairman's Advisory Conference meeting at Wallingford, England, in September 1985. In the notes on this meeting, Kohnhorst is listed as a speaker on several technical topics to be discussed at the 1985 research conference scheduled for November of that year in Rio {1182.01}.

Records of some of the series of meetings held from the mid-1960s through at least 1983 to monitor toxicological (biological) research, including Project Janus, are included in the documents {1164.03 through 1164.26}. B&W personnel participated in three of the meetings for which records are available. R. B. Griffith is listed as a "member" of the Biological Testing Committee in the minutes of the Southampton meeting held in June 1969 {1164.03}; R. A. Sanford is listed as a guest at the same meeting. Dr. Sanford was also present at the May 1970 meeting of this committee {1164.05}, and J. G. Esterle attended the November 1977 meeting {1164.23}.

The documents also include the participant list for the Smoking Behaviour/Marketing Conference held in Montreal in 1983 {1224.01, unnumbered page}. This conference featured major presentations of BAT-sponsored research for marketing personnel of BAT-affiliated companies. B&W personnel in attendance at this conference included the section head of Sensory Evaluation (W. H. Deines), the division head of Product Development (Tilford Riehl), and a representative from Marketing (Andy Mellman).

R&D COST- AND RISK-POOLING AGREEMENT

Additional evidence of the extent to which B&W participated in BAT research can be found in the cost- and risk-pooling agreements between the two companies. According to handwritten notes made sometime in 1980, perhaps by J. K. Wells, B&W's corporate counsel, these agreements dated back at least to April 1958 {1838.01}. At that time, the notes indicate:

> We have been pooling the findings and experience resulting from our joint and separate research programmes. {1838.01, p. 1}

The agreement called for costs to be shared on the basis of B&W sales to BAT sales, and the companies shared reports and findings. In 1961 the 1958 agreement was abrogated (as of October 1, 1960), evidently because the sales formula was not working. In its place, an arrangement was made whereby each company bore the cost of its own research. However, the two companies focused on different areas of concern: B&W was "best suited for research [on] seed to warehouse," while BAT was "better suited for work on processing, smoking, [and] smoke effects" {1838.01, p. 1}. A short entry dealing with March 6, 1962, states:

B&W shall have access to everyone else's [research results]—everyone else shall have access to B&W's. {1838.01, p. 1}

In July 1969 a major cost- and risk-pooling agreement, a copy of which appears in the documents {1810.01}, was entered into by the two companies. The agreement was effective as of January 1, 1969, and was to last five years. According to the notes, among the important aspects of the agreement was the fact that it recognized that the parties had for many years exchanged the product of their R&D work to their mutual benefit. The notes describe the opt-out procedure under the agreement and indicate that the costs were shared on the basis of the sales ratios of the two companies {1838.01, p. 2}.

The 1969 agreement was extended indefinitely in June 1974. It was amended in December 1975, limiting the amount payable by either party to $100,000. In February 1977 the agreement was rescinded, effective as of October 1, 1976, and a new agreement became effective {1838.01, p. 2}. A separate document, evidently a cover letter to the new agreement, written on February 7, 1977, by an unknown person at B&W (only the first page of the letter is available) to the secretary of BAT, discusses the review of the old agreement that led to the decision to formulate a new arrangement. Of particular interest is the following observation:

> This review has served to underscore the importance of the centralized and coordinated research program which is being carried out by BAT in support of long-range overall Group strategy. {1815.01, p. 1}

The notes discussed above indicate that, under the new agreement, central group research was carried out by BAT for the mutual benefit of itself, B&W, and other affiliates. The research included biological, product, smoker, process, and new smoking material areas. B&W contributed 0.15 percent of its net turnover, and received information in return. In 1979 an amendment was proposed to increase B&W's contribution to 0.21 percent, and it was eventually executed in January 1980. Then, on the last day of 1980, everything was canceled. Finally, in a subscript, the notes state that under the 1977 agreement B&W was paying around one million (presumably dollars), whereas, under the increased factor, it would be paying between two and three million {1838.01, p. 2}.

The two companies continued to operate under cost-sharing arrangements after 1980. This fact is shown in the notes to an R&D meeting of BAT affiliates (the CAC Companies, described above) at Wallingford, England, in September 1985 {1182.01}. Under a section entitled "Funding of BATUKE R&D Centre," the notes state:

In view of the pressure from various countries to have some indication of their likely contribution to this laboratory, ALH [A. L. Heard, chairman of the meeting] presented a proposal for funding BATUKE R&D Centre which reflected the BATCo recommendations at least for the next two years.

Despite the considerable reduction in costs of the laboratory, if CAC's were no longer to contribute, the result would be a considerable increase in the sum paid by BATCo (in addition to the individual BATCo companies), with major savings by all CAC's unless they rapidly scale up their domestic R&D costs which looks improbable (with the possible exception of USA). As a guideline for the next two years it is proposed that BATCo will continue to support the laboratory at its current level and that the balance be shared between CAC countries (not Brazil) using a [specified] formula. {1182.01, pp. 6–7}

As indicated in a letter written on August 20, 1970, by attorney David R. Hardy to DeBaun Bryant, general counsel at B&W {1840.01}, these cost- and risk-pooling agreements created a potential legal problem for B&W. In the letter, Hardy discusses the possible adverse effects of statements made by BAT and B&W scientists in a products liability lawsuit against the company. Hardy points out that such statements could be construed as being contrary to the industry's position that there is no proof that smoking causes disease (see the discussion earlier in this chapter regarding concerns of lawyers about scientists' statements). After explaining how the statements could be used by a plaintiff, Hardy notes that the pooling agreement exacerbated the problem:

> Also adding to the need for recognition of the problem created by statements such as those I have described is the existence of the "BAT/B&W R&D Cost and Risk Pooling Agreement" executed in July, 1969. This document creates an inter-relationship (or confirms a relationship which already existed) that would assist a plaintiff's attorney greatly in obtaining information from B&W about BAT research and development work. {1840.01, p. 4}

Later, Hardy notes that:

> The findings and opinions of persons engaged in work covered by the "BAT/B&W R&D Cost and Risk Pooling Agreement" are available to both BAT and B&W. *Carefully framed discovery would certainly force disclosure of the Agreement as well as other documents bearing on smoking and health issues* [emphasis added]. {1840.01, p. 5}

ANTITRUST CONCERNS

One of the tobacco industry's legal concerns was that some of its jointly sponsored research projects might be construed as violating antitrust laws. Antitrust laws are generally designed to preserve competition among sellers of goods and services by preventing or suppressing practices that create monopolies or restrain trade. Evidently, some attorneys in the industry believed that cooperation among the domestic tobacco companies in scientific research that had commercial ramifications, such as the same product modifications by all the companies, could be construed as an anticompetitive practice. For example, the joint effort by the American tobacco companies to sponsor the study of the cigarette additive Chemosol (described in chapter 6) may have created such a concern. Similarly, antitrust implications may be one reason for the evident lack of industry cooperation to produce a fire-safe cigarette. As noted earlier in this chapter, the industry has resisted efforts by Congress to mandate that cigarettes be fire-safe, because the industry does not wish to open the regulatory floodgates. Of course, the very regulatory void that the industry has so assiduously sought has left it with a lack of ground rules on what joint action the companies may safely take and with the concomitant jeopardy of the companies' being accused of collusion when they do act together.

The documents provide two examples of specific expressions of concern over possible antitrust problems. The first has to do with biological research. As subsequently described (in chapter 8), the Council for Tobacco Research funded a series of studies at Microbiological Associates in Bethesda, Maryland, on the effects of cigarette smoke on mice. Most of the studies involved inhalation of tobacco smoke. However, Microbiological Associates also conducted some short-term biological tests on tobacco smoke condensate. The purpose of the work was to attempt to identify specific compounds in cigarette smoke that were responsible for carcinogenesis, the implication being that these compounds, once identified, could be removed as part of the effort to develop a "safe" cigarette. As discussed in chapter 8, the work being conducted at Microbiological Associates aroused concern in tobacco industry lawyers, not only because the tests were "red light" tests that could be used against the industry in court but also because they represented a breach of antitrust laws. In a letter to Addison Yeaman, dated March 10, 1977, Ernest Pepples states,

> I also question whether we come close to an antitrust problem when several companies are funding work in the area of identifying compounds or combination of compounds which may be responsible for biological activity. Certainly that runs away from my concept of the scope of CTR which is etiology and not identification of substances or compounds which ought to be removed from the product. What I have in mind is a contrast between product modification and etiology of diseases. {1816.01, p. 2}

The second example involves research on nicotine analogues (see chapter 3), perhaps the industry's greatest concern in the antitrust area. In a memorandum of April 4, 1978, from Pepples to various persons, which primarily concerns the CTR budget, Pepples notes:

> American [Brands] has also concluded that part of the central nervous system/nicotine work [conducted by CTR] poses a question with respect to the assurances which the companies gave to the Justice Department to the effect that none of the scientific work at CTR would have commercial application. Philip Morris and Lorillard concur in the view that some of the central nervous system (CNS) work has commercial overtones, specifically work which would lead to blocking agents or substitutes for nicotine. {2010.02, p. 1}

CONCLUSION

The documents discussed in this chapter confirm what has been known about the myriad legal problems besetting the tobacco industry in the past few decades. They also shed new light on how the industry has dealt with those problems. Many of the problems are unique to the industry—which is not surprising, since it produces a product that is dangerous when used as intended—and its responses have often reflected that realization. Thus, on the one hand, we have seen that the industry actually welcomed a ban on the broadcast advertising of its products (something that would be unthinkable for the manufacturer of any other legal product); on the other hand, we have seen that the industry adopted a totally uncompromising stance against the settlement of any products liability lawsuits. And we have seen the lengths to which one company apparently went to avoid the discovery of documents that might be useful to an opponent in a lawsuit. Despite its problems, the industry has managed to remain unscathed, considering how much damage some of the attacks against it might have inflicted if they had been more successful.

The industry's charmed existence, however, may not last forever. On the horizon are new legal battles that promise to be even more daunting than those already faced: the possible regulation of cigarettes by the Food and Drug Administration; increased and more comprehensive regulation of smoking in public places and the workplace; class-action products liability lawsuits involving millions of plaintiffs, both smokers and non-smokers; lawsuits by various state governments seeking reimbursement for state medical expenses due to smoking; the possible mandating of fire-safe cigarettes; and the possible ban on or severe restriction of cigarette advertising. It remains to be seen whether the industry's lawyers and public relations experts can weather the impending storm.

REFERENCES

1. Dontenwill W, Chevalier H-J, Harke H-P, Lafrenz U, Reckzeh G, Schneider B. Investigations on the effects of chronic cigarette smoke inhalation in Syrian golden hamsters. *JNCI* 1973;51(6):1781–1832.
2. Hanauer P. Proposition P: Anatomy of a nonsmokers' rights ordinance. *NY State J Med* 1985;85:369–374.
3. Samuels B, Glantz S. The politics of local tobacco control. *JAMA* 1991;266:2110–2117.
4. Traynor M, Begay M, Glantz S. New tobacco industry strategies to prevent local tobacco control. *JAMA* 1993;270:479–486.
5. Cardador TM, Hazan AR, Glantz SA. Tobacco industry smokers' rights publications: A content analysis. *Am J Pub Health* 1995:1212–1217.
6. Levin M. Fighting fire with P.R. *The Nation* 1989 July 10:52–55.
7. Wagner S. *Cigarette Country: Tobacco in American History and Politics.* New York: Praeger, 1971.
8. Food and Drug Administration. Proposed rule analysis regarding FDA's jurisdiction over nicotine-containing cigarettes and smokeless tobacco products. *Federal Register* 1995 August 11:41453–41787.
9. Rabin RL. A sociological history of the tobacco tort litigation. *Stanford L Rev* 1992;44:853.

CHAPTER 8

Lawyer Management of Scientific Research

[T]hese tests [on inducing cancer in mice with tobacco tar]
are so-called red light tests. They have been developed for
use by FDA and other agencies in possibly identifying
harmful ingredients and substances in products which are
available to the consuming public. . . . I do not have to tell
you what Senator Kennedy would do with a finding by a
CTR [Council for Tobacco Research] grantee of red lights in
one of these tests as it applies to cigarette smoke fractions.
We would never be able to explain that we were only
replicating or confirming some other person's work. No
matter what our explanation happened to be the fact of the
red light in our own hands would be a serious burden to
the tobacco industry if it came out in legislative hearings or
in litigation.

> *Ernest Pepples, B&W vice president (law), 1977*
> *{1817.02, p. 1}*

INTRODUCTION

In contrast to the industry's internal research program (discussed in
chapters 3 and 4), which was driven—at least at first—by scientific
concerns, the industry's external research program was driven by the
threats of adverse publicity and litigation. This chapter details the involvement of tobacco industry lawyers in the industry's external scientific research programs. These lawyers encouraged scientific research
to refute the scientific evidence about tobacco, to perpetuate controversy about the health effects of tobacco, and to provide results that
could be used to respond to adverse publicity. To this end, the lawyers selected topics for research and manipulated the publication of
research results through funding mechanisms run by lawyers rather
than scientists.

PROJECTS RUN BY LAWYERS: AN OVERVIEW

Tobacco industry lawyers were involved in several different types of projects. In general, these projects differed in their source of funding and in whether they supported original research or other non-research consultant activities.

CTR Special Projects: These research projects were funded by CTR and did not go through peer review by the independent group of scientists known as the Scientific Advisory Board {1001.01, p. 31}. Instead, CTR special projects discussed in the documents were selected for funding by tobacco industry lawyers.

Law Firm Accounts: These research projects were funded directly by law firms and selected for funding by the lawyers in the firm. "Special Account 4" was administered by Jacob and Medinger. Little is known about "Special Account 5," except for general descriptive information about the projects that were funded through the account.

Consultancies: In addition to funding research projects, lawyers also funded "consultancies," primarily through Special Account 4 but also through CTR special projects as well as directly by the tobacco companies. Consultancies were established for specific tasks (e.g., preparation of expert scientific testimony for a congressional hearing) or for ongoing tasks (e.g., a scientist "on call" to attend scientific meetings or review the scientific literature).

Tobacco Company Projects: These research projects were funded directly by the tobacco companies, sometimes individually by Brown and Williamson and sometimes by pooled contributions from several companies. Grantees were selected by tobacco company executives and lawyers. Projects funded directly by tobacco companies included relatively large and unrestricted grants to universities. Some of these university special projects were not related to tobacco, but were used to support general research.

Between 1972 and 1991, CTR awarded at least $14,636,918 in special project funding. Table 8.1 (on p. 328) contains a list of the CTR special projects, as well as the other types of special projects run by lawyers.

CTR SPECIAL PROJECTS

As described in chapter 2, the tobacco industry has always maintained that the Council for Tobacco Research (and the Tobacco Industry Research

Committee before it) is an independent organization and that its research projects are awarded following peer review by the Scientific Advisory Board (SAB). The documents show, however, that many of CTR's projects were awarded through a special mechanism. Beginning in 1966, shortly after release of the first Surgeon General's report on smoking and health, in 1964, CTR began to fund "special projects" {1000.01, p. 13}. These special projects were awarded by tobacco industry lawyers, rather than the Scientific Advisory Board, and their primary purpose was to produce research that could be used to defend the industry in court or legislative arenas. The money for the CTR, including special projects, came from pooled contributions directly from the tobacco companies according to market share (see chapter 2).

CTR special projects were sometimes used to fund projects that did not get approved through CTR's traditional peer review process but were still desirable to industry lawyers. This arrangement is described in the minutes of a meeting of the general counsels for the six tobacco companies that funded the projects. The meeting was held on December 17, 1965, and the minutes discuss seven projects recommended by the Ad Hoc Committee for immediate implementation. (The precise functions of the general counsels and the Ad Hoc Committee are not known, but they appear to have been groups of industry lawyers and executives, respectively.) The minutes report the following action on one project: "To be submitted to SAB, CTR; if not approved, the project will be carried out by CTR under its 'special projects'" {2000.04, p. 1}. Thus, if this project could not meet the criteria for funding established by the Scientific Advisory Board, it would still be funded by CTR as a special project based on approval by the tobacco company lawyers.

The type of work conducted through CTR special projects awarded to three investigators—Henry Rothschild, Carl Seltzer, and Theodor Sterling—is described in detail below. As the documents show, these three sets of projects were designed to dispute the scientific findings about the adverse effects of tobacco and to produce research that shifted attention away from tobacco as a cause of disease. These three individuals, as well as many others funded through CTR special projects, also received funding directly through law firm accounts (see table 8.1), as described in the next section. We discuss these three CTR special projects in depth because they were funded over extended periods of time, they were awarded large amounts of money, and they are mentioned often and in great detail in the documents.

SPECIAL PROJECTS AWARDED TO HENRY ROTHSCHILD

Henry Rothschild, M.D., Ph.D., has been a professor of medicine at Louisiana State University, New Orleans, since 1972. Between 1977 and 1988 Dr. Rothschild was awarded grants of approximately $250,000 to conduct research on the role of genetics in the causation of cancer (table 8.1). In 1976 Henry Rothschild wrote a letter addressed to "Dear Mister" and sent it to B&W suggesting that his research implicating factors other than tobacco smoke in the causation of lung cancer would be of interest to the tobacco industry {2009.19}. Subsequent correspondence indicates that the tobacco companies were interested in Dr. Rothschild's work and began funding him through CTR special projects in 1977. A 1977 memo from lawyer Timothy Finnegan (at Jacob, Medinger, and Finnegan) to William Shinn (at Shook, Hardy, and Bacon) recommends that Dr. Rothschild be funded to conduct a pilot study "to explore the possibility that peculiar genetic and environmental factors are responsible for this unusual lung cancer pattern [in Louisiana]" {2009.15, p. 1}.

In his progress report about the work conducted in 1977, Dr. Rothschild asks for continued support and states that his work has shown that autopsy and lung biopsy are confirmed in only about 20 percent of deceased patients {2008.04, p. 1}. This finding would be important to the tobacco industry because the industry argues that lung cancer is diagnosed more often than it actually occurs (1). Rothschild also notes that his data will be useful to the industry because "it will allow us to raise several interesting questions concerning the validity of many epidemiologic studies based on Mason and McKay's data" {2008.04, p. 2}.

A 1982 memo from Timothy Finnegan to the counsels for the tobacco companies recommends that Dr. Rothschild be funded through a CTR special project to continue his work related to the genetic aspects of cancer {2015.02}. The 1982–83 funding enabled Dr. Rothschild to complete his work on the association between sugar cane farming and lung cancer. This work did not relate to genetic aspects of cancer, but it supported the tobacco industry's position that environmental factors other than tobacco cause lung cancer. In 1983 Timothy Finnegan again recommended renewing Rothschild's funding for another year to "discover possible genetic markers associated with lung cancers" {2034.02, p. 2}. Rothschild's work was useful to the tobacco industry because it suggested that environmental and genetic factors are associated with lung cancer, thereby shifting attention away from the health dangers of smoking.

The documents contain an example of how Rothschild's work was used by the tobacco industry. First, the work was used for congressional testimony. In the "Statement of Henry Rothschild, M.D., Ph.D. in response to S.772, the 'Smoking Prevention Health and Education Act of 1983'" (cited by Finnegan as a reason for funding Rothschild), Rothschild said that his work "indicates that genetic factors may play a significant role in this excess mortality from lung cancer" and "If we can isolate such genetic markers, it will be a major step toward unraveling another aspect in the mystery of lung cancer causation" {2034.03, pp. 1, 6}.

The documents on Rothschild show that he kept tobacco company lawyers informed about his work, even offering to let them review scientific manuscripts before the manuscripts were submitted for publication. In an April 17, 1979, letter, for example, Dr. Rothschild asks Timothy Finnegan to review a scientific paper:

> Enclosed is a summary of our accomplishments during the past year. A copy of our proposal for the coming year, including the budget, and a preprint of a next to final copy of the paper we would like to submit to the New England Journal of Medicine is also enclosed. (I say the penultimate copy because *I await your comments prior to submission*) [emphasis added]. {2034.18}

The paper in question never appeared in the *New England Journal of Medicine;* the documents do not indicate why. The document demonstrates that a tobacco company lawyer was involved in commenting on a scientific paper before its publication.

In 1979 Rothschild published an article entitled "The Bandwagons of Medicine" (2) in the scientific journal *Perspectives in Biology and Medicine.* The article's basic premise is that physicians "jump on the bandwagon" of whatever therapies are popular and use these therapies even though there is little scientific evidence of their validity. The article criticizes the overwhelming acceptance of unproven but popular ideas—"the bandwagons of medicine." Historical bandwagons cited in the paper include leeches, homeopathy, tonsillectomy, and anticoagulants. When the article was submitted for publication, it contained the sentence:

> Exercise, vitamins, high fiber diet, *and the complete elimination of cigarettes* are all rapidly gaining acceptance among physicians, though at present time there is no definitive evidence to support their value [emphasis added]. {2009.06, p. 13}

Deletion of the phrase referring to cigarettes was suggested by one of the peer reviewers who read the article for the journal that published it. In

the published article the phrase "and the complete elimination of cigarettes" was deleted (2). The editor's acceptance letter stated:

> We will be pleased to publish "The Bandwagons of Medicine". The review-
> ers and I have only one strong suggestion. We are convinced that it would be
> wise to eliminate the comment on cigarettes (p. 13). *Since smoking is known
> to be harmful, your qualification 'complete elimination' will not be carefully
> noted* [emphasis added]. {2009.07}

Rothschild apparently sent the manuscript and the editor's comments to
Timothy Finnegan, who, in turn, circulated the editor's acceptance letter and page proofs of the article to the counsels for the tobacco companies. Finnegan evidently believed that the statement about cigarettes
was an important part of the paper, even though the reference to cigarettes was the only one in the seventeen-page paper.

> Of particular interest is the reviewer's comment about 'complete elimination
> of cigarettes' on page 13 of the manuscript, *which makes the point of the pa-
> per* [emphasis added]. {2009.05}

Thus, the documents reveal that Rothschild cooperated closely with the
lawyers in allowing opportunity for editorial input and in reporting on
professional editing that affected references to tobacco in Rothschild's
work submitted to scientific journals on scientific subjects and that
lawyers at the highest levels followed Rothschild's work closely.

CTR SPECIAL PROJECTS AWARDED TO CARL SELTZER

Carl Seltzer was a professor of public health at Harvard University until
1976. He conducted research related to the constitutional and genetic hypothesis favored by the industry. Specifically, Seltzer's work focused on
countering the evidence that smoking causes heart disease. Like Rothschild's work, Seltzer's work could be used by the tobacco industry to divert attention from tobacco as a cause of disease.

When Seltzer retired from the Harvard University School of Public
Health on June 30, 1976, he continued his research on "constitution and
disease" at the Peabody Museum at Harvard. The Peabody Museum is
a natural history museum, which is an odd place to do tobacco and health
research. Nevertheless, during his retirement Seltzer was awarded grants
of more than $750,000 from 1976 to 1990 through CTR special pro-
jects and Special Account 4 (table 8.1). A 1976 letter from Donald Hoel
of Shook, Hardy, and Bacon describes the arrangements made with Dr.
Seltzer and the Peabody:

Dr. Stephen Williams, Director of the Peabody Museum, has indicated that appropriate arrangements can be made. Such arrangements would be quite similar to those previously maintained at the Harvard University, School of Public Health. The total cost for one year's support from July 1, 1976, through June 30, 1977, would be $50,000. This sum includes a 15 percent "overhead" allocation to the Peabody Museum. Dr. Seltzer's salary, secretarial assistance, purchase or leasing of certain equipment, telephone service, etc., would be paid from the balance of these funds. {2004.01}

An April 4, 1979, memo from Hoel to the counsels for the tobacco companies approved an increase in Dr. Seltzer's annual grant from $60,000 to $70,000 to cover, in part, "increased travel expense for lectures" {2004.09}. As described below, Seltzer traveled extensively to speak about his work and stimulate controversy about the association between tobacco and heart disease.

A 1979 letter from Donald Hoel to the counsels of the tobacco companies describes a trip that Carl Seltzer made to New Zealand and Australia

> [to] meet with scientists, science writers and some industry people concerning his research and opinions on smoking and heart disease. . . . Personal reports from colleagues in Australia and New Zealand indicate that Dr. Seltzer's visit "was a great success." {2004.12}

Eight news clippings and radio transcripts covering Seltzer's visit are attached to the letter. The clippings—with titles such as "Smokers—Take Heart," "Doctor Slams Link between Smoking and Heart Disease," and "Smoking Does Not Cause Heart Disease"—describe Seltzer as a doctor from Harvard University. Only one small clipping discloses that Seltzer was "in Australia at the Tobacco Institute's invitation" {2004.13}. This type of press coverage that is favorable to the tobacco industry is significant because it demonstrates how the industry was quietly paying for scientists to publicize its position that tobacco is not dangerous. Scientists such as Seltzer, who were well-known researchers or had connections to prestigious institutions, lent a patina of legitimacy to the industry's claims that tobacco is not harmful. Seltzer was valuable to the tobacco industry, in part, because it could exploit his connection with Harvard University in press coverage.

Seltzer criticized scientific studies that found an association between tobacco and adverse health effects, and his efforts were monitored by the lawyers. An April 4, 1983, letter from Patrick Sirridge of Shook, Hardy, and Bacon to the counsels for the tobacco companies describes

Seltzer's activities—especially his analysis of a landmark study that found an association between smoking and heart disease (3, 4).

> Dr. Seltzer has been very active in the past year analyzing literature dealing with coronary heart disease (CHD) and advancing his views on the smoking and CHD issue. In particular, he spent a great deal of time reviewing the results of the Multiple Risk Factor Intervention Trial (MRFIT). In this regard, the Journal of the American Medical Association [which published the MRFIT study] recently published his letter [5] commenting on the MRFIT findings. Dr. Seltzer also presented his views about smoking and CHD and MRFIT in a written statement to the Waxman Subcommittee. {2004.21, p. 1}

A 1984 memo from Ernest Pepples to I. W. Hughes, J. Alar, and T. Humber illustrates that researchers funded through special projects were asked to respond to data presented in the lay media as well as in the scientific literature. Seltzer was asked to respond to unfavorable press on tobacco that was aired on the MacNeil/Lehrer television news program. The memo states:

> At B&W's request through Horace Kornegay [chairman of the Tobacco Institute], Carl Seltzer wrote the attached letter to Robin MacNeil taking issue with Dr. Castelli's [an investigator in the Framingham study] comments on the January 11 MacNeil/Lehrer program. My guess is MacNeil will send it to Castelli for rebuttal or he will just chuck it in the waste can. {2004.23}

Carl Seltzer's two-page letter to Robin MacNeil, dated January 31, 1984, states:

> I found some of Dr. Castelli's statements relative to smoking and heart disease to be biased, flawed, and inaccurate. {2004.25, p. 1}

Seltzer's letter criticizes the Framingham heart study, which evidently had been discussed in the interview. This study, the largest population-based study of heart disease epidemiology, had found that smoking is a cause of heart disease (6, 7). In an ad hominem attack on the scientist rather than the science, Seltzer claims that Castelli deliberately misled the "American public":

> I merely wanted you to get some idea of deliberate inaccuracies in the Castelli statements to you and the public, and in the flaws in the works of the Public Health Service's Framingham Study. {2004.25, p. 2}

In the letter to MacNeil, Seltzer devotes a paragraph to describing his own qualifications in an effort to establish that he is a credible, independent scientist. Seltzer does not state that his work has been supported by the tobacco industry during these years, nor does he mention that B&W's lawyers asked him to write the letter to MacNeil.

CTR SPECIAL PROJECTS AWARDED TO THEODOR STERLING

Theodor Sterling is a university research professor at Simon Fraser University in Burnaby, British Columbia. In addition to receiving money through the university, Dr. Sterling also formed a private consulting firm that received funding through CTR special projects. Between 1973 and 1990 CTR special projects provided over $5 million to support Sterling's work, with additional funding through Special Account 4 (table 8.1). The focus of Dr. Sterling's tobacco research has been on examining factors that could potentially confound the association of tobacco smoke and adverse health effects. For example, he has studied the influence of occupational hazards and genetics on lung cancer. This work has been useful to advance the "constitutional hypothesis" of disease (i.e., that cancer is caused by genetic makeup, not smoking) favored by the tobacco industry and provides a distraction from the evidence on the adverse health effects of tobacco.

Documents from tobacco industry lawyers reveal that Dr. Sterling's work became increasingly important to the industry over time because it was used to dispute scientific findings about the adverse effects of tobacco. Dr. Sterling's long history of funding by the tobacco industry illustrates the scientific issues that were important to the industry at different times.

A February 27, 1980, letter {2020.06} from William Shinn of Shook, Hardy, and Bacon to the general counsels of the tobacco companies describes the way in which Sterling was funded both through the university and through his consulting firm, the range of his funded activities, the tobacco industry's use of his work, and the lack of a competitive review procedure to receive continued funding. The projects funded in 1979–80 were directed at refuting the evidence that environmental tobacco smoke is dangerous (see chapter 10). Dr. Sterling's projects were designed to critique published work on environmental tobacco smoke and to draw attention to occupational and other lifestyle factors that might confound an association between environmental tobacco smoke and disease. As described in the lawyer's memo, Dr. Sterling's work was presented at congressional hearings, at scientific meetings, and in scientific publications to support the industry's position that exposure to environmental tobacco smoke should not be regulated.

Dr. Sterling is presently quite busy in at least nine areas. These include: preparation of a review of health effects due to indoor combustion of organic material requested by the National Academy of Sciences; preparation of a paper to present to the American Lung Association on the possible relationship between occupation, smoking and lung disease; completion of work on familial disease among women whose husbands are exposed to irritating dust and fumes; an investigation of the change in employment patterns of women since the 1930's; a study of smoking habits and employment patterns among blacks; completion of an analysis of errors in the [Harold E.] Dorn/[Harold A.] Kahn Study [a study of smoking and mortality among US veterans]; analysis of the use of magnetic techniques to measure long-term lung clearance of particles in smokers and nonsmokers; and an examination of preliminary data from a study of indoor pollutants from gas stoves.

Dr. Sterling has continued to be helpful in frequent consultations about the smoking and health controversy. He testified at Congressional hearings on public smoking in October, 1978; has given several technical papers at professional meetings recently; and has prepared a number of manuscripts, some of which have been published.

. . .

He [Sterling] *has offered to prepare a detailed proposal for the extension, but I am not too concerned about this since we could continue under the old agreement* [emphasis added]. {2020.06, pp. 1–2}

One of the main purposes of CTR special projects funding was to attempt to discredit independent scientific findings about tobacco. A letter from William Shinn at Shook, Hardy, and Bacon to the counsels for the tobacco companies requesting their approval of Sterling's funding credits their funding arrangements with Sterling as enabling the companies to obtain fast responses from Dr. Sterling to dispute scientific results that were not favorable to the industry. In contrast to research grants, which usually focus on a specific topic, the lawyers' correspondence indicates that Dr. Sterling's special projects funding was used to criticize the work of other scientists, such as Cohen's study showing that smoking adversely affects people's ability to eliminate dust from their lungs (described below).

A February 4, 1981, letter from William Shinn of Shook, Hardy, and Bacon to the counsels for the tobacco companies states:

As in the past, Dr. Sterling has used the support received from his grant to develop proposals for other projects. The flexibility inherent in the current arrangement has also provided Dr. Sterling with the ability to respond quickly to new scientific developments.

. . . Dr. Sterling analyzed Cohen's article [8], which appeared in *Science,* May, 1979, and concluded that Cohen's claim that smokers have impaired long-term clearance capabilities compared to nonsmokers' is open to challenge because of his faulty experimental design. Dr. Sterling interested

Dr. Glicksman and colleagues at Brown University in this problem. Subsequently, both Dr. Sterling and Dr. Glicksman presented papers highly critical of Cohen's work at a recent conference. . . . *Dr. Sterling has been informed that Cohen and colleagues have apparently ceased this type of experimental work.* In view of the many claims about the possible interaction of smoking and occupational exposures, Sterling's critical response to Cohen's work seems particularly important [emphasis added]. {2022.06, pp. 1–2}

Cohen and his colleagues (8) had human volunteers inhale a dust that could be traced because of its magnetic properties over a long period of time. They showed that after one year smokers had eliminated only half of the dust from their bodies, whereas nonsmokers had eliminated 90 percent of the administered dose. This work had potentially important implications for setting exposure limits to toxic dusts in occupational and in environmental settings.

Shinn's letter recommending approval of Sterling's funding contains a comment revealing the lawyer's interest in maintaining that Sterling was an independent scientist and not a representative of the tobacco companies:

Dr. Sterling is an independent scientist, of course, and as we have stated in earlier grant requests, there are to be no restrictions attached to his research work. Dr. Sterling's findings are his own, and we are free to agree or disagree with them. {2022.06, p. 3}

A March 1, 1982, memo from Patrick M. Sirridge at Shook, Hardy, and Bacon to the counsels for the companies requesting their approval for further funding of Sterling indicates that the lawyers were directly managing at least some of Sterling's work:

It is further recommended that the extension of Theodor D. Sterling, Ltd. commence May 1, 1982, because of unforeseen expenses *due mainly to additional requests from our office* [emphasis added]. {2037.04, p. 1}

Sirridge's acknowledgment that unforeseen expenses had been incurred by Sterling because Sterling was responding to additional requests from Shook, Hardy, and Bacon presents an ironic contrast with Shinn's insistence a year earlier that Sterling was an independent scientist. Sirridge repeats the point made by Shinn that the companies' funding arrangement with Sterling enabled him to respond quickly, apparently to requests from the lawyers. For example, one special request involved responding to publications on environmental tobacco smoke:

In January, 1982, Dr. Sterling prepared written comments in response to a paper presented by James E. Repace [of the US Environmental Protection

Agency] at the ASHRAE (American Society of Heating, Refrigeration and Air-conditioning Engineers) in Houston. . . . Dr. Sterling's oral presentation at the Houston meeting and the written comments which will be published in the ASHRAE Transactions this summer provide the first public criticisms of the deficiencies in Repace's scientific methodology. Further, Dr. Sterling pointed out that Repace's reliance on studies such as Hirayama's [Takahishi Hirayama published a paper in 1981 demonstrating that environmental tobacco smoke increases the risk of lung cancer in nonsmokers] was misplaced and that his conclusions were at variance with many published reports and Dr. Sterling's own research on indoor air pollution.

The flexibility inherent in Dr. Sterling's ongoing project enables him to respond within a short time to scientific developments. His willingness to prepare written comments on Repace's paper with only a few weeks notice is a good example. Dr. Sterling also responded to the publication of Hirayama's article early last year with a highly critical letter to the *British Medical Journal*, a copy of which is enclosed as Appendix D. Most recently, Dr. Sterling has prepared responsive materials on the scientific aspects of legislative proposals (Waxman and Hatch bills) pending in Congress [emphasis added]. {2037.04, p. 2}

Sirridge then points out that Sterling's work will be useful for stimulating controversy about the health effects of environmental tobacco smoke:

[Sterling] has written an extensive critical review of the literature on indoor by-product levels of tobacco smoke which is scheduled for publication in March. This paper will serve as *a useful critique of previous studies in this area, as it points out their deficiencies and emphasizes the need for more careful work* . . . [emphasis added]. {2037.04, p. 2}

In 1984, at the request of Ernest Pepples, B&W vice president for law, Sterling began to receive funding directly through the law firm of Shook, Hardy, and Bacon to continue his work reviewing epidemiological studies that demonstrated a link between smoking and disease {2037.01}. In a January 24, 1984, letter to Sirridge at Shook, Hardy, and Bacon, Pepples agrees that Sterling should be funded at the budget levels set forth but also states:

I do not think, however, that we should continue burdening CTR with such programs, and instead suggest that they be handled as law firm projects. {2037.01}.

Table 8.1 shows that in 1985 Sterling began to receive funding through Special Account 4, which was administered by the law firm of Jacob and Medinger.

In 1984, two years after Sirridge wrote the memo describing the usefulness of Sterling's work {2037.04}, that work continued to be useful to the industry by stimulating controversy and refuting scientific findings about tobacco. A January 23, 1984, memo from Patrick Sirridge of Shook, Hardy, and Bacon to the general counsels of the tobacco companies summarizes some of Dr. Sterling's accomplishments for the tobacco industry:

> He [Sterling] has also been concerned with selectivity in reporting in government reports such as the Surgeon General's. His conclusions have been presented at scientific meetings. . . . Dr. Sterling and members of his staff have appeared before scientific and professional groups such as BOCA, ASHRAE [American Society of Heating, Refrigeration and Air-conditioning Engineers], and the California Energy Commission. . . .
> During the past year, Dr. Sterling attended international meetings in Geneva and Turin to present reports on environmental conditions in office buildings. Based on his research results, Dr. Sterling reported that there was no difference in the prevalence of complaints about health or environment among smokers and nonsmokers working in offices where smoking was permitted versus those where it was prohibited. Dr. Sterling continues to publish papers in scientific journals and make presentations at scientific meetings. . . . Dr. Sterling has also provided assistance in responding to the 1982 and 1983 proposed legislation regarding new warning labels. He appeared before Congressman Waxman's Committee in 1982 and submitted statements in 1983. {2015.04, p. 2}

BOCA, ASHRAE, and the California Energy Commission are organizations involved in creating ventilation standards for buildings that are directly affected by environmental tobacco smoke. Sterling's presentations had the potential to influence regulation of environmental tobacco smoke exposure directly. The meeting in Geneva was a tobacco industry–sponsored symposium (9). Like those of other industry-sponsored symposia, the published proceedings of the Geneva conference featured the work of industry-funded scientists and contained articles that support the tobacco industry's position that tobacco smoke is not harmful (9). The industry-sponsored symposia are often cited by the industry as if they are peer-reviewed scientific journal articles that support the industry's position (1).

Sterling and Harold Perry were also funded under a CTR special project from 1978 through February 1982 to conduct an environmental study entitled "Retrospective Analysis of Environmental Contacts of Patients with Respiratory Cancer, Other Cancers, and Other Diseases" {2020.01}. In 1980 Sterling was funded under a CTR special project to conduct a study of indoor environments ("Feasibility Study on Office

Environments" {2022.10}). Robert Northrip (of Shook, Hardy, and Bacon), in a letter to the general counsels recommending funding, states:

> It is our opinion that this work could be extremely useful in view of the intense activity we are witnessing in both legislatures and referendums to restrict indoor smoking. {2020.03, p. 2}

This study led to the development of a proposal entitled "Office Building Syndrome," with the purpose of examining

> [the] dependence of this syndrome on building design and ventilation features, and investigating the syndrome's relationship, if any, to life-style factors, such as smoking. {2022.03, p. 1}

Theodor Sterling and his son, Elia Sterling, were coinvestigators on the $200,160 special project {2022.02}.

The documents show that Sterling has continued to receive funding through CTR and law firm special projects through at least 1993. The publication of Sterling's criticisms was part of a broad industry strategy to stimulate controversy about the adverse health effects of environmental tobacco smoke (1, 10, 11). Sterling's publications also gave the tobacco industry supportive material that could be cited in testimony before Congress, in court, in the medical literature, and in response to government documents in support of their position that the links between active and passive smoking and disease were "controversial."

MICROBIOLOGICAL ASSOCIATES

Although lawyers appear to have been primarily involved with CTR's special projects, in at least one case they became involved with a project that had been awarded as a contract through CTR. The contract was approved by the Scientific Advisory Board, but CTR had control over the data and publication of the results. The documents describe a contract during the 1970s with Microbiological Associates to conduct studies on the effects of cigarette smoke in mice.

Microbiological Associates was conducting inhalation studies, in which mice were placed in small chambers and breathed smoke-laden air for part of the day. Other studies were short-term biological tests to determine the carcinogenicity of cigarette smoke condensate. Tobacco industry lawyers were unaware that CTR had been funding the biological tests until 1977, when one of the scientists at Microbiological

Associates (a Dr. Gardner) requested additional funding from CTR to study smoke fractions in the biological tests. The ultimate purpose was to identify the compounds within tobacco smoke that are responsible for its carcinogenic effects.

The lawyers were apprehensive about this work because its results might give rise to lawsuits if the tests showed that certain elements in tobacco smoke were carcinogenic and also because the tests might constitute a breach of antitrust laws (discussed in chapter 7). These concerns are described in a memo from Ernest Pepples of B&W to Addison Yeaman, another B&W lawyer, dated March 10, 1977.

> I did not understand until I talked with Arthur Stevens [CEO of B&W] that CTR in the last several years has tested cigarette smoke condensate fractions in the following tests: (1) in the Ames microbiological screen for mutagenic activity; (2) for possible tumorigenic activity in a tissue culture assay; and (3) for promoting activity by using subcutaneous injections in mice. The fractions were originally produced by someone at the USDA for CTR under what has been called the "Stedman procedure." Most of the assay work has been carried out at Microbiological Associates.
>
> Let me say parenthetically that years of cherishing Dr. [Robert] Hockett's [of the CTR] oft quoted comment about mice tests—the wrong animal, the wrong tissue, etc.—*I confess that I was somewhat jarred by the revelation to me about tests on mice through the CTR* [emphasis added]. {1817.02}

Pepples says that he has discussed the tests with several other tobacco industry lawyers, and none of them knew that CTR was engaged in this sort of work.

> We all think these tests are so significant that members of your [CTR] Board and people who attend the scientific sessions as I have off and on for the last couple of years should be better informed. Pursuing the thought just a bit further, *these tests are so-called red light tests.* They have been developed for use by FDA and other agencies in possibly identifying harmful ingredients and substances in products which are available to the consuming public. At best they show only a probability of trouble but they are used as a signal in such things as whether Red Dye No. 7 or cyclamates or hexachlorophene should be yanked off the market. *I do not have to tell you what Senator* [Edward] *Kennedy* [D-MA] *would do with a finding by a CTR grantee of red lights in one of these tests as it applies to cigarette smoke fractions.* We would never be able to explain that we were only replicating or confirming some other person's work. *No matter what our explanation happened to be the fact of the red light in our own hands would be a serious burden to the tobacco industry if it came out in legislative hearings or in litigation* [emphasis added]. {1817.02}

One of the short-term tests being done at Microbiological Associates was a test to see whether tobacco smoke caused chromosomal abnormalities in laboratory animals. Such a study had been done by the Food and Drug Administration in its investigation of cyclamates (see chapter 7). Pepples recommended that the inhalation program at Microbiological Associates should continue until completion, but that the short-term biological tests should not be funded through CTR {1817.03, p. 1}.

The final action taken on the research at Microbiological Associates is described in a memo from Ed Jacob, of the Jacob and Medinger law firm, to Pepples. The memo is dated June 22, 1978, and is titled "Current Status of CTR's Consideration of Microbiological Associates Contract Proposals."

> Following the visit by the SAB [Scientific Advisory Board] Task Force and staff to Bethesda regarding status of Microbiological Associates (MA) contract and later discussions between SAB and staff, CTR has now proposed the following action to MA with regard to the MA proposals for the contract year July 1, 1978 through June 30, 1979:
>
> 1. CTR would like to continue, subject to receiving from MA appropriate protocols and contract, the inhalation work, using various strains of mice, whole smoke, and whole smoke together with BaP [benzo(a)pyrene, a carcinogen in cigarette smoke].
>
> . . .
>
> 2. CTR has expressed to MA *a lack of interest* in contracting for the following:
>
> (i)   Deposition studies employing laboratory carcinogens such as MCA aerosolized in smoke.
>
> (ii)   Studies of biochemical markers such as ODC, aimed at testing the possible [cancer] promotional effects of whole cigarette smoke condensate and its various fractions.
>
> (iii)   Certain initiation studies, especially those using DNA damage assays.
>
> (iv)   Studies aimed at detection and quantitation of possible carcinogenic metabolites in mouse urine as a lead to bladder cancer.
>
> (v)   Whole smoke experiments testing the immune system's prevention of lung cancer and the susceptibility to lung cancer as a function of age.
>
> (vi)   In the area of so-called "initiation" studies, studies aimed at evaluating the initiating capacity of whole cigarette smoke condensate and its various fractions by variations of Ames-type tests [italic emphasis added]. {1820.04, pp. 1–2}

The studies that CTR declined to fund include short-term biological tests. Although the documents do not indicate the reasons for CTR's decision, the decision is consistent with Pebbles's recommendation. Ed Jacob's memorandum on CTR's final action was transmitted to eight industry lawyers (at both tobacco companies and outside firms) in a memo describing it as "a most interesting report" {1820.02}. The degree of industry lawyer participation and interest in CTR's action on the Microbiological Associates work is particularly noteworthy because the work at Microbiological Associates was funded through CTR's Scientific Advisory Board, not through its special projects division.

ADDICTION RESEARCH FOUNDATION: A CASE STUDY OF A SPECIAL PROJECT THE INDUSTRY WAS *NOT* INTERESTED IN FUNDING

The documents contain at least one instance in which an applicant for funding considered the lawyers as the court of last resort in attempting to procure tobacco industry funding for research. In December 1976 the Addiction Research Foundation, directed by pharmacologist and Stanford University professor Avram Goldstein, M.D., submitted a formal grant application to CTR requesting $400,000 for the purpose of constructing a new research facility. The Addiction Research Foundation had been studying the mechanism of opiate addiction, and the new facility would enable it to expand its work to include the mechanism of nicotine addition.

Dr. Goldstein was told by CTR that it would consider proposals "directly related to tobacco and health, but that it was not in a position to provide funds for structuring the Addiction Research Foundation" {1913.08}. He then pursued funding from individual tobacco companies. Correspondence alerting the individual companies that Leonard Cornell of the Addiction Research Foundation would be contacting them was circulated by Shook, Hardy, and Bacon to Brown and Williamson, American Brands, Liggett & Meyers, Lorillard, Philip Morris, R. J. Reynolds, and US Tobacco. The letters stated that Cornell would be writing the tobacco companies to request funding and that CTR had already rejected the Addiction Research Foundation's application for funding. Cornell did approach the individual companies seeking funding. Only Lorillard responded to his letter, and it issued a terse denial of funding that offered no reason for its decision.

In a final attempt to receive funding from the individual companies, Cornell wrote William Shinn, attorney at Shook, Hardy, and Bacon, on August 9, 1978. Cornell argued that the tobacco industry should be interested in funding the Addiction Research Foundation because the foundation's work could be directed to developing a "safe cigarette"—i.e., a cigarette that "could create the nicotine effect that smokers enjoy without the toxicity of nicotine" {1913.04}.

> Perhaps the term 'addiction' turns them [the tobacco companies] off. That is
> no obstacle. We're willing to establish the tobacco research under a separate
> name: 'The RJ Reynolds Program . . .' or whatever. {1913.04, p. 2}

Although Cornell wrote that his appeal was "attuned to the needs and
desires of the tobacco industry in terms of public relations and accelerating profits" {1913.04, p. 2}, he did not realize that the tobacco industry would not fund any proposals that acknowledged that nicotine
is addictive.

The document shows that Shinn transmitted Cornell's letter to the
general counsels for several tobacco companies as well as to other outside lawyers {1913.04}, but the lawyers showed no interest in approv-
ing Cornell's request. The tobacco companies refused to fund the Addiction Research Foundation because of their starting assumption about
nicotine; at the same time, BAT's internal research program had come to
similar conclusions about nicotine and addiction fourteen years earlier
(see chapter 3). The reason that the Addiction Research Foundation did
not receive support from the industry is summed up in a memo from
C. L. Waite to H. R. Kornegay (of the Tobacco Institute):

> Mr. Cornell's foundation actually assumes tobacco (nicotine) is addictive and
> costs the U.S. citizen 42 billion dollars a year! He also believes tobacco causes
> 300,000 premature deaths each year. And he wonders if this is why we might
> not be interested. {1913.01}

LAW FIRM ACCOUNTS

The documents contain information about two special accounts, Special
Account 4 and Special Account 5. (We have no information about Special Accounts 1, 2, 3, or numbers above 5, or even whether such accounts
existed.) Special Accounts 4 and 5 supported research projects and consultancies with money provided directly by law firms. Special Account
4 was administered by Jacob and Medinger. It was one of several special
accounts maintained by law firms and administered by lawyers. These
accounts funded research by expert witnesses in preparation of testimony directly related to a particular case, or prepared witnesses to testify at congressional or other hearings, or supported other research
deemed useful by the lawyers {1000.01, p. 44}.

In a 1978 memo to the counsels for the tobacco companies, William
Shinn of Shook, Hardy, and Bacon explains how Special Account 4 is
administered:

> This account is administered by Jacob & Medinger and Ed Jacob and I have reviewed the enclosed report. I also enclose a memorandum with regard to funding of projects and would appreciate your advice if you find this to be incorrect in any way. There is probably no need for you to retain those notes once you have satisfied yourself of the current situation. {2010.01, p. 1}.

The notes are not among the documents.

As shown in table 8.1, seventy-two projects (forty-nine research projects and twenty-three consultancies) were funded between 1976 and 1993 through these special accounts. The documents describe only one project funded through Special Account 5 (table 8.1) and do not contain a clear explanation of the difference between Special Accounts 4 and 5. The Special Account 5 project appears to have been a consultancy, because two individuals received $637,000 between 1979 and 1983 to analyze policy issues dealing with control and regulation of routine behavior in a democratic society. The analyses generated from this project may have been used for the tobacco industry's smokers' rights campaigns.

SPECIAL ACCOUNT 4: PROJECTS AND CONSULTANCIES

Most of the research projects funded through Special Account 4 described in the documents are related to environmental tobacco smoke (table 8.1). For example, the purpose of four of the Special Account 4 research projects was to measure levels of tobacco smoke in the environment. Other Special Account 4 research projects studied potential confounding factors for adverse health effects associated with smoking. For example, projects examined genetic factors associated with disease or the influence of low-protein diets or psychological stress on pregnancy outcomes. Funding research projects such as these, which divert attention from research on the adverse health effects of tobacco, has been a long-standing tactic of the tobacco industry (1, 11).

Twenty-four of the consultancies funded through Special Account 4 were to support the preparation of statements for hearings on public smoking restrictions (table 8.1). Individuals were paid from $2,500 to $4,000 to prepare these statements. As described later in this chapter, the statements favored the tobacco industry's position that smoking in public places should not be regulated. The Special Account 4 consultancies also supported the preparation of reviews of the scientific literature on topics ranging from the "tobacco habit" to lung retention of particulate matter. As was noted earlier, tobacco industry–sponsored reviews published in symposia proceedings consistently favor the industry's position that tobacco is not harmful (9). Some individuals were also paid for "continuing consultancies" for unspecified purposes. These continuing consultancies ranged from $500 to $1,500 per month and up.

SPECIAL ACCOUNT 4: DOMINGO AVIADO

The documents describe in detail the Special Account 4 consultancy that was awarded to Dr. Domingo Aviado. Domingo Aviado was a faculty member (rising from assistant professor to professor) in the Department of Pharmacology at the University of Pennsylvania from 1953 through 1977. A well-respected researcher on the effects of various airborne pollutants on health, he published extensively and served on numerous government committees. A May 9, 1977, letter from William Shinn of Shook, Hardy, and Bacon to the counsels for the tobacco companies indicates that Dr. Aviado received grant support from CTR during his years at the University of Pennsylvania, but that he is now requesting funding directly from the companies while he is in his new position:

> Dr. Aviado was supported until January 1 of this year by the Council for Tobacco Research—U.S.A. but has been advised that his latest application for funds was not approved. {2007.02, p. 1}

Shinn recommends that Aviado's request for $85,000 be approved for the period July 1, 1977, to June 30, 1978.

In 1977 Dr. Aviado left the University of Pennsylvania and became senior director for Biomedical Research Corporate Medical Affairs, Allied Chemical Corporation. In an October 24, 1979, letter Shinn tells the counsels for the tobacco companies that Dr. Aviado plans to leave Allied Chemical and proposes that he be supported by the tobacco industry in an amount equal to his annual total compensation at his previous position.

> Dr. Aviado is planning to leave Allied Chemical. . . .
>
> Dr. Aviado is currently earning $75,000 in salary. He also receives an annual bonus, fringe benefits and a travel account that bring his total compensation to over $100,000.
>
> I seek authority to make a grant or set up some other arrangement with Dr. Aviado for an estimated total cost of $100,000. . . .
>
> Dr. Aviado has been most helpful in evaluating research proposals, suggesting various projects and conducting a continuing literature search in several important areas such as carbon monoxide and "dependency." {2007.05, pp. 1–2}

Letters from Patrick Sirridge of Shook, Hardy, and Bacon to the counsels for the tobacco companies indicate that Dr. Aviado formed his own consulting organization in 1980 and that this organization was supported by Special Account 4 through 1985. In addition, the letters describe the importance of Dr. Aviado's work to the industry. This correspondence provides an instructive chronology of work of interest to the industry. The letters confirm that the tobacco industry sought to benefit from Aviado's good reputation as a retired scientist and from his membership on government committees, such as the EPA Clean Air Advisory Committee. Excerpts from the letters, outlining the chronology of his support, are given below:

Letter dated February 6, 1981:

A grant of $80,000 was given to Dr. Domingo Aviado during 1980. . . .

During 1980, Dr. Aviado formed his own consulting organization named Atmospheric Health Sciences, Inc. He devoted approximately 150 days of the working year to projects related to smoking and health. His projects included an ongoing review of smoking and health literature, preparations of recommendations re research projects, several site visits to research institutions and the preparation of materials relating to our work on various smoking and health related matters. Without question, Dr. Aviado's efforts were of immense benefit to us. {2007.08, p. 1}

Letter dated February 8, 1982:

In 1981, a grant of $92,000 was given to Dr. Domingo Aviado. . . .

During 1981, he devoted approximately 160 days of the working year to projects related to smoking and health. These projects included an ongoing review of smoking and health literature, preparations of recommendations regarding research projects, several site visits to research institutions and the preparation of statements and critiques relating to our work on various smoking and health related matters. Dr. Aviado was especially active in the areas of public smoking, self-extinguishing cigarettes and occupation-related diseases.

Dr. Aviado remains an extremely important resource for us in our smoking and health work. *He also is a valuable source of information by reason of his membership on the EPA Clean Air Advisory Committee . . .* [emphasis added]. {2007.10, p. 1}

Letter dated January 26, 1983:

For the past three years, Dr. Domingo Aviado has received a Special Fund 4 grant for the support of his consulting activities in the smoking and health area. In 1982, the amount of the grant was $102,000. . . .

During 1982, he devoted approximately 190 days of the working year to projects related to smoking and health. These projects included an ongoing review of smoking and health literature, preparation of recommendations regarding research projects, several site visits to research institutions, *the preparation of statements (including one for the Waxman/Hatch hearings)*, and the analysis of ongoing technical issues related to our work in the smoking and health area. . . .

Dr. Aviado *continues to be a valuable source of information by reason of his work for the EPA Clean Air Advisory Committee . . .* [emphasis added]. {2007.13, p. 1}

Letter dated February 1, 1984:

For the past four years, Dr. Domingo Aviado has received a Special Fund 4 grant in support of his consulting activities in the smoking and health area. In 1983, the amount of the grant was $102,000. . . .

During 1983, he devoted approximately 195 days of the working year to projects related to smoking and health. These projects included an ongoing review of the relevant literature, preparation of recommendations regarding research projects, the preparation of statements (including *two* for the Waxman/Hatch hearings), *attendance at various scientific meetings,* and the analysis of ongoing technical issues relating to our work in the smoking and health area. Dr. Aviado was especially busy in the areas of public smoking, occupation-related diseases, and the possible effects of tobacco smoke constituents/ingredients.

Dr. Aviado continued his technical association with the EPA Clean Air Advisory Committee. . . .

As you may remember, *Dr. Aviado attended both the Fifth World Conference on Smoking and Health and the Rylander Symposium during 1983* [emphasis added]. {2007.16, pp. 1–2}

(Aviado does not appear to have made a presentation at the Fifth World Conference.) The Rylander symposium was a tobacco industry–sponsored scientific meeting on environmental tobacco smoke; participants presented research criticizing the data on passive smoke and suggesting that passive smoke is not harmful (9).

Letter dated February 8, 1985:

For the past five years, Dr. Domingo Aviado has received a Special Fund 4 grant in support of his consulting activities in the smoking and health area. In 1984, the amount of the grant was $102,000 for professional time and expenses. We recommend that Dr. Aviado be given support in 1985 in the same amount ($102,000) to be funded again through Special Fund 4.

During 1984, he devoted approximately 204 days of the working year to projects related to smoking and health. These projects included his ongoing review of generally relevant literature, special reviews of literature relating to bronchogenic carcinoma, environmental carcinogenesis and pulmonary metastases, *analysis of environmental tobacco smoke materials and preparation of related critiques, attendance at various scientific meetings, work on the smoking aboard aircraft issue and participation at a CAB* [Civil

Aeronautics Board] *hearing,* and analysis of studies involving atherosclerosis and smoking behavior. Dr. Aviado has been especially busy in the last few months working with the newly formed industry committee on environmental tobacco smoke.

Dr. Aviado *continued his informal association with the EPA Clean Air Advisory Committee and other governmental groups. . . . He also continues to be helpful in identifying possible medical consultants in the New Jersey area* [emphasis added]. {2007.18, pp. 1–2}

The chronology of Aviado's work illustrates a common tobacco industry technique to bootstrap its consultants' work into scientific authority that is used to try to influence legislation and smoking policy. Aviado was hired by industry lawyers to do work including critiques of evidence on tobacco's health dangers, which were presented at scientific meetings. In addition, Aviado's work included presentation of papers at symposia on tobacco and health sponsored by the tobacco industry that, not surprisingly, questioned the evidence linking tobacco to disease. The papers at the symposia were then cited in congressional testimony and other forums without featuring the fact that the symposium at which the papers were presented was industry funded. In addition, when Aviado submitted critical comments to the EPA regarding its risk assessment of environmental tobacco smoke and lung cancer, he did not mention his tobacco industry connections (1); we do not know whether he had disclosed his industry connections in earlier comments submitted to the CAB.

UNIVERSITY SPECIAL PROJECTS

Some research projects were funded directly by the tobacco companies, rather than through CTR or the law firms. Some of these projects were funded individually by Brown and Williamson and some by pooled contributions from companies. Projects funded directly by tobacco companies apparently included relatively unrestricted grants to universities {2003.01}. The motivation for funding these projects is not revealed in the documents.

In contrast to projects funded through CTR or the law firms, these university projects did not focus exclusively on research related to tobacco use. There was debate among the tobacco companies concerning whether or not projects that were not directly related to tobacco should be funded. For example, some of the companies declined to join in support of a diabetes research project at Washington University ($8,100,000 from April

1, 1971, through March 31, 1991 {2003.01}) or research at UCLA on genetic markers, host defenses of the lung, and immune action in the body ($2,750,000 from June 1, 1974, through May 31, 1982 {2003.01}).

As with CTR and law firm special projects, lawyers and high-level tobacco industry executives were intimately involved in funding decisions for university projects. For example, in 1980 William Shinn of Shook, Hardy, and Bacon organized a site visit to review Washington University's request for continued support {2019.01}. The site visit committee consisted of the executive officers of Brown and Williamson, Liggett & Myers, Philip Morris, R. J. Reynolds, Tobacco Associates, the Tobacco Institute, and US Tobacco {2019.09}. There is no indication that the lawyers and executives were accompanied by scientists or that the funding was subject to the scientific peer review process.

INVOLVEMENT OF LAWYERS IN RESEARCH DESIGN

One example of the way in which lawyers influenced the design of research projects is the Response Analysis Corporation project, which involved the measurement of environmental tobacco smoke (ETS). A November 10, 1976, letter from Donald K. Hoel of Shook, Hardy, and Bacon to the attorneys of five tobacco companies describes a meeting at which the Response Analysis Corporation's questionnaire for assessing annoyances in indoor air was discussed:

> Concern was expressed that the questionnaire's list of annoyance items, which included several related to tobacco products, did not have a modern empirical foundation. . . . In order to strengthen the study in the above regard, a two-step effort was proposed by the Response Analysis staff. First, a national sample of approximately 200 persons would be asked essentially to list items that they find annoying. Then a different national sample of 200 persons would be asked to rate the annoyances obtained in the first step as to their frequency of occurrence and intensity. {2006.03, pp. 1–2}

In a later letter to the attorneys, Hoel discusses the results obtained from this modified proposal:

> [The results point to] a new and potentially profitable direction to pursue. Specifically, of the total of 852 annoyances or irritations reported by the 207 respondents, only 26 (about 3%) were annoyances related to cigarettes, smokers or tobacco smoke. In the judgment of those in the Public Smoking Research Group, if the above results were obtained from a national sample of approximately 750 respondents, its impact in the public smoking controversy would be substantial. {2006.05, p. 1}

The rest of the letter requests approval of the Response Analysis Corporation's request for money to conduct the larger survey. In this project a seemingly minor change in design—a switch from a closed questionnaire (better design) to an open-ended questionnaire (poorer design)—gave the tobacco industry the results it wanted. The project also shows that the tobacco industry's lawyers were aware of the importance of ETS as an issue long before the mainstream health community appreciated its importance.

SMOKELESS TOBACCO COUNCIL

The Smokeless Tobacco Council (STC) is a tobacco industry–sponsored research organization that concentrates on smokeless tobacco. Like CTR, the Smokeless Tobacco Council is supported by contributions from individual tobacco companies (see chapter 2). Also like CTR, the STC appears to fund many proposals not on the basis of scientific peer review, but on the basis of interest to tobacco company lawyers.

In September 1978 Ernest Pepples, counsel for B&W, recommended that B&W join the Smokeless Tobacco Council:

> I think it would be polite to join and would recommend contributing $5000 per annum. . . . The primary purpose of such membership, however, would be to know what the Smokeless Tobacco Council is doing as a protective measure both for our interest in that product area and against the possibility that some research they do could impact on our cigarette business. {1500.06}

B&W appears to have joined the STC because it wanted to keep abreast of what the STC was doing. Furthermore, as described in more detail below, the individual companies were concerned that research on smokeless tobacco might indicate that the smokeless tobacco products were less hazardous than cigarettes.

J. K. Wells, a B&W lawyer, attended an STC meeting after B&W joined. In a November 9, 1979, memo to Ernest Pepples {1502.01}, Wells summarizes what went on at the meeting.

> Tim [Finnegan of the law firm Jacob, Medinger, and Finnegan] reported that *Dr. H. Russell Fisher appeared at the annual meeting of the AMA* [American Medical Association] *in Chicago and protested on the floor the adoption of an AMA resolution which urged the media to refuse smokeless tobacco advertising, especially television and radio.* [Dr. Fisher also received roughly $2,500 through a Special Account 4 consultancy to prepare testimony for the Waxman/Hatch hearings in 1982.]

Dr. Fisher's appearance was cleared beforehand with Fred Panzer [a public relations expert with CTR].

. . . efforts had been made to find scientists in other areas of the country [outside the southeast] willing to do research in the area of health and smokeless tobacco, but . . . no interested scientists had been found.

. . .

Tim gave an update on the *Douglas v. US Tobacco* [case], now pending in Ft. Smith, Arkansas. . . . Tim believes the plaintiff will have a difficult time winning the wrongful death claim [involving Red Seal snuff] because the cause of death was listed as secondary, but primary site pelvic cancer [*sic*].

The approach to research used by the STC is based on the concept that the only serious line of scientific attack on smokeless tobacco at the present time in the United States is clinical observation studies (in contrast to epidemiological studies). [The memo goes on to give the usual attacks on epidemiology.]

. . .

I discussed with Tim privately whether research had been or was being done to identify the constituents or by-products of smokeless tobacco and whether any research was planned dealing with NNN [N-nitrosonornicotine, a laboratory carcinogen present in smoke and smokeless tobacco]. Tim said that . . . *[n]one is planned because the prevailing theory is that the best position for the STC is on the question of the effect on the human body of the whole product and to identify various constituents, many of which might be defined as tumorigenic in other contexts[,] would weaken the industry's position. In other words, it is 'the other side's' duty to produce allegations that certain constituents result from the use of smokeless tobacco and are harmful* [emphasis added]. {1502.01, pp. 1–2}

As Wells's report indicates, the STC funded scientists who would work closely with the industry to combat policies to regulate smokeless tobacco and to attack and dispute scientific findings about smokeless tobacco. Furthermore, the STC steered away from funding research, such as that on NNN, that might have suggested a harmful effect of tobacco. The STC's refusal to fund work on NNN, an obligatory component of tobacco with a high likelihood of being harmful, was particularly significant. The STC meeting also served the purpose of keeping the participants informed about ongoing litigation related to smokeless tobacco.

In 1985 the STC responded to a request by Joseph W. Cullen, of the US Public Health Service, for scientific evidence on the health consequences of using smokeless tobacco. Cullen was chairman of the Advisory Committee on the Health Consequences of Smokeless Tobacco, which was preparing a Surgeon General's report on the topic. A letter to Dr. Cullen from Michael Kerrigan, president of the STC, contains the same arguments that are being used today to combat the EPA risk assessment of environmental tobacco smoke (1, 11) (see chapter 10).

> [T]he industry is concerned that the conclusions and resulting report by the Advisory committee are preordained. . . .
>
> Enclosed are statements submitted in those forums [of Waxman's subcommittee] by many eminent scientists who, after close review of the literature and, in many cases, from their own work, have concluded that smokeless tobacco has not been scientifically established to cause human disease and is not addictive. . . .
>
> [T]o date no one knows the cause or causes of oral cancer and . . . much more research is needed before any conclusions can be drawn. . . .
>
> The need to identify the areas where more knowledge is required is important. . . . [T]he industry is continuing to fund independent research into questions of smokeless tobacco and health. . . .
>
> [E]nclosed is a compilation of citations to a substantial portion of the world's literature pertaining to smokeless tobacco and oral cancer. {1503.02, pp. 1–3}

In short, the STC, using the same strategy that CTR was using, paid scientists to produce data that would dispute scientific findings on tobacco, to review and criticize the scientific literature on tobacco, and to perpetuate controversy about the adverse effects of tobacco. Nothing in the documents suggests that the STC would support research that could possibly contradict the industry position that smokeless tobacco is not harmful. The research by the STC-supported scientists revealed in the documents was used in attempts to influence policy makers involved in regulating tobacco and to inform lawyers involved in litigation.

THE KENTUCKY TOBACCO AND HEALTH RESEARCH INSTITUTE

The state of Kentucky established the Tobacco and Health Research Institute at the University of Kentucky to conduct a program of research on smoking and health issues. The institute is financed through the state excise tax on cigarettes, and its external grants are approved by the Kentucky Tobacco Research Board. The board's membership includes a representative of the tobacco product manufacturers, and B&W General Counsel Ernest Pepples held that seat in 1984 {1602.01}. The Kentucky Tobacco and Health Research Institute was publicized as an independent taxpayer-funded program that supports research on tobacco. However, the documents suggest that tobacco company lawyers were involved in the administration of this program.

In a November 6, 1980, letter, Ernest Pepples asks attorney Timothy Finnegan to check the background of a Dr. David Justus, of the University of Louisville, who has requested funding from the Tobacco and Health Research Institute {1600.01}. Justus had written Dr. Gary Huber, then the director of the Institute, to ask if the institute would be interested in funding his work on tobacco hypersensitivity {1600.01}. Pepples forwarded the request to Finnegan and asked Finnegan:

> I wish you would find out, *without tipping over any cans,* what Dr. Justus has done in the tobacco allergy field. At this point all I would like to have is a search of the literature to see if Dr. Justus has published on tobacco and how *we* assess his work. *I would not want him to become worried that a tobacco company somehow is reviewing his request for continued assistance from the* [Kentucky Tobacco and Health Research] *Institute* [emphasis added]. {1600.01}

This is a most interesting episode. The kind of preliminary enquiry regarding funding for a possible research project would normally be answered by the agency staff with a letter encouraging or discouraging a proposal. Only after such a formal proposal had been received and favorably reviewed would the proposal normally be submitted to a policy-making board for final approval of funding. The documents do not indicate how Pepples came into possession of the Justus letter to Huber, the institute director. Pepples's request for discretion in checking Justus's background indicates that he wanted to keep quiet the active role that he and the other industry lawyers were playing in the selection of grantees. In any event, transmission of Justus's request to a lawyer from an out-of-state law firm suggests funding requests to the institute were subjected to influences other than scientific peer review.

The documents reveal that Pepples also asked William Shinn, a lawyer at Shook, Hardy, and Bacon, to evaluate the scientific work done by the Kentucky Tobacco and Health Research Institute. Following the September 1984 meeting of the Tobacco Research Board, Pepples wrote Bill Shinn at Shook, Hardy, and Bacon with some concerns about the research program the institute had developed.

> Looking at the Kentucky Institute's Annual Report of Research, it seems to cover an impressive amount of work in many disciplines. Most, if not all of it, however, has been published before by others. . . .
> I believe Layten Davis [director of the institute at the time] is interested in positive aspects of smoking. He has encouraged the work in stress abatement and good people are working in the area. Dr. Martin and his colleagues have been looking at the effect of nicotine on the dog's brain. They are seeking to

identify effects on the brain and then to selectively mimic those effects with
new compounds. Both Martin and Fell appear to be on the leading edge of
positive research.

I would be interested in hearing your views on the credits and debits of
the current research at the Kentucky Tobacco and Health Research Institute.
{1603.01}

(The discussion of Martin's research indicates that the institute, like BAT
and Philip Morris, was engaged in research on nicotine analogues. The
"positive" research referred to in the letter is research that would demonstrate a benefit of smoking—e.g., stress abatement.)

The Kentucky Tobacco and Health Research Institute also turned to
the industry and its lawyers for help in preparing congressional testimony. In a letter dated September 28, 1983, Ernest Pepples informs John
Rupp, an attorney at Covington and Burling, about one such request:

> Dr. Layten Davis, Director of the Kentucky Tobacco & Health Research In-
> stitute, has just received a letter from Congressman Larry Hopkins seeking
> comment on Moakley's self-extinguishing cigarette bill [see the discussion of
> fire-safe cigarettes in chapter 7].
>
> Layten called me for help in replying to Hopkins's letter. He wants to say
> something about better fabrics and better ashtrays and something about the
> need for deliberate care and study before tinkering with cigarette construc-
> tion. He is particularly concerned about the biological effects of newfangled
> "self-extinguishing" cigarettes.
>
> I said that Spears [Alex Spears, research director at Lorillard Tobacco]
> had prepared a good state-of-the-art summary, which Davis said he'd like to
> see. Could you send me the Spears paper and any other testimony you think
> should be provided to Dr. Davis. He also asked about MORE and the Nat Sher-
> man cigarettes [two brands of cigarettes that were relatively fire-safe], of
> course. {1601.01}

The episodes revealed by the documents betray an unusually close
working relationship between the institute, which presented itself as an
independent arm of a publicly funded university, and industry lawyers,
both in the evaluation of the institute's research and the institute's participation in public policy formulation.

USE OF RESEARCH FROM SPECIAL PROJECTS

Although CTR's publicly stated purpose was to conduct scientific research, it actually served purposes related to public relations, politics,
and litigation.

PRODUCING GOOD PUBLICITY

The tobacco industry used CTR to create a public image as a benevolent funder of science. In "Cigarette Smoking and Health: What Are the Facts?" TIRC-funded research is touted as contributing "to the fund of knowledge about lung cancer and other diseases" {1903.02, p. 4}. The document also boasts that "300 papers have been published in medical and scientific journals and societies which credit TIRC for support in whole or part" {1903.02, p. 4}.

A "Report to CTR Annual Meeting," dated January 31, 1975, describes 1974 as a "good year" for CTR because the work of its grantees was covered favorably in the lay press {1908.01}. The report specifically mentions that a paper published by Carl Seltzer (a special projects researcher, discussed earlier in this chapter) on the effect of smoking in lowering blood pressure "was reported on the front page of the Chicago Daily News and moved on CDN [Chicago Daily News] newswire" {1908.01}. The report also describes CTR's reaction when it did not receive credit for its sponsored research:

> A CTR grantee last month had an article in an AMA journal that did not credit CTR for support. The article was brought to the attention of certain writers who were told of CTR's sponsorship. There was some followup on my part [the unnamed person who wrote the memo] and the science writer of the Pittsburgh Post-Gazette interviewed the scientist and wrote a nice piece. {1908.01}

SUPPORTING THE INDUSTRY'S PUBLIC POLICY POSITIONS

An undated, unsigned document labeled "Privileged Attorney Work Product" and entitled "CTR Special Projects" shows that CTR and Special Account 4 special projects were used to fund researchers to testify at legislative hearings.

> Dr. LGS Rao also received Special Account 4 money for testifying in the Hatch-Packwood, Waxman hearings. {2005.01, p. 1}

Rao's research, funded, in part, from 1977 through 1984 from Special Account 4, supported the tobacco industry's position that poor fetal outcome is associated more with poor nutrition than with smoking (table 8.1).

> [Dr. Henry Rothschild] also testified at Hatch-Packwood, Waxman Hearings and probably received Special Acct 4 money. {2005.01, p. 2}

Rothschild's work, discussed above, was funded as a special project from 1977 through 1984, and was designed to support the tobacco industry's position that cancer is genetically determined (table 8.1).

> Dr. [Gerhard] Schrauzer also testified in hearings re: Comprehensive Smoking Prevention Act of 1982. {2005.01, p. 3}

The memorandum does not specifically say whether Schrauzer was paid for this testimony. Schrauzer received support through CTR special projects to study selenium in tobacco and tobacco smoke (1981–83) and to conduct statistical and epidemiological studies on lung cancer (1983–85). He also was paid on a date not revealed in the documents through a Special Account 4 consultancy to prepare a statement on public smoking (table 8.1).

The undated, unsigned document described above summarizes studies that support alternate hypotheses for disease (e.g., the constitutional and genetic hypotheses):

> CONCLUSION: Low protein intake (poor nutrition) associated with poor fetal outcome more than smoking habits. (NUTRITIONAL HYPOTHESIS) [From a summary of L. G. S. Rao's Special Project through Account 4.] . . .
>
> SALVAGGIO/LEHRER PROJECT: All studies deal with rebutting contention that ETS [environmental tobacco smoke] aggravates allergies. . . . [These investigators were funded through CTR special projects from 1981 to 1983 and from 1985 to 1988 (table 8.1).]
>
> RESULTS: Challenge studies showed that exposure to cigarette smoke did not cause a significant decline in lung function among "smoke sensitive" individuals. Found that ETS did not impair lung function in asthmatics. . . .
>
> RESULTS: Preliminary clinical [trials] suggest that there are little, if any, human allergens in tobacco smoke. {2005.01, pp. 1–4}

This same document also cites a special project that could actually suggest positive health benefits of tobacco:

> INVESTIGATORS: Drs. Henry and Linda Russek (Father and daughter) [They received funding through a CTR special project between 1979 and 1981 (table 8.1).]
>
> SUBJECT: Relationship between psychological factors and disease. . . .
>
> Henry and Linda Russek have long investigated the link between stress and heart disease using prospective epidemiological studies. *Have also found that smoking may be an effective means of coping with stress. . . .*
>
> RESULTS: Proposal approved, and *expected results to show that cigarette smoking is the best mechanism for smokers to cope with stress. Expect to show benefits of smoking (i.e. to reduce risk of stress-related heart disease)* [emphasis added]. {2005.01, p. 3}

CREATING A FALSE CONTROVERSY AMONG SCIENTISTS

The tobacco industry's strategy of perpetuating controversy about the adverse effects of tobacco took place on two levels. One was to generate controversy among the lay public as discussed above. The other was to generate controversy among scientists. The controversy among scientists could then be publicized in the lay press. As mentioned in the previous sections of this chapter, special projects were often used to support scientists to prepare talks for conferences and to send scientists to conferences.

Sponsoring scientific conferences was identified early on as a way of publicizing results favorable to the tobacco industry's position. Support "in conducting conferences of scientists" is first mentioned in a document describing the formation of TIRC in 1954 {1903.03, p. 2}. Sponsoring and publishing the results of scientific conferences has been used as a strategy by both the pharmaceutical and the tobacco industries to publicize research that supports their interests (9, 12). For example, the tobacco industry has sponsored at least six symposia on ETS. These symposia present research articles that are primarily unbalanced reviews of the medical literature, rather than original work. In general, the symposia articles, many of which are authored by industry-affiliated individuals, suggest that ETS is not harmful or that other factors contribute more to health problems than ETS does (9). Furthermore, once the symposia articles are published, they can be cited in a misleading fashion by the industry as if they were peer-reviewed medical or scientific journal articles. For example, articles from symposia proceedings were cited frequently by tobacco industry–affiliated individuals who reviewed the EPA risk assessment of ETS (1).

The tobacco company lawyers encouraged industry-supported scientists to attend scientific meetings in order to counter the results presented by the general scientific community. In 1978 William Shinn, an attorney at Shook, Hardy, and Bacon, wrote in a memo that it "may also be important to evaluate the desirability of increased attendance at scientific meetings" {1910.05}. Shinn then summarized the work of four non-industry-funded scientists who would be presenting data unfavorable to the industry at meetings, such as evidence that smoking is an addiction. The memo then notes that Dr. Gary Huber, then director of the CTR-supported research facility at Harvard University, will conduct a session at another meeting:

> Dr. Huber has agreed to conduct a two-hour presentation at an American Thoracic Society/American Lung Association meeting in May. There will be

several participants, who will discuss the status of tobacco research in the fields of cancer, cardiovascular disease and chronic obstructive pulmonary disease. Dr. Huber also contemplates a section on the nonsmoker and tobacco smoke. {1910.05, p. 2}

Shinn's letter spends six paragraphs reporting on various aspects of Dr. Huber's work, including that Huber was concerned about the appearance that he had become closely identified with the tobacco industry:

> Sometime ago Dr. Huber asked that a committee be formed at Harvard to critique the scientific aspects of the smoking and health programs. Dr. Huber, as you know, is very proud of the caliber of work done and wanted to lay to rest any accusations (completely unfounded) that the industry had control over the research. {1910.05, p. 3}

The lawyers also monitored the performance of industry-supported researchers at scientific conferences. It may be fairly inferred that if an industry-supported researcher presented data that were unfavorable to the industry, his or her chances for future industry funding would decrease. For example, an April 22, 1981, letter from attorney William Shinn to the counsels for the industry describes a meeting attended by special projects grantee Theodor Sterling:

> At a meeting on occupational health, held earlier this month, he gave a presentation titled "Job Discrimination Based on Exposure Consideration and Smoking." *This meeting was monitored by one of our research analysts*; she felt that Dr. Sterling's manner of presentation put his potentially hostile audience in a receptive mood and that the audience paid close attention to what Dr. Sterling had to say. He reviewed published evidence contrary to the idea that smoking heightens the risk of disease by interacting with certain substances to which workers are occupationally exposed. He also stated that the questions of whether other people's tobacco smoke is hazardous to non-smoking workers, and whether smoking workers represent an additional cost to industry, are not settled and that the published reports in these areas are based on data which can be questioned on sound scientific grounds [emphasis added]. {2022.03, pp. 2–3}

Researchers supported through special projects also reported back to the law firms and tobacco companies on the scientific conferences they attended. A January 19, 1978, memo from Donald Hoel at Shook, Hardy, and Bacon to Ernest Pepples states:

> I enclose herewith a copy of a program for the International Symposium on Mechanisms of Airways Obstruction to be held in South Africa during March 28–31 of this year. You will note that Dr. [Domingo] Aviado [who was funded through special projects] is making a presentation at this symposium. I am

sure that upon his return, Dr. Aviado will be giving us a general report on the papers and presentations given at the symposium. {2007.03}

The tobacco industry sometimes sponsored conferences through an independent foundation, so that its sponsorship of the conference would not be disclosed. For example, in 1972 Dr. Theodor Sterling wrote to William Shinn asking for $5,000 to fund a panel on "Effects of Pollutants on Human Health at the International Meeting of the Society of Engineering Science in Tel Aviv, Israel." Sterling also suggested that the grant be awarded to the ALEPH Foundation, to "enable us to manage the arrangement of support in a proper and desirable manner" {2002.02}. It is advantageous for the tobacco industry to hide its sponsorship of scientific conferences because it makes the results that are presented at the conferences appear independent of the industry. In a memo to other industry lawyers, Shinn recommends that Sterling's request be approved and that it be funded through a "special project non-CTR" {2002.05}. Shinn believed that the conference proposed by Sterling would be valuable for advancing the industry's position that ETS is not dangerous because Sterling had been effective in this way in the past:

> The work which Dr. Theodor Sterling has been doing in connection with air pollution became unusually valuable following the President's transmission on January 31 of an air pollution message to Congress, which you have received, that attempted to implicate cigarette smoking in 95% of lung cancer and 90% of chronic obstructive lung disease. {2002.05, p. 1}

Sterling's work was used to criticize this message.

The tobacco industry continues to fail to disclose its sponsorship of conferences; of the six conferences on ETS known to be sponsored by the tobacco industry, only four openly mentioned industry funding (9).

REACTING TO "UNDESIRABLE" RESULTS

According to the principles of academic freedom, researchers who work at universities are free to publish the findings of their research in the scientific literature regardless of the outcome of the research. Although tobacco industry–sponsored research organizations have maintained publicly that they do not restrict publication by their researchers, the documents show that they actually did attempt to influence scientific publication.

A document (undated) describing the organization and policy of TIRC, and later CTR, contains the following statement about scientific publication:

Recipients of Tobacco Industry Research Committee grants are *assured complete scientific freedom in conducting their investigations and reporting the results of their research in the accepted scientific manner through medical and scientific journals* and societies. The investigators receiving grants from the Committee are alone responsible for publishing or reporting their research results [emphasis added]. {1920.01, p. 6}

CTR's behavior regarding publication of results unfavorable to the tobacco industry, however, did not always follow these ideals.

When CTR-sponsored research that was unfavorable toward the tobacco industry was published, CTR had to defend the research to the tobacco companies. In a 1977 memo from Robert C. Hockett, assistant scientific director of CTR, to Addison Yeaman, president of CTR, Hockett attempts to undermine the conclusion of a paper published by C. G. Becker in the *Journal of Experimental Medicine* (13). Becker's paper concluded that glycoproteins isolated from tobacco leaves produce a substance known to cause allergic reactions and blood clotting. In his memo Hockett claims that Becker did not provide evidence showing that tobacco contains glycoproteins. Therefore,

[A]ll their work on rutin [a glycoprotein] has an obscure and doubtful relevance to the effects of smoke exposure on human subjects. . . .

I regard the Becker-Bauer publication, as it appeared, to be very unfortunately premature.

Some of the observations might have been reported legitimately, in a different form, if the extensive speculations had been modified appropriately. {1910.01, p. 2}

Hockett also notes that CTR cannot be held responsible for the publication of Becker's results:

The present paper was seen here [at CTR] only after its submission to and acceptance by the journal. It represented a wide digression from the subject of the grant as we understood it. Our request that credit lines to The Council and to individual persons be deleted was reported to be 'too late' and the paper, with press releases, was published shortly thereafter, to our discomfort. {1910.01, p. 3}

CTR also attempted to turn a CTR-sponsored publication that was unfavorable to the industry into a public relations advantage. When such a publication came out, the tobacco industry publicized the fact that it had encouraged the author's research; it also prepared a response to the work. For example, in response to a paper on smoking as a cause of heart disease, published by CTR grantee Gary Friedman in the *New England Journal of Medicine* (14), CTR issued the following public statement:

> Grantees are always encouraged to publish their findings. This study reports relationships between various factors and death rates. There isn't any suggestion of cause-and-effect. . . . This and so much else in the medical literature just shows that we have a great deal more to learn before we can reach any solid conclusions about smoking. It may or may not be hazardous, and that's where we are. {1916.01}

INFLUENCING GOVERNMENT POLICY

The documents reveal at least one instance where a CTR contract monitored by industry lawyers funded work that attempted to directly influence future publication of government documents on public policy related to tobacco and health. In 1967, the US Public Health Service published a study on the health effects of tobacco entitled *Cigarette Smoking and Health Characteristics*. The documents contain corre-spondence among industry lawyers in which the CTR contract is described as calling "for recommendations concerning the feasibility of a review *and public analysis* of the PHS report [emphasis added]" {2001.02, p. 1} that would criticize the methods used to collect the data for the PHS report. According to the documents, Theodor Sterling, then at Washington University, convened an "Advisory Panel" to for-mulate such recommendations, funded by a CTR contact to Washington University.

A December 26, 1968, letter from David R. Hardy of Shook, Hardy, and Bacon to the counsels for the tobacco companies describes a letter from Sterling and enclosures. (Neither the letter from Sterling nor the enclosures are among the documents.) Referring to the advisory panel, Hardy states: "I believe that this is perhaps the best work that Professor Sterling has done and it appears that we now have several other distinguished scientists who were members of the panel and who concur in our long held position that the Government's work in these various surveys is not reliable" {2001.01}.

One of the enclosures with Sterling's letter described by Hardy is a summary of the advisory panel's analysis of the PHS study. Sterling states:

> It is worth quoting the concluding paragraph in [the summary of the advisory panel's analysis]:
>
>> "There can be no doubt, however, that the claims made by Cigarette Smoking and Health Characteristics cannot be justified. Neither are the

data of adequate validity and reliability, nor is the analysis of these data properly designed and executed. The problems raised by these unjustified claims ought to be reviewed with the authority of a public body, properly constituted to do so, behind it."

Final recommendations of the [e]valuation group were delayed because of an apparent loss in the mail of comments from one member. These have just been received by me and are enclosed. . . . It contains (a) the actual recommendations of the "Advisory Panel", (b) the principal justifications for such recommendations (*Cigarette Smoking and Health Characteristics and PHS claims based on it are examples used to demonstrate why a review procedure is needed*) and (c) minutes of the group's discussions ("*not* to be distributed outside the sponsoring agency") which bear on many problems in the health area.

The group which Dr. Sterling convened saw little use in going forward with a "definitive evaluation" of the morbidity study, preferring, in the words of the "Status Report" enclosed, to recommend that "*a permanent commission needs to be formed for the purpose of establishing a consensus on the results of various studies and what they mean.*"

This is an extremely ambitious undertaking and is not dissimilar to other recommendations made in the past. Dr. Sterling feels, however, that *simply attacking the morbidity study alone would not cause the Government to withdraw the report nor make any headlines. Sterling believes that a top level advisory group (perhaps working with the* [US] *President's Science Advisory Committee or under its auspices, for example) would have the necessary prestige to prevent the future publication of documents such as Cigarette Smoking and Health Characteristics* [italic emphasis added]. {2001.02, pp. 1–3}

Hardy's description makes it clear that the CTR contract was not funded simply to critique the PHS morbidity study; it was intended to stimulate a "public analysis" of the PHS study—an analysis with a government imprimatur. Judged against this goal, Hardy's assessment of Sterling's success is understandable—Sterling's panel went beyond recommending a public analysis of the PHS report, and instead (apparently justifying the recommendation on the basis of alleged flaws in the PHS study) recommended the creation of a high-level government agency (perhaps in the White House) that would divert scientific efforts in an attempt to establish a "consensus on the results of various studies and what they mean" {2001.02, p. 2}. It was Sterling's judgment that such an agency would prevent the publication of future studies on tobacco and disease like the PHS study.

Although Hardy was enthusiastic about the boldness of the advisory panel's recommendation, he was also concerned that creation of a high-level agency could have adverse repercussions for the industry. He stated:

> Obviously, there are problems involved in setting up any advisory group where conclusions might be binding on industry. There would certainly be implications involving the present industry-government dialogue. In any event, the very recommendations by Sterling's panel appear to be a condemnation of publication quality control at PHS. {2001.02, p. 3}

The advisory panel's recommendation that the process by which the report was generated be criticized, as well as the data in the report, is similar to a strategy that the tobacco industry has used to criticize the EPA's risk assessment of ETS (15). Seven tobacco industry–affiliated individuals who reviewed the risk assessment criticized the government procedure used to assess risk. In contrast, the independent EPA Science Advisory Board concluded that the risk assessment of ETS was "fully consistent with the risk assessments that [the EPA has] done for many other carcinogens" (1).

CONCLUSION

The tobacco companies funded special projects through three different funding mechanisms; each funding mechanism was subject to extensive lawyer management of scientific research. The special projects included research projects and consultancies that were for writing critiques of scientific studies on tobacco and health and were not limited to providing expert testimony for the tobacco companies. In addition, the documents reveal that lawyers on occasion influenced research that was not funded by the special projects.

The extensive attorney participation in management of the special projects' research on tobacco and health raises some profound and troublesome questions. Industry attorneys may be expected to participate—as advocates—in arranging and presenting expert scientific testimony in lawsuits, law-making proceedings, and regulatory proceedings regarding tobacco and health. The documents show that the role played by lawyers in scientific research went far beyond their customary roles. Industry lawyers were extensively involved in research and symposia that were not directly related to any particular legal or governmental proceeding. Since lawyers are advocates for a position, the broad (and publicly unacknowledged) participation of lawyers in funding, selecting, monitoring, and evaluating research is strong evidence of the extent to which the industry was, in fact, result oriented in its funding and support of nominally independent scientific work and actively sought to obtain favorable (or "positive") results from research that was presented as independent scientific work. The result-oriented approach to scientific research revealed by the documents contrasts rather dramatically with the public statements of the industry, which fostered a benevolent image of supporting independent scientific research without attempting to influence the outcome. More fundamentally, the broad role played by lawyers in secretly directing nominally independent scientific research with no apparent relation to particular legal proceedings raises disturbing questions about distortion of the scientific process in order to influence legislators, regulators, and juries who are charged with making decisions based on scientific knowledge. Furthermore, the documents reveal instances in which tobacco industry support was not disclosed by researchers funded by special projects.

The CTR special projects received preliminary judicial scrutiny in a 1992 wrongful death action, *Haines v Liggett Group, Inc.*, discussed in chapter 7. The court ruled, based in part on the CTR special projects, that the plaintiffs had presented *prima facie* evidence of fraud by the tobacco companies for purposes of permitting discovery of allegedly privileged tobacco company documents. In discussing the evidence supporting the plaintiff's fraud case, the court's opinion stated:

> It now appears that there were a series of research grants designated as "special projects" which were developed in a manner so as to receive the protection of the attorney-client privilege. The "special projects" division was under the auspices of the CTR, although defendants insist that the "special projects" division was managed entirely separately from the CTR. . . . The claimed purpose of the "special projects" division was to sponsor research relevant to the links between smoking and disease in order to develop a field of expert witnesses for defensive litigation in tort suits. Consistent with this purpose, defendants' counsel were substantially involved in strategic and specific decision-making within the "special projects" division.
>
> Although defendants represented to the public that research conducted under the auspices of the CTR would be made public, the "special projects" research was not publicized, nor was the existence of the "special projects" division disclosed. In addition to this nominal association between the CTR and tobacco industry, the channelling of selective research proposals into either the CTR or the "special projects" division and the shared research between the two belies defendants' public representations and ongoing defense that the CTR was an independent, objective body [*Haines v Liggett Group, Inc.*, 140 F.R.D. 681, at 688 (D.N.J. 1992)].

Later, in analyzing the significance of the evidence presented, the court stated:

> In the court's opinion, the factual inference arising from the segregation of the "special projects" program and its avowed purpose of generating re-

search for use in defendants' litigation is highly suggestive of the public fraud which plaintiff alleges. The fact that selective research was "siphoned off" into "special projects" protected against disclosure due [to] the claims of privilege, strongly implies that the CTR "special projects" division was an integral part of the CTR's general practice of sponsoring and reporting selective research. Moreover, sharing the special projects, litigation oriented research with the CTR directly counters defendants' representations that CTR published research was independently selected and monitored. According to defendants themselves, the attorney involvement in the special projects program included proposing and monitoring research consistent with defendants' litigation interests. Such commingling of special projects with CTR research directly implicates the special projects program in the alleged ongoing public fraud for which this court has found *prima facia* evidence [at 694].

The court then noted that the disputed documents themselves constituted even more persuasive evidence of fraud:

This court's own *in camera* [private] inspection of selected documents has revealed the most explicit admissions that defendants used the special projects program to further the alleged ongoing fraud and deception surrounding the advertised function and operation of the CTR [at 695].

Finally, the court summarized its findings with regard to the special projects documents:

Given plaintiff's theories of fraud, which, if believed by a jury based on the evidence presented, would give rise to liability, after an *in camera* review of these selected documents, the court is convinced that the only possible conclusion is that the crime/fraud exception applies to these documents. The court finds that there is *prima facie* evidence that defendants were engaged in an ongoing fraud, and that defendants obtained attorney assistance in furtherance of that fraud through the use of the special projects division [at 697].

This case was later vacated by the US Court of Appeals because of a procedural error unrelated to the specific findings as to fraud [*Haines v Liggett Group, Inc.*, 975 F.2d 81 (3d Cir. 1992)].

The decision-making process revealed in the documents is unheard of in research programs funded by other sources, such as the National Institutes of Health. The documents confirm that scientific merit played little role in the selection of special projects or consultancies. Instead, grantees were selected by tobacco industry lawyers on the basis of their potential legal or political usefulness to the tobacco industry. Projects or investigators that had the potential to produce data unfavorable to the industry were not funded.

TABLE 8.1 SPECIAL PROJECTS AND CONSULTANCIES, 1972–1991

Investigator	Type of Project	Project Title	Dates Funded	Total Funded (dollars)
ACVA Atlantic, Inc.	CTR Special Project	Pilot study to assess residential air quality	1985	13,800
Aviado, Domingo	CTR Special Project	Cardiopulmonary and renal vascular effects of constituents of tobacco smoke	1977–78	85,000
Aviado, Domingo	SA 4 Consultancy	Continuing review of relevant smoking and health topics	1981–86	488,000
Aviado, Domingo	SH&B Consultancy	Continuing review of relevant smoking and health topics	1986–90	187,500
Bahnson, Claus	CTR Special Project	Project studying personality and social factors related to smoking and health	1972–73	8,000
Battelle Columbus Laboratories	SA 4 Research Project	Research to quantify the exposure of the nonsmoker to environmental tobacco smoke	1981–82	83,000
Battelle Columbus Laboratories (cotinine project)	SA 4 Research Project	The experimental determination of nicotine to particulate mass ratios and levels of cotinine in ambient smoke	1982–83	69,000
Berkson, Joseph	SA 4 Consultancy	Continuing consultancy	unknown	1,500/ month est.
Bick, Rodger L.	CTR Special Project	A prospective five-year epidemiological study of lung cancer in Kern County [California]	1983–89	159,754
Bick, Rodger L.	SA 4 Consultancy	Biological testing of TGP [tobacco glycoprotein?]	unknown	9,718
Blau, Theodore	SA 4 Consultancy	Analysis and evaluation of literature on the "tobacco habit"	1981–86	120,000
Booker, Walter	SA 4 Consultancy	Continuing consultancy	unknown	500/ month
Booker, Walter	SA 4 Consultancy	Preparation of public smoking statement	unknown	2,262
Booker, Walter	SA 4 Consultancy	Continuing consultancy	unknown	
Bowers, Evelyn J.	SA 4 Research Project	Data analyses and related expenses to complete dissertation exploring a possible genetic component in disease by gathering historical data on mortality by age and cause in the Orkney Islands	1979	2,500

Name	Account	Description	Dates	Amount
Brooke, Oliver	SA 4 Research Project	Effects of smoking on fetal growth. Study A: Smoking and nutrition; Study B: The effects of psychosocial stress in pregnancy on birth size	1980–86	265,780 pounds
Brotman, Richard/ Freedman, Alfred	Special Account 5	Analysis of policy in issues dealing with control and regulation of routine behavior in a democratic society	1979–83	637,000
Brown, Barbara	SA 4 Consultancy	Consultancy	unknown	1,500/ month
Buhler, Victor	CTR Special Project	Spend about 40 hours a month reviewing current literature of interest	1977	18,000
Carter, John R.	CTR Special Project	Autopsy study designed to examine accuracy of lung cancer diagnoses (investigators checking autopsy records of university hospitals for period extending from 1948 to 1974 for errors in diagnoses)	1974–76	92,085
Cline, Martin J.	SA 4 Consultancy	Library research and review re: lung retention of particulate matter	unknown	600
Cosentino, Anthony	SA 4 Consultancy	Preparation of statement re: public smoking	unknown	2,500 est.
Cox, Gertrude	SA 4 Consultancy	FDA/OC review; preparation of statement for hearing	unknown	4,000
DiNardi, Salvatore	CTR Special Project	Assessing the contribution of environmental tobacco smoke to the respirable suspended particulate levels in the indoor environment	1986–88	688,878
Dunlap, Charles	SA 4 Consultancy	Preparation of statement re: public smoking	unknown	2,500 est.
Evans, Frederick J.	SA 4 Research Project	Correlates and medical implications of smoking: differences between nonsmokers and quitters vs. chronic smokers and unsuccessful quitters	1981–82	74,434
Eysenck, H. J.	SA 4 Consultancy	Consultancy	1977–80	85,116 (pounds?)
Eysenck, H. J.	SA 4 Research Project	Survey analyzing alternative satisfactions sought by former smokers after they quit	1978–79	5,000 or 6,000 pounds
Eysenck, H. J.	SA 4 Research Project	Study of stress and cardiac disorders in twins	1980–82	25,000 pounds

TABLE 8.1 *(continued)*

Investigator	Type of Project	Project Title	Dates Funded	Total Funded (dollars)
Eysenck, H. J.	CTR Special Project	Maintenance of twin registry	1978–86 (1986–89 pending)	133,600 pounds (135,000 pounds pending)
Eysenck, H. J.	CTR Special Project	Study of the relationships among smoking, personality, and lung cancer on a cross-cultural basis	1983–86	127,000 pounds
Farris, Jack Matthews	SA 4 Consultancy	Preparation of statement re: public smoking	unknown	2,500 est.
Feinhandler, Sherwin J.	SA 4 Consultancy	Preparation of statement re: public smoking	unknown	3,042
Feinhandler, Sherwin J.	SA 4 Consultancy	Review of 1979 Surgeon General report	unknown	unknown
Feinstein, Alvan R.	CTR Special Project	Support biostatistician to assist Dr. Feinstein	1976–78, 1981	67,284
Feinstein, Alvan R.	CTR Special Project	Basic epidemiological research studies	1985–86, 1988–90	700,960
Finley, T. N.	CTR Special Project	Construct "lung" model consisting of lipid layer, enzyme, and protein to test activities of lipid monolayer, especially effects on enzyme activity	1977	30,000
Finley, Theodor	SA 4 Consultancy	Preparation of statement re: public smoking	unknown	2,500 est
First, Melvin	SA 4 Research Project	Methods for environmental tobacco smoke measurement	1983	10,000
Fisher, Edwin R.	SA 4 Consultancy	Preparation of statement re: public smoking	unknown	2,500 est.
Fisher, H. Russell	SA 4 Consultancy	Preparation of statement re: public smoking	unknown	2,500 est.
Franklin Institute	CTR Special Project	Isolate 5 g of tobacco glycoprotein from tobacco smoke condensate and tobacco leaf	1978	51,650
Franklin Institute	CTR Special Project	Determination and characterization of tobacco glycoprotein as an artifact	1979	20,130

Name	Type	Description	Years	Amount
Franklin Institute	CTR Special Project	Generation of 25 milligrams of artifact	1979	10,000
Friberg, Lars/Cederloff, Rune	CTR Special Project	Preparation of comprehensive monograph on twin methodology and on highlights of their research on Swedish Twin Registry	1975	23,300
Furst, Arthur	CTR Special Project	Study the effects of combined asbestos and benzo(a)pyrene on lungs of mice	1977–79	64,500
Furst, Arthur	SA 4 Consultancy	Preparation of statement re: public smoking	unknown	2,500 est.
Furst, Arthur	SA 4 Research Project	Review of scientific literature	1979–84	108,000
Gibbons, Jean	SA 4 Consultancy	Review of smoking and health articles	unknown	per diem
Gibbons, Jean	SA 4 Consultancy	FDA/OC review; preparation of statement for hearing	1978	1,005
Gorlin, Richard/Klein, Lloyd	Other Special Project	Clinical study of the relationship between smoking and other activities and myocardial ischemic events	1983–86	431,503
Gruhn, John G.	CTR Special Project	Preparation of a monograph, "A History of Lung Cancer"	1985–87	31,200
Gutstein, William	CTR Special Project	Study of neural factors on coronary spasm and atherogenesis	1983–85	271,015
Gutstein, William	CTR Special Project	Hypothalamic stimulation and cardiovascular disease	1985–87	319,545
Harvard Medical School	SA 4 Consultancy	Occasional accounting expenses	unknown	unknown
Hecht, Frederick	CTR Special Project	The nature of fragile sites and their possible relation to cancer	1985–86	35,985
Heimstra, Norman	SA 4 Consultancy	Consultancy and preparation of statement re: public smoking	unknown	1,610
Hickey, Richard J.	CTR Special Project	Epidemiological and etiological studies on the relation of air pollution, smoking, and other environmental variables to human chronic diseases	1976–86	579,849
Hickey, Richard	SH&B Consultancy (see note)	Continuing consultancy	1986–90	24,000
Hickey, Richard	SA 4 Consultancy	Preparation of statement re: public smoking	unknown	2,500 est.
Hilado, Carlos	SA 4 Consultancy	Continuing consultancy	1983–84	48,000
Hine Inc.	SA 4 Research Project	Review literature relating to public smoking	1978–79	unknown
Huber, Gary L.	SH&B Consultancy	Review and analysis of chronic obstructive lung disease literature with focus on pre-1966 literature; review literature on other pulmonary diseases	unknown	computer/staff expenses
Husting, E. L.	CTR Special Project	Methodological study of the effects of control selection and exposure ascertainment bias in the case control context	1986–88	198,034

TABLE 8.1 (*continued*)

Investigator	Type of Project	Project Title	Dates Funded	Total Funded (dollars)
Hutcheon, Duncan	CTR Special Project	A pilot project to investigate the environmental pharmacology of industrial inhalants	1979–80	89,870 (additional 35,000 pending)
Hutcheon, Duncan/ Regna, Peter	CTR Special Project	Laboratory studies of the cardiovascular effects of carbon monoxide inhalation	1982–83	99,250
Hutcheon, Duncan	CTR Special Project	Electrophysiological properties of the heart following acute and chronic exposure to carbon monoxide	1983–84	79,355
ITT Research Institute	CTR Special Project	Investigation of self-reporting questionnaires for environmental tobacco smoke	1985–86	70,000
IT Corporation	SH&B Research Project	Collaborative pilot study on indoor air sampling	1986–87	25,000
Janis, Joe	CTR Special Project	Statistical model of lung cancer mortality	1979–80	12,800
Jenson, A. Bennett	CTR Special Project	Search for papillomavirus structural antigens in premalignant and malignant squamous cell lesions of the oral cavity and upper and lower respiratory tracts	1982–90	493,853
Knoebel, Suzanne	CTR Special Project	Determine reliability of noninvasive technique to measure changes in cardiac function, if any, during inhalation of tobacco smoke	1977–78	23,825
Knoebel, Suzanne B.	SA 4 Consultancy	Preparation of statement re: public smoking	unknown	2,500 est.
Kupper, Lawrence/ Janis, Joseph/ Greenberg, Bernard	CTR Special Project	Verification of a statistical age-period-cohort analysis of lung cancer	1982–87	247,500
Kupper, Lawrence/ Janis, Joseph	CTR Special Project	Pilot study of causality	1984–85	31,300
La Via, Mariano	CTR Special Project	Support for graduate student to assist in basic research in field of immunopathology	1978–80	24,000

Name	Category	Description	Years	Amount
Langston, Hiram	SA 4 Consultancy	Preparation of statement re: public smoking	unknown	2,500 est.
Lieberman, G. J.	SA 4 Consultancy	FDA/OC review	unknown	1,600
Macdonald, Eleanor	CTR Special Project	Regional patterns of cancer of major sites in five large regions of Texas and regional patterns of mortality in Houston, 1940–69 (study of factors associated with high cancer rates in states or regions of US)	1974–81	390,043
Macdonald, Eleanor	CTR Special Project	Completion and publication of book *Cancer in Focus* (tentative title)	1982	35,000
Mancuso, Thomas F.	CTR Special Project	Demographic studies of mortality in Ohio (step-by-step progression of identification of high-risk population subgroups and attempts to determine specific causes for high risk)	1975–76	38,700
Mancuso, Thomas F.	CTR Special Project	Low-level radiation study	1979	10,000
Meckler Engineers Group	SA 4 Research Project	Review of literature on ventilation/air quality models	1983–84	10,000
Meckler Engineers Group	SA 4 Research Project	Preparation of scientific reports on ventilation/air quality models for legislative and engineering forums	1984	60,000
Mello, Nancy/ Mendelson, Jack	SA 4 Research Project	Review of scientific literature	1982–84	30,000
Micozzi, Marc	SA 4 Consultancy	Consultancy	1982	11,000
Moser, Kenneth	CTR Special Project	Investigation of potential role of polymorphonuclear leucocyte elastase concentration in pathogenesis of emphysema	1977–79	198,000
Moser, Kenneth M.	SA 4 Consultancy	Preparation of statement re: public smoking	unknown	15,100 est.
Niden, Albert	SA 4 Consultancy	Preparation of statement re: public smoking	unknown	2,500 est.
Nylander, Lee R.	SA 4 Consultancy	Preparation of statement re: public smoking for Chicago hearing 9/12/78	1978	3,129
O'Lane, John	SA 4 Consultancy	unknown	unknown	153
Oak Ridge National Laboratory	CTR Special Project	Methodology for quantitating exposure to inhalable ambient tobacco smoke	1985–87	855,000
Ogura, Joseph	CTR Special Project	Effects of tobacco and air pollution on the lung	1974–75	24,000
Okun, Ronald	SA 4 Consultancy	Preparation of statement re: public smoking	unknown	2,500 est.
Olkin, Ingram	SA 4 Consultancy	FDA/OC review	unknown	1,600

TABLE 8.I (continued)

Investigator	Type of Project	Project Title	Dates Funded	Total Funded (dollars)
Olkin, Ingram	CTR Special Project	A study of the models used in the analysis of certain medical data (review of the appropriateness of treating biomedical data with the multivariate techniques of assumed normality)	1976–78	12,000
Puglia, Charles/Roberts, Jay	CTR Special Project	Adaptation to components of tobacco smoke (a study of the response of the lung to oxidants contained in cigarette smoke; adaptation of the heart to nicotinic effects)	1979–80	44,014
Rao, L. G. S.	SA 4 Consultancy	Consultancy	unknown	2,500 est.
Rao, L. G. S.	CTR Special Project	Research relating to correlation of plasma steroid levels in urine of lung cancer patients and controls	1974–77	30,000
Rao, L. G. S.	SA 4 Research Project	Research related to effects of maternal smoking during pregnancy.	1977–86	455,000
Ratcliff, Herbert	CTR Special Project	Cardiopulmonary lesions in zoo animals	1975–76	15,275
Response Analysis	SA 4 Research Project	The response of the nonsmoker to cigarette smoke and smoking behavior (survey of annoyances and irritations that are part of the everyday life of American adults)	1976	45,000
Rigdon, R. H.	SA 4 Consultancy	Consultancy	unknown	2,500 est.
Riley, Vernon	CTR Special Project	Three-year program of studies on stress physiology	1981–82	155,000
Spackman, Darrel (formerly Riley project)	CTR Special Project	Modified one-year proposal for studies on stress physiology	1982–83	86,000
Roberts, Jay	CTR Special Project	The effect of exposure to cigarette smoke on atrial and ventricular pace-maker activity	1982–83	49,511
Rothschild, Henry	CTR Special Project	Pilot study of disproportionately high mortality in respiratory tract cancer in southern Louisiana to determine if genetic and environmental factors are possible causes	1977–80	79,328
Rothschild, Henry	CTR Special Project	Genetic aspects of lung cancer	1982–88	160,705

Name	Type	Description	Years	Amount
Russek, Henry/ Russek, Linda	CTR Special Project	Behavior patterns and strategies for the mastery of stress, anxiety reduction, and perceptual functioning (a comparison of the efficacy of different methods of relaxation in the face of stress; differences between Type A and Type B individuals)	1979–81	48,500
Russek, Linda	SA 4 Research Project (Also listed as SH&B Research Project)	Follow-up study of Harvard alumni and their psychological and physiological profiles	1984–86	50,000
Salvaggio, John	CTR Special Project	Investigation of physical, chemical, and immuno-chemical properties of components present in tobacco smoke	1976–81	283,777
Salvaggio, John/ Lehrer, Samuel	CTR Special Project	Provocative inhalation challenge testing: the exposure of "smoke-sensitive" individuals to the actual inhalation of sidestream tobacco smoke	1981–83	132,664
Salvaggio, John/ Lehrer, Samuel	CTR Special Project	The pulmonary effects of passive cigarette smoke exposure on atopic smoke-sensitive asthmatics	1985–88	263,117
Savage, I. Richard	SA 4 Consultancy	FDA/OC review	unknown	1,720
Schilling, R.	SA 4 Consultancy	unknown	unknown	1,685
Schrauzer, Gerhard N.	SA 4 Consultancy	Preparation of statement re: public smoking	unknown	2,500 est.
Schrauzer, Gerhard N.	CTR Special Project	Determination of selenium concentration and nature in tobacco products and tobacco smoke	1981–83	20,000
Schrauzer, Gerhard N.	CTR Special Project	Statistical and epidemiological studies on the etiology of lung cancer	1983–85	30,000
Seltzer, Carl	CTR Special Project	Constitutional differences between smokers and nonsmokers	1976–87	650,000
			1989–90	70,000 pending
Seltzer, Carl	SA 4 Consultancy	Preparation of statement re: public smoking	unknown	2,500 est.
Seltzer, Carl	SA 4 Consultancy	Continuing consultancy based on specific projects	unknown	per diem
Seltzer, Carl	SA 4 Research Project	Examination of Kaiser-Permanente data on ex-smokers' CHD rates in relation to continuing smokers' CHD rates	1978–79	7,000
Seltzer, Carl/ van den Berg, Bea	CTR Special Project	Study of smoker/nonsmoker differences	1981–89	597,000
Senkus, Murray	SA 4 Consultancy	Consultancy	1981–82	62,400

TABLE 8.1 *(continued)*

Investigator	Type of Project	Project Title	Dates Funded	Total Funded (dollars)
Solmon, Lewis	SH&B Research Project	Preparation of a review paper on smoking and absenteeism in the workplace	1986–87	8,000
Spielberger, Charles	SA 4 Research Project	The origins and correlates of smoking behavior—attempt to replicate major findings from laboratory work of Dr. Eysenck relating to origins and maintenance of smoking behavior with American subjects	1978–83	172,381
Stanford Research Institute	SA 4 Research Project	Develop unobtrusive instrument package for analyses of atmospheric carbon monoxide, nicotine, and total suspended particulate matter (suitcase air-monitoring device)	1976	172,400
Stedman, R. L.	SA 4 Consultancy	Consultancy/preparation of statement re: public smoking	unknown	2,500 est.
Stein, Arthur	SA 4 Consultancy	Review of public smoking bill	unknown	500
Sterling, Theodor	CTR Special Project	A continuing critical review of the major factors in the etiology of lung cancer and other lung diseases emerging from statistical studies	1973–90	5,214,253
Sterling, Theodor	CTR Special Project	Evaluation of the interaction between geographical, geocultural, smoking, and health variables and indices	1979–81	54,710
Sterling, Theodor	CTR Special Project	The study of architectural, ventilation, and lighting factors in relation to office building illness	1981–83	207,913
Sterling, Theodor	SA 4 Research Project	Critical assessment of draft OTA [Office of Technology Assessment] report "Smoking-Related Deaths and Financial Costs"	1985	42,000
Sterling, Theodor	SA 4 Research Project	Critical evaluation of current environmental tobacco smoke health risk models	1985	49,720
Sterling, Theodor D.	SA Consultancy	Preparation of statements re: public smoking	unknown	7,520 est.

Name	Type	Description	Years	Amount
Sterling, Theodor/ Perry, Harold/ Glicksman, Arvin	CTR Special Project	Retrospective analysis of environmental contacts of patients with respiratory cancer, other cancers, and other diseases	1979–82	235,686
Valentin, Helmut	SA 4 Consultancy	Preparation of paper re: literature review on public smoking and health	unknown	4,000
Wakefield, James A.	CTR Special Project	(1) Preliminary study of interrelationships and causal paths linking smoking, personality, and health variables; and (2) assessment of the relationship between methodological quality of previous smoking and health studies and their results	1985–87	76,000
Washington University	Other Special Project	Funding for the cancer immunology laboratories	1984–91	2,200,000
Zeidman, Irving	SA 4 Consultancy	Analysis and evaluation of literature primarily in the lung cancer area	1983	7,500

NOTE: This table represents a compilation of the special projects and consultancies funded by the tobacco industry from 1972 to 1991. As described in this chapter, special projects and consultancies were funded either through the Council for Tobacco Research (CTR) or through the law firms of Jacob and Medinger (Special Account 4, SA 4) or Shook, Hardy, and Bacon (SH&B). The table is based on a series of pages in the documents that appear to have been compiled by and for lawyers; many pages are marked "Confidential—For Counsel Use Only." This table probably does not list all the special projects and consultancies that have been funded by the tobacco industry, because it began funding CTR special projects in 1966, and our table begins in 1972. The information in the documents suggests, however, that the tobacco industry spent more than $20 million on special projects and consultancies from 1972 to 1991.

SOURCE: Compiled from {2048.01} through {2048.29}.

REFERENCES

1. Bero L, Glantz S. Tobacco industry response to a risk assessment of environmental tobacco smoke. *Tobacco Control* 1993;2:103–113.
2. Cohen L, Rothschild H. The bandwagons of medicine. *Perspectives in Biology and Medicine* 1979;Summer:531–538.
3. Ockene J, Hymowitz N, Sexton M, Broste S. Comparison of patterns of smoking behavior change among smokers in the Multiple Risk Factor Intervention Study (MRFIT). *Prev Med* 1982;10:476–500.
4. Hughes G, Hymowitz N, Ockene J, Simon N, Voght T. The Multiple Risk Factor Intervention Trial (MRFIT): V. Intervention on smoking. *Prev Med* 1981;10:476–500.
5. Seltzer C. Effect of stopping smoking after unstable angina and myocardial infarction (letter). *Brit Med J Clin Res Ed* 1983;287(6401):1301–1302.
6. Castelli W. Epidemiology of coronary heart disease: The Framingham study. *Am J Med* 1984;76(2A):4–12.
7. Castelli W, Garrison R, Dawber T, McNamara P, Feinleib M, Kannel W. The filter cigarette and coronary heart disease: The Framingham story. *Lancet* 1981;2(8238):109–113.
8. Cohen D, Arai SF, Brain JD. Smoking impairs long-term dust clearance from the lung. *Science* 1979;204:514–517.
9. Bero L, Galbraith A, Rennie D. Sponsored symposia on environmental tobacco smoke. *JAMA* 1994;271:612–617.
10. Glantz S. Tobacco industry response to the scientific evidence on passive smoking. In *Proceedings of the Fifth World Conference on Tobacco and Health, 1983* (pp. 287–292). Winnepeg, Canada: Canadian Council on Smoking and Health, 1983.
11. Durbin R. The tobacco industry strategy: New subject, same tactics (editorial). *Tobacco Control* 1993;2:8–9.
12. Bero L, Galbraith A, Rennie D. The publication of sponsored symposiums in medical journals. *N Engl J Med* 1992;327:1135–1140.
13. Becker C, Dubin T. Activation of factor XII by tobacco glycoprotein. *J Exp Med* 1977;146:457–467.
14. Friedman G, Dales L, Ury H. Mortality in middle-aged smokers and nonsmokers. *New Engl J Med* 1979;300:213–217.
15. USEPA. *Respiratory Health Effects of Passive Smoking: Lung Cancer and Other Disorders.* Indoor Air Division, Office of Atmospheric and Indoor Programs, Office of Air and Radiation, US Environmental Protection Agency, 1992. EPA/600/6-90/006F.

CHAPTER 9

Stonewalling: Politics and Public Relations

We have a responsibility—both legal and moral—as a cigarette manufacturer to ensure that people are aware of the <u>facts</u> relating to our products, that a factual and balanced picture is presented, and that inaccuracies and imbalance are corrected [emphasis in original].

Anne Johnson, BAT attorney, 1985 {1828.02, p. 4}

INTRODUCTION

The attorneys at B&W and BAT were instrumental in establishing the companies' public relations posture toward the growing evidence on the health dangers of smoking. The public relations statements had to be carefully crafted to avoid creating liability problems. The attorneys had to walk a fine line between not saying anything and saying too much about the alleged health dangers of tobacco. At the same time, the tobacco industry continued to develop increasingly sophisticated marketing strategies to promote tobacco use and maintain the social acceptability of smoking. In addition to traditional advertising, these efforts included product placement of B&W brands in movies and on television. The companies directed their efforts not only at the general public but also at physicians, so that they would encourage smokers to switch to low-tar cigarettes, instead of simply stopping smoking. The documents also reflect efforts by the tobacco industry to use its considerable economic clout with suppliers and the media, as well as important community-based organizations, to obtain favorable treatment.

INFLUENCE OF ATTORNEYS OVER PUBLIC RELATIONS

On November 2, 1985, Anne Johnson, a member of the BAT legal department, wrote a lengthy memo containing a detailed discussion of what BAT's stance should be with regard to smoking and health {1828.02}. Her memo is labeled an "Attorney Work Product" and is divided into sections titled "Smoking and Health Issues," "Scientific Information," "Reasons for Making Public Statements on Smoking and Health," "Areas for Response," and "Proposed Response." The basic premise of Johnson's memo is that BAT cannot afford to remain silent on issues related to the health effects of tobacco. By remaining silent, the company will be implying that it agrees with claims that its products are hazardous to health. Under the heading "Reasons for Making Public Statements on Smoking and Health," Johnson states:

> If we fail to make the facts and our views known on smoking and health, we run the risk of seeing the introduction of more and more restrictions—some unacceptable and unwarranted—on our products, our commercial objectives and our freedom to operate. If we have no statement to make, then we lose credibility with government, and the public (including shareholders and employees).
>
> *We have a responsibility—both legal and moral—as a cigarette manufacturer to ensure that people are aware of the facts relating to our products, that a factual and balanced picture is presented, and that inaccuracies and imbalance are corrected.*
>
> This applies not merely to the BAT Companies, but also to the National Manufacturers Associations in each country. The NMA's are often seen and indeed are set up to be the spokesman for the industry as a whole and, even more than individual companies, are expected by government and other institutions to respond effectively on smoking and health issues. In the case of the N.M.A.s other member companies may wish to take some action or make a response and we need the ability to participate with those companies [italic emphasis added]. {1828.02, p. 4}

Nevertheless, Johnson notes, even discussing causation might be dangerous in view of the ongoing lawsuits in the United States:

> Since the New Jersey Law Suits [probably a reference to the *Cipollone, Haines,* and other cases] and the RJ Reynolds campaign were commenced we have effectively taken no action and made no response in deference to the US legal constraints.
>
> *We recognize that there are legal constraints in the US which we must observe and we appreciate the practical problems of discussing causation and in particular the possible impact of causation on the voluntary assumption of risk defence* [emphasis added]. {1828.02, p. 6}

This position precluded any objective discussion of the scientific evidence that smoking causes disease; such a conclusion was simply not acceptable on legal grounds.

Johnson is acknowledging that comments made by BAT officials might have an impact on lawsuits against the industry in the United States. She is concerned that the industry's assumption of risk defense, which depends on the plaintiff's knowing the risks of his or her actions, might be endangered if it were to be revealed that the industry actually possessed information about the causes of smoking-related diseases and had not shared that information with the public. In that event smokers, in fact, could not have known the full risks of smoking or, at least, could not have known the extent of those risks. As noted in chapter 7, this defense has been largely responsible for protecting the industry from liability in the wave of lawsuits that began in the mid-1980s. Johnson continues:

> We have no wish or intention to "overplay" the causation argument or to mislead consumers (or anyone else) into thinking that smoking is free of risk, or that the risks are minimal, or that they can ignore the potential risks or health warnings.
>
> However for the reasons mentioned above the effective silence which the BAT Companies have maintained over the last few months cannot be sustained.
>
> As science is the basis for the smoking and health arguments, we wish to put third parties in possession of a balanced view of smoking and health issues based on the scientific information set out in the appendix [discussed below]. {1828.02, p. 6}

Thus, although Johnson recommends that BAT not remain silent, she also advises that the company should not take an aggressive stand regarding the health effects of smoking. Instead, the company should provide third parties (presumably, scientists, politicians, the media, and the general public) with a "balanced" view of the issues, a tobacco industry euphemism for making the public believe that there is a controversy as to whether cigarettes are dangerous. The implication here is that BAT should provide third parties with scientific research supporting the position that the causal relationship between smoking and disease has not been proven. As discussed in chapter 8, the industry has funded research through its lawyers that was specifically designed to develop this sort of contradictory scientific evidence.

The memo then provides a general outline of the argument that BAT should make about the health effects of smoking:

> There is a lot of evidence which links smoking statistically with certain diseases . . .
>
> Statistics alone cannot prove cause and effect . . .
>
> Research is needed to clarify the situation. {1828.02, pp. 6–7}

These are the same arguments that the tobacco industry has been making since the 1950s, when it established the Tobacco Industry Research Committee (discussed in chapters 2 and 8). They are also the same arguments that the tobacco industry is using in current discussions over the health effects of environmental tobacco smoke.

The memo ends with an interesting cautionary note:

> The views expressed above[,] which incorporate warnings to the consumer, creates [sic] problems in countries where warnings are not required on packs or advertising and this situation should be reviewed. {1828.02, p. 7}

This afterthought by Johnson suggests that the tobacco industry might be more vulnerable to products liability lawsuits in countries that do *not* require warning labels on cigarette packages. In the industrialized world, where warning labels are required, the tobacco industry has been protected against claims that it has failed to warn smokers about the health effects of its products. In other countries, however, the industry may have a much harder time proving that it has given smokers adequate warnings.

Johnson's memo contains two appendices. The first, titled "Scientific Information," summarizes the scientific position of Dr. Ray Thornton, the smoking and health adviser at BAT's research center {1828.02, pp. 8–10}. It provides the scientific underpinnings for the tobacco industry's argument that causation has not been proven.

Thornton notes that a large number of epidemiological studies have shown a statistical association between smoking and a variety of diseases, particularly lung cancer. However, he states, it has never been formally established through experimental studies that smoking actually causes these diseases. After listing various other potential causes of cancer, Thornton concludes:

> It is therefore impossible to claim as a fact that smoking is the only or main cause of lung cancer and other diseases. On the other hand the views of the medical profession and the judgement they have made cannot be ignored and the reverse has not been established either—*it is equally impossible and quite wrong—factually and morally—to suggest or imply that smoking is safe or free from risk or that the risks are not particularly great.*
>
> Smoking may be implicated in the inception or development of some diseases—it may not—whether it is and/or the extent to which it is or may be is not known. Other factors appear to be implicated as well.
>
> The theory that smoking has been established as the main cause of lung cancer has become "conventional wisdom" and is accepted both in medical and scientific journals, and in the media generally without question—information is used selectively and other potential causes and evidence which conflict with the "traditional" view may be and often are ignored.

> As has been pointed out . . . there is risk that the real causes of diseases
> may be "missed" by ignoring "non traditional" research [emphasis added].
> {1828.02, pp. 9–10}

Again, this argument—that the causes of lung cancer and other diseases
normally associated with smoking are not really known and that further
research is necessary to determine those causes—is the same argument
used during the 1950s, when the Tobacco Industry Research Committee was formed. Yet, by the mid-1980s there was universal agreement
among scientific and medical authorities around the world that a causal
link between smoking and disease had been established conclusively.
Also, the suggestion that "non-traditional" research may be needed to
discover the "real causes" of diseases is in keeping with the industry's efforts to fund research projects that it knew would be unavailing, for the
purpose of distracting scientists and the public from the worthwhile research being conducted (see chapter 8).

The second appendix to the memo is titled "Summary of BAT's Approach to Smoking and Smoking Issues" and is dated May 21, 1984
{1828.02, p. 11}. It appears to provide an explanation for why BAT
would produce low-tar cigarettes when it claims that it does not believe
the tar produced by smoking is dangerous. The document states that, although there is a statistical association between smoking and disease, "the
question of cause continues . . . to be a controversy" {1828.02, p. 11}.
It then notes that many government agencies and physicians have advised the public to switch to low-tar brands, and that the industry has
simply responded by meeting the public demand.

> The tobacco industry has responded quickly to this changing demand, and
> to published government advice, by marketing an expanding range of ciga-
> rette products—so that each consumer can make his own informed choice of
> product. {1828.02, p. 11}

Of course, the consumer is hard pressed to make an "informed choice,"
since the tobacco industry has not provided the information it had that
smoking is dangerous, regardless of the amount of tar in the cigarettes.
This behavior is still another example of the industry's trying to have it
both ways: maintaining that there are no health dangers in smoking but
providing "healthier" cigarettes to those people who are worried about
possible dangers.

B&W's lawyers were also involved in setting public relations policy
for the company. Some of the issues that particularly concerned them are
discussed in a memo from Ernest Pepples, who was then B&W's senior

vice president and general counsel, to E. E. Kohnhorst, vice president of research, development, and engineering (RD&E) at B&W {1831.01}. The memo, dated August 16, 1984, and marked "Privileged," discusses Pepples's concerns over a report titled "The Functional Significance of Smoking in Every Day Life." Pepples states that use of the report for public affairs purposes, either by B&W or by the industry, would be inappropriate and inadvisable.

> Even the theme of the report, which promotes the concept of "the psychological benefits of smoking," is not appropriate or advisable as a public affairs position. {1831.01, p. 1}

This concern about promoting "the psychological benefits of smoking" is another indication of just how much the industry's attitudes toward cigarettes had changed since the 1960s, when research on nicotine as a stress reducer was being conducted because of the fear of competition from new tranquilizing drugs (see the discussion of Project Hippo II, in chapter 3). Pepples also voices his concern that some of the authorities cited in the report might not agree with its conclusions.

> [N]amely they might maintain that cigarette smoking is a [sic] not a suitable "coping aid" in everyday life. {1831.01, p. 1}

Unfortunately, we do not have a copy of the report itself, so we do not know which authors Pepples is referring to or what the report actually said.

Pepples then points out "more serious problems" with the report {1831.01, p. 1}. Specifically, it essentially concedes that nicotine is an addictive drug.

> In developing and carrying forward the position that a "simple" addiction model cannot explain smoking behavior, the report seems to concede that many potential criteria for addiction identification are met by smoking behavior. For example, the report urges the position that the primary motivation for smoking is ultimately tied to a pharmacological "psychoactive" function of nicotine. Some of the scientists who consult with B&W in connection with health litigation would not agree with this approach. *Accordingly, the report presents some potential for an apparent inconsistency among B&W's scientists, which could cause some difficulty in court.*
>
> Throughout the report, unfortunate concessions appear regarding "tolerance and withdrawal". . . . The report frequently expresses the view that smoking has certain "therapeutic properties" and nicotine is compared to the action of tranquilizers, alcohol, etc. In addition, smoking is referred to as one form of "drug usage", "psychoactive substance abuse", or "psychoactive drug usage".
>
> The authors of the report attempt to draw a fine line between "addiction" and "functional" behavior. . . . Our opponents would probably disregard

such a distinction and contend that this was an acceptance by the authors of the report of the basic allegation that cigarette smoking is addictive [emphasis added]. {1831.01, pp. 1–2}

Pepples then discusses the danger to the tobacco industry of admitting that nicotine is addictive. He specifically mentions that such an admission could be used against the industry in court as well as by the Food and Drug Administration (FDA) to justify regulation of tobacco products.

> *As you know, in the current legislative and litigation environment, claims of addiction have been and will be used against Brown & Williamson and the other companies by our adversaries. Such claims have been vigorously opposed in order not to give a claimant an unjustified weapon to use against the company or the industry.*
>
> In addition, the *possibility for FDA involvement would be heightened by company or industry promotion of the theme of this report, as it will be generally perceived* [emphasis added]. {1831.01, p. 2}

These memos written by attorneys for B&W and BAT clearly indicate that the companies were carefully monitoring their public statements in order to avoid making any claims that could be used against them in court or regulatory actions. The BAT attorney advises the company to maintain that a causal relationship between smoking and disease has not been proven, while the B&W attorney warns the company not to admit the addictiveness of its products. These are the same positions that all the tobacco companies have publicly held. Again the position of the lawyers has changed since the early 1960s, when they were encouraging the companies to develop a "safe" cigarette as the best way to stave off litigation (see chapter 4).

There is an interesting contrast between these two memos, indicating the different approaches to public relations problems in England and the United States, which, in turn, probably reflect the different levels of concern about potential lawsuits. Whereas the BAT attorney focuses on the need for the industry to be more forthright and willing to engage in public discussion of the health issues, the B&W attorney is more concerned about covering up any possibly damaging scientific material. Specifically, Pepples evidently believed that tobacco industry public relations statements must never even cite scientists who disagree with the industry's basic positions on the health issues, even though they may support the specific statements made. To do so would lend credibility to the scientists and thereby undermine the industry's attack on the scientific evidence indicating that there is a link between smoking and disease. (A particularly striking example of this attitude is discussed in the following section.)

The B&W attorney also evidently wanted to impose a rigid uniformity on the scientific opinions expressed by B&W scientists, so that no untoward scientific opinions would come to light and be used against the company in court (also discussed in chapter 7).

THE BLACKMAN PAPER: REWRITING SCIENTIFIC DOCUMENTS

The extent to which lawyers for B&W were concerned about having damaging scientific statements linked to the company is conveyed in a letter dated October 25, 1984, from J. Kendrick Wells, III, B&W's corporate counsel, to H. A. Morini, a lawyer at BAT {1833.01}. The letter contains Wells's comments on a draft paper titled "The Controversy on Smoking and Health—Some Facts and Anomalies," which had been written by Dr. L. C. F. Blackman, executive director of research and development for BAT (figure 9.1) {1833.02}. The paper presents the industry's view on the "controversy" over the health effects of smoking. As it was originally written, the Blackman paper contained a reasonably complete presentation of the evidence that smoking causes disease, and then used quotes from various scientists and scientific reports to support the claim that a causal link between smoking and disease had not been proven. However, as Wells's letter shows, even merely acknowledging the existence of some evidence pointing to such a link was unacceptable.

The title page of the Blackman paper indicates that it contains "Notes on talks given at the BAT Management Centre, Chelwood, by Dr. L. C. F. Blackman" {1833.02}, suggesting that the paper was intended to be a primer for BAT executives on issues related to smoking and health. The introduction states:

> This booklet is not a comprehensive review of all the research on the issues, but it sets out some of the reasons for stating that a controversy exists, and gives examples of some of the research reports which are inconsistent with the view that smoking has been proven to be a cause of disease. {1833.02, p. 3}

Wells made comments on virtually every page of Blackman's thirty-three-page paper, some of which are written in the margins of the draft. He also made forty-five detailed comments, including line-by-line recommendations regarding items that he thought should be deleted or included in the final report. These comments were too long to be written in the margins and are instead enumerated in his letter to Morini. Many of the suggested changes involve deletion or reconsideration of scientific authors cited in the paper, usually because the scientists cited had published work (sometimes not even cited in the paper) that did not support the tobacco industry's position. In other instances Wells suggests that material be rewritten so that it will conform to the company's stated positions, rather than the published scientific evidence.

Wells's comments on the draft paper are prefaced with a cautionary note:

> Recent developments have reaffirmed the need for the attention we customarily have given to proposed BAT publications. The smoking and health litigation in the U.S. has demonstrated that plaintiffs' lawyers are aggressive in questioning tobacco CEOs about published company statements, as we had predicted they would be. Peter Taylor's *Smoke Ring* [1] demonstrated that BAT publications which may be intended for limited distribution can be obtained and scrutinized by our most articulate adversaries. {1833.01, p. 1}

This comment suggests that attorneys for B&W routinely reviewed BAT documents prior to publication, even if they were only intended for "limited distribution" within BAT.

Wells began by changing the titles of some of the chapters (figure 9.1). Some of his revisions appear to have been designed to reinforce the idea that there is a "controversy" over the dangers of smoking. For example, Wells recommended changing the chapter on "Background to the Medical Concern" to "Background to the Scientific Dilemma." Interestingly, Wells also recommended deleting the word "facts" from two of the chapter titles: "Some Facts and Anomalies in the Literature Regarding Cancer" was changed to "Some Anomalies in the Literature Regarding Cancer." A similar change was made in the chapter on heart disease.

Wells seemed particularly interested in removing references to researchers who had published any findings that did not agree with the tobacco industry's position. For example, the original document contained the following quote from Sir Richard Doll and Richard Peto, who conducted one of the first epidemiological studies showing that smoking is associated with lung cancer and heart disease:

> To say that these conditions were related to smoking does not necessarily imply that smoking caused (or prevented) them.
> The relation may have been secondary in that smoking was associated with some other factor, such as alcohol consumption or a feature of the personality, that caused the disease. {1833.02, p. 8}

In his letter to Morini, Wells suggests that this reference be deleted:

> 8. Delete Doll and Peto reference. Doll and Peto have published a table which shows "cancer of the lung" is "caused by cigarette smoking" and have

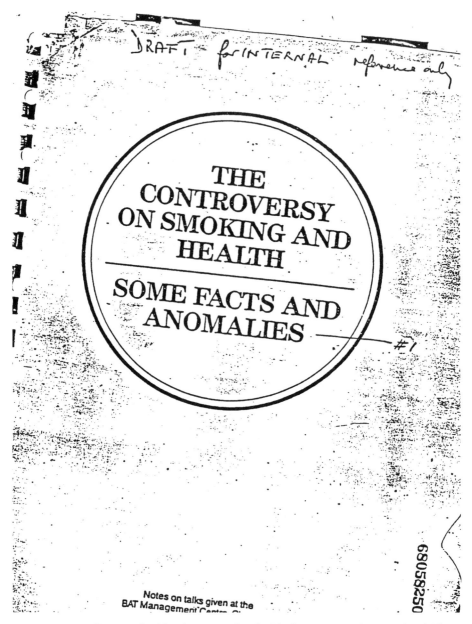

DRAFT for INTERNAL reference only

THE
CONTROVERSY
ON SMOKING AND
HEALTH

SOME FACTS AND
ANOMALIES

#1

680582250

Notes on talks given at the
BAT Management Centre

FIGURE 9.1. Cover and table of contents for the Blackman report {1833.02}, which was based on talks given at the BAT Management Centre by Dr. L.C.F. Blackman. Note that the editing by the lawyer J.K. Wells {1833.01} changed "medical concern" to "scientific dilemma," deleted the term "facts," and emphasized the use of the term "causality."

THE CONTROVERSY · ON SMOKING AND HEALTH

SOME FACTS AND ANOMALIES

CONTENTS

FIGURE 9.1. *(continued)*

concluded that "much of the excess mortality in cigarette smoking can be attributed with certainty to the habit . . ." {1833.01, p. 2}

Later in his comments, Wells notes that any mention of Doll should be handled with care.

> 35. . . . Parenthetically, any reference to Doll must be crafted carefully because he is a dedicated advocate of the causal hypothesis. {1833.01, p. 6}

Wells also recommends deleting a reference to research conducted by Drs. Friberg, Cederloff, and Lundman, who had compared disease rates in smoking and nonsmoking twins. Interestingly, this research had been funded by the tobacco industry for years in an attempt to prove the "constitutional hypothesis." The constitutional hypothesis, which had originally been proposed by Sir Ronald Fisher in 1957, essentially argues that some people are genetically predisposed both to being the type of person who smokes and to developing diseases such as lung cancer and heart disease. Friberg and his colleagues all but disproved the constitutional hypothesis when they showed that a person who smokes is more likely to develop smoking-related diseases than his or her nonsmoking identical twin, even though they have the same genetic makeup and therefore the same genetic predisposition to disease. The Friberg group's work was referred to in the original draft of the Blackman paper in a quote taken from the 1979 *Bibliography on Smoking and Health* (published by the federal government):

> The results from the twins study clearly demonstrate the importance of genetic, behavioural and psychosocial factors which have not been considered in conventional epidemiologic studies. {1833.02, p. 18}

Wells states in his letter that the reference to Friberg, as well as the reference to the bibliography, should be deleted.

> 21. Recommend delete references to Friberg and the Bibliography on Smoking and Health. Unfortunately, Friberg, Cederloff and Lundman published a monograph in 1977 which stated that "lung cancer is closely related to the amount smoked . . . ," that associations were confirmed between smoking and respiratory, cardiovascular and other symptoms of disease or ill health, that there is no doubt about a causal link between smoking and lung cancer, and that the results from the Swedish monozygotic twin studies are contrary to the constitutional hypothesis advanced by Fisher.
> The problem carries over into the quote from the Bibliography on Smoking and Health. . . . The same article states that "the well documented evidence of a causal association between smoking and lung cancer found in other studies has been further supported." {1833.01, p. 4}

Ironically, the monograph of the Friberg group's work mentioned by Wells was actually funded as a CTR special project (table 8.1).

A quote from Dr. Lawrence Garfinkel, vice president for epidemiology of the American Cancer Society, and an author of one of the early papers on environmental tobacco smoke (ETS) and lung cancer that had produced equivocal results (2), was included in the draft:

> Passive smoking may be a political matter, but it is not a main issue in terms of health policy. {1833.02, p. 31}

The tobacco industry had widely used this quote in its efforts to create controversy about the early evidence that ETS causes lung cancer (see chapter 10, particularly figure 10.1 and the associated discussion). Wells, however, notes in his comment that Garfinkel later retracted this statement after his second study on ETS and lung cancer showed an increased risk (3) and criticized the tobacco industry for continuing to use Garfinkel's first study in industry advertising.

> 40. Delete. Dr. Garfinkel has published a letter in the *New York Times* (June 5, 1984) which protests R. J. Reynolds' use of the passage quoted in the Draft and states:
>> It is irresponsible of Reynolds to attempt to create a false sense of security about the potential dangers of passive smoking, especially at a time when incriminating evidence continues to accumulate. {1833.01, p. 7}

Wells left unchanged quotations from an international symposium in Vienna in 1984, which was organized by an individual affiliated with the tobacco industry (4) and exonerated ETS as a cause of disease.

In his letter to Morini, Wells even recommends deleting a short subsection of the paper dealing with chronic obstructive lung disease (COLD). The subsection presented a table from the fourth report of the Royal College of Physicians. The data in the table suggested that COLD might be associated with social class. However, Wells notes,

> 26. ... The same paragraph in the fourth Report which presents the table reprinted in the Draft states "it must be emphasized that at present only the effects of tobacco are reliably known to be of substantial importance." {1833.01, p. 4}

Table 9.1 (on p. 377) summarizes some of the changes suggested to the Blackman paper. These editorial changes would have effectively removed any reasonable presentation of the then-current state of scientific information from the paper and turned it into a purely public relations piece. Given that the paper was apparently prepared for "limited

distribution" within BAT to review the "smoking and health controversy," it is remarkable that B&W evidently did not want its employees
to be presented with arguments contrary to the company position, even
when those arguments appeared in a document designed to discredit
mainstream scientific opinion.

SCIENCE AND PUBLIC RELATIONS FROM
A LAWYER'S PERSPECTIVE

On June 16, 1981, in response to a request from Ernest Pepples, William
Shinn, an attorney at Shook, Hardy, and Bacon, sent a "Confidential
Memorandum" to Pepples, listing various events in the area of smoking
and health over the past few years and categorizing them as either "plus"
or "minus" items {2130.02}. Two days later, Pepples sent the same material, essentially verbatim over his own signature, with the list of items
reformatted, in a "Privileged Memorandum" to C. I. McCarty, BATUS's
chairman and chief operating officer, with a copy to Dr. I. W. Hughes,
B&W's chairman and CEO {2130.01}. The complete text of the memorandum follows:

> The following list of what I am calling "plus" and "minus" items is certainly
> not complete (nor in any particular order) but should be illustrative of smok-
> ing and health "events" over the past few years, sometimes having a great
> deal of coverage and sometimes not. I know you asked for "science" only but
> I have included a few other items for completeness. The designation of "plus"
> in some cases should probably read "mixed".

PLUS

1.   Paper by Samuel S. Epstein and others at a meeting of the American Public Health Association late last year reported as contradicting the hypothesis that smoking is the overwhelming causal factor for lung cancer and explaining that occupational exposure was not adequately recognized when the major statistical studies on lung cancer were commenced.

2.   Defeat of 1978 and 1980 initiative propositions in Dade County [Florida] and in California.

3.   Articles by McDonald and Bea van den Berg on women and lung cancer (may have appeared only in the *Tobacco Observer* for February 1980).

MINUS

1.   White/Froeb, Hirayama and Greek paper on non-smokers—(much publicity).

2.   Surgeon General reports.

3.   Federal Trade Commission reports.

4.   Fourth World Conference on Smoking and Health (not much publicity).

5.   Gary Friedman paper on quitting smoking and reduction of heart disease.

6.   Louisville *Courier* articles on smoking.

7.   Stories on fires reportedly caused by cigarette smoking.

PLUS

4. Wharton study on financial impact of tobacco (1980)—(Not smoking and health).

5. Hirayama error and Garfinkel paper.

6. Seltzer editorial on heart disease and smoking.

7. Sterling letter re series in *Courier-Journal*.

8. Gori comments re "Less Hazardous Cigarettes" (1978).

9. Other reports (e.g., Hammond) on low "tar" and nicotine cigarettes.

10. Dr. Peter Bourne statement on smoking [special circumstances].

11. Dr. Huber letters and comments on smoking and health made after going to University of Kentucky [caveat re later developments].

12. Jones hearing (1978)—lack of evidence tobacco smoke harmful to the average non-smoker (but little publicity).

13. 1978—Superdome decision by Judge Gordon upheld by Federal Court of Appeals.

14. Eysenck's recent book emphasizing personality traits as accounting for susceptibility to cancer. After a review of literature concluded that smoking is not clearly linked to cancer. (Dr. Eysenck is a psychologist at the London Institute of Psychiatry.) His book has generated a number of articles about the "rekindling of the smoking debate."

15. Washington University research (St. Louis coverage)—General research.

16. Court opinion cigarettes are not under FDA.

17. Letters re Aronow—(no publicity).

MINUS

8. State Mutual Life Assurance Company study (1979) purporting to show that smokers die younger than non-smokers.

9. January 1978—Califano unveils his anti-smoking plan.

10. CAB hearings on smoking in aircraft.

11. Senator Kennedy introduces bill on smoking including program to deter children from smoking (1978).

12. Birth control pill warning.

13. FTC CO testing.

14. Government report on smoking as an addiction and inclusion of tobacco in DSM III under "tobacco use disorder".

15. Smoking and byssinosis.

16. AMA-ERF report.

17. Aronow on CO and non-smokers.

18. Smoking and asbestos.

19. Queries re "advantage" of low "tar" and nicotine cigarettes.

20. Additives inquiries. {2130.01, pp. 1–2}

Many of the "positive" scientific developments involved publications by individuals who were being quietly supported by the tobacco industry (e.g., Seltzer, Sterling, Gori, Huber, Eysenck; see chapter 8). In addition to providing an insight into the wide range of issues facing the industry at the time, this memorandum once again demonstrates the extent to which the lawyers were dominating B&W's corporate affairs. As the memorandum indicates, the original request for information was for "'science' only," and yet the information was sought from an attorney rather than a scientist. Of course, there was a good reason for this: as discussed in chapter 8, the lawyers were directing much of the scientific research, and Shinn was one of the principal actors in that endeavor. Again, even assuming a scientist should not have compiled such a list, one might expect that a public relations person would have done so, but then the lawyers were pretty much in charge of that aspect of the business as well. One item in the list stands out as an example of the inconsistency that exists between the tobacco industry's internal and public pronouncements on smoking issues. Despite the consistent claims by the industry that it does not advertise to attract children and that it believes smoking is an adult custom that children should not adopt, the memorandum lists a congressional bill, which included a program to deter children from smoking, as a "minus."

SWAYING PUBLIC OPINION

The documents show that Brown and Williamson—and probably the other tobacco companies—was not above using its significant economic clout to try to sway public opinion. Several documents from the 1970s and 1980s describe discussions about, or actual involvement in, manipulating corporations, the media, and physicians.

INFLUENCING CORPORATIONS

As the tobacco industry faced increasing government regulation, it turned to the corporate world, particularly the corporations with which it had business ties, for assistance. Such corporate friends could obviously be useful to the industry in various ways, but, if nothing else, they could at least refrain from taking actions that were detrimental to the industry. A memo from the late 1970s discusses a proposal to use B&W's economic relationships to convince various corporations to maintain a more favorable attitude toward smoking and the tobacco industry. The memo, dated February 3, 1977, was sent from Ernest Pepples to C.I. McCarty.

> *A question has arisen in different forms about approaching companies we do business with who are prominent in association with the American Cancer Society or with other forces against the tobacco industry, or who happen to be involved in some other way with aspects of the anti-smoking campaign.* Three examples: the Chairman of the St. Regis Paper Company is lending his name to the anti-smoking press release put out by the American Cancer Society; TWA [Trans World Airlines] would not let their premises be used by persons who were seeking petition signers in support of the industry's position before the CAB [Civil Aeronautics Board]; and the Chase Bank in New York is permitting a stop smoking clinic on their premises.
>
> *I favor the idea of raising with our friends in such companies the points which we consider are being used unfairly and falsely against tobacco and giving our side of the story.*
>
> *It is imperative that we do not apply overt economic pressure in carrying our message. It is also essential that we operate this program solo. If it is done in collaboration with other companies or through the* [Tobacco] *Institute, in my opinion a serious question arises under various trade regulation laws which prohibit boycotts and other joint economic action.*
>
> Just as a rule of thumb, we have considerably greater latitude in deciding who [*sic*] we will deal with than we do in deciding when we will stop dealing with someone. Both areas must be approached with great caution.
>
> If properly structured, however, Brown & Williamson can certainly tell its side of the story in the smoking and health controversy and refute the false claims made against cigarettes. It goes without saying that communications to our friends in other industries should be done deliberately, carefully and tactfully in order to have maximum impact. If we follow that common sense approach, we will not stray off the path into the thicket of unfair trade practices and boycotts [emphasis added]. {2116.01}

In view of the industry's consistent public posture that smokers can quit if they so wish, it is hard to understand Pepples's concern over the existence of a stop-smoking clinic at the Chase Bank. In any event, the memo was written just as an initiative campaign was being launched in California to limit smoking in workplaces and public places (see chapter 10), and the tobacco industry in fact did exert enormous influence on restaurants and small business associations, as well as other corporate entities, to oppose that initiative. However, although the industry was able in the early days of the nonsmokers' rights movement to wield great influence with corporations, it gradually lost much of its corporate support as the dangers of secondhand smoke and the costs of smoking to employers became more evident. For example, when a law to regulate smoking in the workplace was proposed in San Francisco in 1983, it was supported by the Bank of America.

INFLUENCING THE MEDIA

Like any other industry whose products are the subject of public debate, the tobacco industry has always attempted to curry favor with the media. As discussed in chapter 5, during the "safe" cigarette era of the 1960s, the industry enjoyed some strong support in the media. However, by the 1980s much of that support had eroded, and the industry often had to struggle to find a sympathetic media voice. As several memos from the early 1980s indicate, the industry attempted to influence media coverage of proposed legislation on cigarette labeling and advertising by Congressman Henry Waxman (D-CA) and Senators Orrin Hatch (R-UT) and Robert Packwood (R-OR).

On February 8, 1983, Horace Kornegay, chairman of the Tobacco Institute, wrote to Ernest Pepples at B&W stating:

> First, the project to determine in each company who is personally acquainted with the publisher, editor or business manager of any of the newspapers on the list which was distributed at the meeting of the Executive Committee and to set up a meeting with the publisher, editor or business manager for the purpose of informing him of the great dangers contained in the Waxman-Hatch-Packwood bills. I would urge you to move as soon as possible on this undertaking inasmuch as the Congressional committees could begin action on these bills within the next few weeks. {2131.02, p. 1}

This project appears to have been part of an industry-wide effort to approach all major media. Thus, a letter dated February 8, 1983, from C. H. Judge, who was in the office of the president of Lorillard Tobacco, to Samuel D. Chilcote, Jr., president of the Tobacco Institute, states:

> Have met with Dick Monroe, Chief Executive and Cliff Grum, Executive V. P. of Time, Inc. Agreement reached for presentation to Editor-in-Chief of Time, Inc. and Managing Editors of all Time, Inc. Magazines. Presentation to be mainly rebuttal of upcoming Surgeon General's Report and a plea for fairness and objectivity.
>
> . . .
>
> cc: TIEC [Tobacco Institute Executive Committee] Members. We need help. Key city newspapers (eg. NY Times, LA Times, Wash. Post, Houston Chronicle, etc., etc.) key. If you can set up and attend a similar meeting, please let Sam [probably Sam Chilcote] know. {2131.03, p. 1}

In a memo to Dr. I. W. Hughes, B&W chairman and CEO, also dated February 8, 1983, Tom Humber, B&W assistant director of corporate affairs, discusses the possible pitfalls involved in attempting to influence the media:

> I have persistently criticized the industry and TI [Tobacco Institute] for not taking a pro-active stance with regard to article placement in what I call, for lack of a better umbrella term, the popular press. By that I mean the mass circulation magazines, ranging from *Ladies Home Journal* to *Playgirl*. That, I believe, is where the attack is headed. Having lost our advantage of positive pursuit during relative quiet, we must now fight a rear-guard action with limited hopes.
>
> . . .
>
> Given the proclivities of several companies, I believe there is significant danger of pressure tactics that could easily backfire and make matters worse. If we've got what we say we've got, then the authoritative, coherent presentation of information is the best course. The seminar approach is substantive and clean; it can, to some extent, be better controlled. It can provide more information to more people in a shorter time. We will be attacked for whatever we do, but the open approach has a better chance of being regarded as honest and straightforward, even gutsy, than private meetings in parking garages [perhaps a reference to "Deep Throat" of Watergate fame] or French restaurants.
>
> Our message should be simple: We shall not use our advertising dollars to influence editorial material. In fact, we believe that the smoking and health controversy mandates more public discussion, not less, just as it mandates increased research. But the discussion should be informed, balanced and accurate, not based on anyone's propaganda. *To that end, here are scientists, here are films, here are documents, here are resources for you to call on when you have questions* [emphasis added]. {2131.04, p. 2}

Some of the same concerns are expressed in a February 14, 1983, "restricted" memorandum from Pepples to Dr. Hughes, regarding "industry contacts with editors":

> The gist of what I said was as follows. While contacts to media by CEO's do make sense in the present circumstances, they need to select the ground carefully and coordinate with the appropriate advisers. I suggested that the better ground was the Waxman-Hatch-Packwood legislation on cigarette labeling and advertising because it presents First Amendment concerns which are so dear to the heart of publishers. I further suggested that the footing would not be as good on the alternative ground, heart disease and the Surgeon General's Report. [The 1983 Surgeon General's report dealt with smoking and heart disease.]
>
> . . .
>
> *Finally, a concern was mentioned to* [Arthur] *Stevens about a potential backlash, legal and otherwise, if the publishers see our contacts as either solo or joint* underline*coercion* *to influence news and editorial content.* I mentioned the *Wall Street Journal* article of some several weeks back as well as the recent

contact from a Milwaukee reporter, raising the issue of advertising dollars and the press' freedom to express antismoking views. This is merely a caveat, not a bone-breaker. The industry has a good, respectable position to present. It is just a matter of keeping it in mind and saying it to the publishers. No company uses its advertising dollars in a coercive way. Indeed, the industry urges that the public deserves <u>more</u> not less discussion of the smoking and health controversy. But the discussion should be balanced and accurate and it should be free of the rhetoric and one-sided propaganda which sees no good in cigarettes and only great harm.

. . .

Curt [Judge] then informs his listener that if such legislation [providing for rotational warnings on cigarette packs] passes, litigation will wipe out the cigarette industry and the publishers will not have a customer for their advertising space. Arthur [Stevens] indicated that Curt Judge would use this approach as part of his presentation to the editors of *Time Magazine*. Stated another way, he would get into the Waxman/Hatch/Packwood situation even though it is extraneous to the central subject of heart disease and the Surgeon General's Report [italic emphasis added]. {2131.01, pp. 1–3}

That both Humber and Pepples would state that the industry does not use its advertising dollars in a coercive way is remarkable. Not only does the industry apply pressure through its advertising clout to forestall criticism in the media, but, as was discussed in chapter 5, the industry occasionally buys favorable media coverage by paying people to write articles supporting the industry without disclosing their ties to the industry.

INFLUENCING PHYSICIANS

The tobacco industry's efforts to influence physicians began with the publication in 1954 of a booklet entitled *A Scientific Perspective on the Cigarette Controversy* (5). The booklet was merely one part of a large-scale public relations campaign being organized on behalf of the industry by the firm of Hill and Knowlton to counteract the emerging evidence of the health dangers of smoking (see chapter 2). According to a May 3, 1954, memorandum from Hill and Knowlton to the Tobacco Industry Research Committee (TIRC), the publisher of the booklet, it was released on April 14, 1954, and 205,000 copies were printed. It was sent to 176,800 doctors (general practitioners and specialists as well as the deans of medical and dental colleges), members of Congress, and 15,000 members of the press. As noted in a "Confidential" memorandum from Hill and Knowlton to the TIRC on August 17, 1954 (reporting the firm's activities through July 31, 1954), the booklet contained quotations from three dozen research and medical authorities, culled from both domestic and foreign sources. The booklet "was held necessary and urgently timely to present to leaders of public opinion the fact that there was no unanimity among scientists regarding the charges against cigarettes" (5).

The documents contain evidence of continuing efforts by the tobacco industry to influence physicians over the next few decades. An untitled and undated document, apparently from about 1970, summarizes various proposed advertising strategies for the tobacco industry and B&W's analysis of them (see chapter 5); one item relates to "Communications with Physicians":

> The need was felt for directing printed material to MDs on research efforts and studies which cast doubt on anti-smoking theory. Talk centered on reinstituting the [Tobacco] Institute's "Tobacco and Health Research" publication [which was distributed quarterly to more than 100,000 physicians in the late 1950s and early 1960s]. Our [i.e., B&W's] opinion was that a better approach would be to run a paid insert in some medical journals (particularly the well-read "Medical Economics" [a "throw-away" journal that focuses on how physicians can increase their incomes]) rather than direct mail pieces, which would probably end up in wastebaskets. We were in favor of a pilot study to determine the best method and, indeed, the feasibility of this type of communications. {2112.04, p. 2}

Thus, as in 1954, the tobacco industry was not content to influence physicians by passively responding to inquiries or communicating with them through the media. Rather, the industry was considering proactive steps, at substantial expense, to communicate directly with physicians.

Brown and Williamson also studied physicians' attitudes about cigarette smoke, to see what physicians were telling their patients and what their attitudes toward a safer cigarette would be. In March 1979 Dugan/Farley Communications Associates presented a report to B&W on a series of interviews with physicians {2127.01}. The emphasis the interviewers placed on "gasses" suggests that this was a marketing study for the Fact brand, which B&W had on the market at that time (see chapter 4). The interviewers found that doctors generally had poor success encouraging people to quit smoking, and that virtually all physicians were aware of conditions besides lung cancer linked to cigarette smoking. Despite this knowledge, fewer than one-third were aware that carbon monoxide is a problem or that other gases are linked with other diseases. Dugan/Farley's report concludes:

> The "concept" of a cigarette that is low in tar and nicotine with a filter that greatly reduces known deleterious gasses was exposed to them [the doctors]. It was generally well received.
>
>   . . .

> At this early stage in our research there seems to be hope for an educational program that would lead to acceptance by the medical profession of a "safer" cigarette. {2127.01, pp. 10, 11}

Medical textbooks at the time advised physicians to recommend low-tar cigarettes if a patient was not able to stop smoking. The marketing company's interviews with physicians introduced them to the concept of toxic gases in cigarette smoke, a problem they had not usually considered. Once confronted by this new problem with tobacco smoke, physicians responded favorably to the idea of a low-tar cigarette that also reduced "deleterious gasses." As it happened, B&W had such a product already on the market, Fact cigarettes, and the competition did not. However, B&W apparently was unable to capitalize on this insight, since Fact never attracted enough sales to warrant continued support. Indeed, this marketing study may have been part of a last-ditch effort to revive the brand. Nonetheless, the vignette well illustrates the underlying health benefit B&W promised in a low-delivery cigarette and, if the market research was, indeed, for Fact, it also shows that, with the Purite filter of Fact, the company made an additional health claim: that lower levels of certain toxic gases are better for the consumer.

Two years later, on April 29, 1981, G. E. Stungis, B&W's director of marketing research services, sent a "Limited" memorandum to Dr. I. W. Hughes, J. Alar (president and chief operations officer), and Ernest Pepples. In this memo Stungis discusses the possibility of marketing low-tar cigarettes through a Medical Communications Program {2129.01}. First, Stungis presents some background:

> Up to now we have bits/pieces of how "Medical Communications Program" (MCP) may operate. Several optional and indeed variations within options exist . . . all with cost structure implications.
>
> Currently a number of assumptions exist . . . by necessity at this stage. In this document Benefits Research will not be dealt with directly; consequently, we take as a given that:
>
> There is [sic] indeed benefits associated with smoking along the lines of stress/mastery.
>
> There is a stable, sound and controllable benefits research team that is operative.
>
> The output of the Benefits Research is technically sound.
>
> Appropriate information channels with associated controls are indeed "assets in place".
>
> Opposition counter measures developed [emphasis in original].
> {2129.01, p. 1}

Using a communications diagram and an explanatory text, Stungis next describes an "MCP Model." In both the diagram and the text, he distinguishes between the "General Smoking Public" and "Extreme Concerned Smokers." The diagram pictures communications running among "Health/Medical," "Benefits Research Program," "Extreme Concerned Smokers," and "General Smoking Public." The text, which is written in shorthand form, reads as follows:

> Benefits Research conducted in conjunction with <u>credible asset</u>. Results of Benefits Research are communicated through two controlled information channels . . . devices for physician[s] and extreme concerned smokers. Physician community, accepts/refers in an interactive sense with smoking public and initiates information diffusion or so-called word of mouth process. To operate, the entire system must be <u>continually</u> driven. At introductory stage (time period?) referred smoking product would be only distributed through outlets <u>associated closely</u> with Health/Medical System [emphasis in original]. {2129.01, p. 2}

In conjunction with the model, Stungis notes that the following assumptions operate:

> 1)   Physicians realize they are not successful in achieving/inducing "quit smoking" posture for substantial numbers of their patients.
>
> 2)   Physicians are gravitating toward "Behavioral Medicine" in route toward "holistic treatments" . . . eg. accepting that given environments, lifestyle, genetics, etc. alternative consumable products with "acceptable" risk/benefit profiles can and should be recommended if not prescribed for certain patients.
>
> 3)   Physicians will accept the concepts of Type A, Type B behavior implications of stress to disease through autoregulation of the human nervous system.
>
> 4)   Smokers, through recommendation by physicians (directly or indirectly) would respond to smoking alternatives readily . . . eg, switch rather than quit.
>
> 5)   Members of Health/Medical System, pharmacists, nurses, etc., would respond positively to smoking alternatives with benefits. {2129.01, p. 3}

However, these assumptions are far from exhaustive:

> Our earlier work (qualitative) with physicians provided clues . . . no more, no less. We should pursue fairly rapidly to tighten up loose points above as well as uncover latent issues. Suggested further research work is:
>
> > Quantitative Study among Physicians . . . primary objective would be to determine willingness on part of physicians to consider alternatives to consumables that affect patients' <u>health</u> and <u>well being</u> . . . eg., cigarettes, coffee, etc. . . . Properly designed study should confirm/refute assumption 1 through 3.

Qualitative Studies—Peripheral Health/Medical Systems (Pharmacist[s], Nurses, etc.) . . . primary objective is to determine attitudes toward alternative risk/benefit consumables. This phase similar to early qualitative physician study. Would in all probability require quantitative follow up.

Consumer Qualitative Study . . . primary object would be to obtain clues as to how effective physicians would be in convincing patients to use alternative products for improving his/her lifestyle management. Would require quantitative follow up [emphasis in original]. {2129.01, pp. 3–4}

Finally, Stungis outlines the cost estimates of the proposal {2129.01, p. 4}.

By 1981 several epidemiological studies had demonstrated that the tar reductions of the previous generation did not markedly reduce the risk of lung cancer (6), and internal BAT studies beginning around 1974 had shown that smokers of low-tar cigarettes compensate for the weaker smoke by smoking more intensively, in order to maintain their accustomed nicotine levels, and thereby lose much of the supposed benefit of low-tar brands (see chapter 3). Despite these findings, B&W apparently continued its efforts to sell low-tar cigarettes through the medical profession. Stungis's proposed Medical Communications Program may have been organized around the Barclay brand, B&W's "99% tar free" cigarette. Whatever specific brand, though, the concept belies any pretense that low-tar cigarettes are not about health. The MCP was organized to influence physicians to recommend certain types of cigarettes, if not specific brands, on the basis of their perceptions of health benefits.

These documents corroborate the impression that low tar and "low gas" were intended as a health benefit and demonstrate that B&W at least considered marketing these benefits to physicians. The documents do not indicate whether the MCP was ever actually put in practice. Its existence as a concept and the physician survey about "deleterious gasses," however, reveal that B&W, at least internally, considered marketing particular types of cigarettes as intended to prevent disease. This intent to provide health benefits (whether or not the products actually provided any), in turn, would have made the brands that were to be detailed through the MCP, as well as the "low gas" brand (probably Fact), drugs under the Food, Drug and Cosmetic Act.

BUYING FRIENDS

The Brown and Williamson documents include the confidential budget for state and local activities performed by the Tobacco Institute for 1987 {2229.01}. The proposed budget allotted $10,096,000 for state lobbying activities, including campaign contributions and donations to a wide variety of organizations that play a role in determining public policy (table 9.2, p. 385). In many cases the connection to tobacco is not obvious; the industry simply seems to be opening doors and buying friends who can be called on to oppose controls on tobacco sales and use, taxation, and other issues handled politically.

ADVERTISING

From the late 1970s through the mid-1980s, Brown and Williamson was investing in two new forms of mass advertising. First, the company bought on-screen advertisements in movie theaters, so-called trailers, that run before the movie itself is shown. Second, it contracted for product placements in movies themselves as well as in television shows. Both types of advertising reach large numbers of children. As discussed below, in one instance the placement of a cigarette ad in a movie particularly attractive to children proved to be a bad idea.

ON-SCREEN ADVERTISING AND THE
SNOW WHITE CONTROVERSY

The on-screen advertisements used by B&W were coordinated by Cinema Concepts, a company based in Nashville, Tennessee, and were distributed to movie theaters throughout the country. For example, as of January 24, 1984, advertisements for the Kool Jazz Festival, a nationwide series of jazz concerts sponsored by Kool cigarettes, were being shown on 1,235 screens at virtually every large theater group in the United States, with a combined yearly attendance of 93.8 million people (table 9.3, p. 387).

B&W's campaign backfired when its ads for Kool ran prior to screenings of Walt Disney's *Snow White and the Seven Dwarfs* in Newton, Massachusetts, and attracted protests by a grass-roots nonsmokers' rights organization, Massachusetts GASP (Group Against Smoking Pollution), because it was shown before a children's movie. The Brown and Williamson advertising department's reaction to this incident is summarized succinctly in an August 4, 1983, memorandum from N. V. Domantay, B&W's vice president of brand management, to Dr. I. W. Hughes, the company's chairman and CEO.

> In line with your request to be kept informed of all complaints re: cinema advertising, attached is a copy of Mr. Sutton's attorney's letter, which summarizes the KOOL incident in Newton, Mass.

Our response is also attached. Please note that Mr. Sutton is not directing his complaint at us but rather at the theater owner.

Nevertheless, if this becomes a firestorm (apparently thanks to GASP's efforts in alerting other newspapers to the story), it could impact the acceptance rate of our ads among other theater owners. *Worse yet, it could get Washington into the act.*

Screenvision, our theater distributor, has already taken steps to avoid this kind of mistake in the future. The KOOL/BARCLAY film reels now carry a warning sign: "DO NOT EXHIBIT AD TRAILER WITH A G-RATED FEATURE." In addition, Screenvision is soliciting input from theater owners as to how they could absolutely avoid these mistakes in the future [emphasis added]. {2400.15}

Most likely because of the negative publicity surrounding the *Snow White* incident, and potential further public relations problems, B&W ultimately discontinued its cinema advertising program. The decision to discontinue the program is set forth in a letter written on February 21, 1984, by Ernest Pepples, B&W's senior vice president and general counsel, to Cinema Concepts {2400.12}. According to a memorandum of March 8, 1984, to Pepples from B. H. Freedman, B&W's marketing counsel, Brown and Williamson had by then extracted itself from its contract with Cinema Concepts by settling for $545,000. Freedman indicated that a Jim Adams needed to know whether the payment should be charged to law or marketing, and recommended it be charged to marketing. In a handwritten note, Pepples agreed {2405.06}. That there was a question as to where the charges belonged may indicate that liability concerns played a role in the company's decision.

Thus, an extensive B&W advertising program using trailer advertisements in movie theaters was derailed by the protest of a small grass-roots organization. This incident illustrates the potential effectiveness of strong grass-roots action against tobacco promotion activities.

PRODUCT PLACEMENT IN MOVIES AND ON TELEVISION

Product placement refers to the practice of having a specific product, or the product's brand name or logo, appear conspicuously during the course of a chosen movie or television show. Such placement is considered especially effective when an actor or actress playing the part of a hero or a sympathetic character personally uses the product in a conspicuous manner on screen. This is a relatively recent phenomenon; not only did older movies not contain product placements, but the producers and directors deliberately avoided having any identifiable product names appear in the movies. Of course, many products other than cigarettes are now advertised in this manner, such as candy and soft drinks. However, such advertising of cigarettes raises obvious ethical concerns not associated with the advertising of other products; when the advertisements are placed on television, there may be legal ramifications as well, because of the ban on television advertisement of cigarettes, which went into effect on January 2, 1971.

Brown and Williamson hired Associated Film Promotion (AFP), a firm in Century City, California, to obtain product placement for B&W in motion pictures and television programs. B&W eventually became dissatisfied with the placement of its product by AFP and felt that other companies, particularly Philip Morris, were getting better exposure. In addition, B&W concluded that even Philip Morris often did not get its money's worth. According to an October 26, 1983, "Limited" memorandum from D. R. Scott, B&W's director of auditing, to N. V. Domantay,

> The relationship with AFP or Mr. Robert Kovoloff, President of AFP, apparently began in 1979, and was prompted by the Company's desire to *remain competitive* in the "movie placement" arena [emphasis added]. {2400.01}

This statement suggests that tobacco industry advertising by product placement predated 1979 and was a widespread activity in the industry at the time. According to the audit report itself, between the inception of the contract with AFP in July 1979 and August 1983, B&W paid a total of $965,500 to AFP, which included $687,500 for special movie placements (summarized in table 9.4, p. 387) and $278,000 in retainer fees {2400.23, p. 1}.

In one of the most important deals arranged by AFP, it received firm written commitment for use of Brown and Williamson's products from Sylvestor Stallone (figure 9.2). In a letter dated April 28, 1983, and addressed to Kovoloff, the actor guaranteed in writing to smoke Brown and Williamson cigarettes in five of his upcoming films for payment of $500,000. Stallone wrote:

> As discussed, I guarantee that I will use Brown & Williamson tobacco products in no less than five feature films.
>
> It is my understanding that Brown & Williamson will pay a fee of $500,000.00. {2404.02}

The agreement between Brown and Williamson and Stallone (via AFP) was consummated shortly thereafter. On June 14, 1983, James F. Ripslinger, senior vice president of AFP, wrote Stallone:

> In furtherance of the agreements reached between yourself and Associated Film Promotions, Inc. representing their client Brown & Williamson Tobacco

Sylvester Stallone

April 28, 1983

Mr. Bob Kovoloff
ASSOCIATED FILM PROMOTION
10100 Santa Monica Blvd.
Los Angeles, CA   90067

Dear Bob:

**As discussed, I guarantee that I will use Brown & Williamson
tobacco products in no less than five feature films.**

It is my understanding that Brown & Williamson will pay
a fee of $500,000.00.

Hoping to hear from you soon;

Sincerely,

Sylvester Stallone

SS/sp

FIGURE 9.2.   Letter from star Sylvester Stallone agreeing to smoke B&W products in five upcoming movies in exchange for a $500,000 fee. Source: {2404.02}

Corp. (B&W), I wish to put in summary form the various understandings and details regarding B&W's appearances and usage in your next five scheduled motion pictures. B&W is very pleased to become associated with the following schedule of films and to have you incorporate personal usage for all films other than the character of Rocky Balboa in Rocky IV, where other leads will have product usage, as well as the appearance of signage (potentially ring).

The following is the current list of the next five (5) minimum films for B&W's appearance. It is understood that if production commitments change the order or appearance of any of the group of films to be released, B&W will appear in a substituted film. The only nonappearance for B&W will be by mutual consent of both parties in which case another Sylvester Stallone movie will be arranged for substitution.

The initial schedule of films is:

A). <u>Rhinestone Cowboy</u>

B). <u>Godfather III</u>

C). <u>Rambo</u>

D). <u>50/50</u>

E). <u>Rocky IV</u>

In consideration for these extensive film appearances of B&W products, Brown and Williamson agrees to forward to Robert Kovoloff and Associated Film Promotions, Inc. their initial deposit to you of Two-Hundred-Fifty-Thousand Dollars ($250,000.00). This represents a fifty percent (50%) deposit of the total financial commitment by B&W. The subsequent Two-Hundred-Fifty-Thousand Dollars ($250,000.00) is agreed to be forwarded in five (5) equal payments of Fifty-Thousand Dollars ($50,000.00) each payable at the inception of production of each participating film. {2404.01}

As discussed below, B&W terminated its contract with AFP before all the films were made, because of disappointment with the lack of prominent placement achieved. A file note, written on February 8, 1984, by J. M. Coleman, manager of media services, with a copy to T. P. McAlevey, media director, indicates that B&W discussed settlement with Stallone for $110,000, although it is not clear whether such a settlement was made or whether Stallone actually smoked B&W brands in any of the planned films {2400.07}.

Some motion picture producers were actively soliciting product placement in their films as a way to increase the overall profitability of the project. For example, Alta Marea Productions, a motion picture production company, sent promotional material to B&W soliciting product placement for its planned movie *Supergirl,* specifically mentioning the effectiveness of placements that had appeared in *Superman II.* The material, which is undated but refers to the release of *Superman III* "this June" (1983), states:

> *Audiences everywhere will recall watching the titanic battle over Metropolis between Superman and the Arch Villains, which occurred in front of gigantic Coca Cola and Cutty Sark signs, and will be able to tell you that a truck bearing a prominent Marlboro logo played an important role in the sequence.* The advertising opportunities on the Midvale Street [in *Supergirl*] will be equally as memorable.

> In addition to the outdoor billboard advertisements, exposure can be provided on storefronts, bus shelters, neon signs and trade vehicles. We are also offering a variety of promotional and premium opportunities, and are developing plans for advertiser tie-in promotions, in conjunction with the United States Government programs on Drug and Alcohol Abuse and Highway Traffic Safety [emphasis added]. {2400.24, p. 2}

Although B&W did not respond to this solicitation, Liggett & Myers apparently did. Liggett's placement was one of many that were later highlighted in congressional hearings in 1989 on a bill (H.R. 1250) to, among other things, ban product placement of cigarettes. At the opening hearing, on July 25, before the Subcommittee on Transportation and Hazardous Materials of the Committee on Energy and Commerce of the House of Representatives, Thomas A. Luken (D-OH), a cosponsor of the bill, described the various methods by which "the merchants of addiction advertise and promote" cigarettes. One such method, he noted, was to

> [spread] their message in ways that do not appear even to be advertisements, such as paying to have cigarettes in the movies. The subcommittee's investigation in recent months has revealed, for example, Philip Morris paid $42,500 in 1979 to have Marlboro cigarettes appear in the movie "Superman II" and paid $350,000 last year to have the Lark cigarette appear in the new James Bond movie, "License to Kill." Liggett told the subcommittee that in 1983 it paid $30,000 to have Eve cigarettes appear in the film "Supergirl", and American Tobacco told us that in 1984 it supplied more than $5,000 and other props to have Lucky Strike appear in the movie "Beverly Hills Cop." Philip Morris told us in 1987 and 1988 it supplied free cigarettes and other props for 56 different films. {2406.01, p. 2}

The tobacco industry realized that one of the benefits of placing tobacco products in films was that people would also be exposed to the product if they saw the movie on video or on television. As a letter from Kovoloff to Ted Parrack, vice president for brand management at B&W, dated August 4, 1981, makes clear, the placement of tobacco products in films was treated as a mechanism for getting around the broadcast ban on tobacco advertising:

> Pursuant to our telephone conversation this morning, I believe that it would be most beneficial for the Barclay Brand to take advantage of the placement of two Barclay Billboards in the soon to be produced, Columbia Feature, The Tempest.
>
> The Tempest, produced and directed by Paul Mazursky, will star Mr. John Cassavetes, Ms. Gina [sic] Rowlands, Ms. Susan Sarandon and Mr. Victorrio [sic] Gassman. The two principal characters, Mr. John Cassavetes and Ms. Gina Rowland [sic], will both use Barclays [sic] cigarettes in such a way that the packages will be readily identified by movie-goers, *as well as future cable television, video cassette, video disc, and network viewers.*
>
> The total investment to Brown & Williamson for the above service is seventy-thousand dollars ($70,000.00), payable upon the commencement of production of The Tempest [emphasis added]. {2400.16}

This proposal generated an enthusiastic response from B&W. The letter {2400.16} includes a handwritten note from someone stating, "Tom: follow up immediately I would do." "Tom" was probably Thomas Neville, B&W's director of marketing services. On August 13, 1981, Neville wrote back to Kovoloff:

> Confirming our August 12 conversation, we will proceed with the Tempest project. As you requested we will forward four 30-sheet billboards to your office. Additionally, I am enclosing two BARCLAY lighters which might be appropriately used in the movie.
>
> Also we are getting together a list of new materials for the various brands and this will be forwarded to you as soon as possible. We are looking into creating a new KOOL T-shirt that can bee [sic] worn by appropriate people. {2400.17}

Despite Kovoloff's representations, Brown and Williamson was not pleased with the results of the *Tempest* project. On March 22, 1982, Neville wrote Kovoloff:

> Thank you for your recent letter explaining what we will receive for our $70,000 dollar commitment to your company. However, I am still at a loss as to what happened in 1981. I was under the impression that we would also get some placement in the film, The Tempest. While I now understand that the placement was not as originally presented, there was something for BARCLAY or was there?? The attached letter also indicates that two BARCLAY lighters were to be used. If so, can you let me know how? {2400.19, p. 1}

In 1983 B&W conducted an audit of its relationship with AFP, and a report on the results of the audit was transmitted from D.R. Scott to Domantay on October 26, 1983 {2400.23}. The audit was requested by Domantay and Coleman. Its principal objectives were stated to be:

> (1) review of current and past contractual agreements, (2) review of Company internal control systems, and (3) review of performance of AFP. {2400.23, p. 1}

In his October 26, 1983, memorandum accompanying the audit report, Scott raised serious questions about the sufficiency of B&W's procedures for documenting the product placements specified in its contract with AFP.

> Based on the audit findings and recommendations, I have concluded that the Company's internal controls and procedures for documenting intended movie placements and performance have not been and are not currently adequate. {2400.01, p. 1}

Perhaps more troubling to B&W, however, was the fact, as noted in the audit report, that AFP had a practice of keeping two sets of books and of distributing payments in the form of cash, jewelry, or cars, rather than in the form of checks.

> During a field visit we were informed by AFP personnel that AFP keeps two sets of books for its movie placement activities. One set of books is for their daily operations (commissions earned and ordinary business expenses) and the "second set of books" is for all their special movie placements (e.g., the Sylvester Stallone movies).
>
> Mr. Robert Kovoloff, President of AFP, and Mr. James Ripslinger, Senior Vice-President, are primarily in charge of operations. They told us the following concerning the monies involved with the special placements:
>
> (1) They are the only two individuals at AFP who know that a "second set of books" exists.
>
> (2) AFP does not profit from the special placements. They act only as "middlemen" between B&W and the movie studios.
>
> (3) AFP distributes payments based upon the instructions of the movie producer.
>
> (4) The producers normally do not want payments in the form of checks to individuals. They prefer cash, jewelry, cars, etc.
>
> It should be noted that this "second set of books" appeared to have been prepared solely for the auditor's visit. {2400.23, p. 3}

According to the audit report, the practice of keeping two sets of books violated the provision in the contract between the parties requiring AFP to maintain proper accounting procedures {2400.23, pp. 3, 4}. As is indicated in an audit of the AFP payments to actors, producers, and other people associated with the films where B&W products were placed (see table 9.5, p. 388), B&W's auditors did not question the use of noncash payments. (After release of the documents, the *Los Angeles Times* found that many of these goods never reached the stars; Kovoloff told the *Times* that Sean Connery never got any jewelry, and that Paul Newman, Sylvester Stallone, and Clint Eastwood never got cars [7].)

As part of the audit, B&W did a detailed analysis of several of the films, similar to Hazan, Lipton, and Glantz's research on smoking in the movies (8), except that it was much more detailed and focused on looking for specific brand imagery. The B&W auditors were not pleased with what they found:

> No procedures have been in place at B&W to ensure that AFP actually has been placing our products in movies. Because of this, we viewed seven movies in which AFP has indicated that they have made placements for B&W (two of which involved special payments). Our observations are as follows:

Body Heat—We observed a Kool poster on a wall in a restaurant. It appeared three times in the movie. The first time it was on screen for approximately a minute, but was blurred except for a couple of seconds. The other two times the sign was blurred. We also observed the two lead characters in the movie smoking Marlboro throughout the movie.

First Blood—We observed a Kool lights billboard on screen for a couple of seconds. We saw a glimpse of a Raleigh billboard and a Barclay poster.

Jinxed—The top half of a Barclay pack appeared on screen momentarily.

Only When I Laugh—We observed a blurred pack of Kool on the front of a vending machine. The lead character of the show bought a pack of Marlboro from the machine. She smoked Marlboro throughout the movie.

Nine to Five—We observed no B&W products or advertising in this movie. We did see a cigarette vending machine in the movie.

Never Say Never Again ($20,000 special payment)—We observed what appeared to be a pack of Kool Super Lights on screen for one or two seconds. The word Kool could not be seen. A pack of Winston appeared briefly in this film.

Tempest ($70,000 special payment. The Company also was to receive a bonus placement in Traces. We were unable to obtain a copy of Traces.)—We observed what appeared to be a pack of Barclay on screen for a second. The word Barclay could not be seen. Mr. E. T. Parrack (Vice President of Brand Management when the Tempest was released) stated that Mr. Kovoloff called shortly after Tempest was released and told us that B&W did not receive much exposure and he promised to provide placement in two or three other movies as a "make good". Records currently available at B&W do not indicate which movies were to be utilized.

With the exception of the Sylvester Stallone movies, there is virtually nothing in writing at B&W which indicates what specifically B&W is to receive. The agreement involving the Sylvester Stallone movies only specifies that he will be smoking our products in four of the five movies and that B&W signage will be included. The agreement does not specify the length of time or frequency of [sic] which our products will appear nor does it assure that the visual clarity of the product logo will be acceptable to B&W. {2400.23, pp. 5–6}

Despite these concerns, as late as November 8, 1983, Tom Humber, B&W's assistant director of corporate affairs, wrote to J. M. Coleman, manager of media services, and recommended continuing the product placement program:

Confirming our conversation of yesterday, I support the continuation of product placement in movies made for theatrical release, provided that correct business practices are followed, there is a concerted effort to restrict the program to adult-interest films and characters, we have greater knowledge than I believe currently exists about context, and each project is commercially sound. {2402.06}

In any event, disappointment with AFP's performance and growing political pressure—fueled in part by the *Snow White* controversy—led Ernest Pepples, B&W's senior vice president and general counsel, to recommend getting out of product placement. He explains his reasons in detail in a "Restricted and Privileged" memorandum to Coleman on November 8, 1983:

> Brown & Williamson should discontinue the [AFP] program in an orderly way.
> Of the four points listed under RATIONALE [in a draft statement of issues on the AFT matter], I agree only with the statement that "control weakness can be corrected". In my opinion:
>
> 1.   The embarrassment to BWT [B&W Tobacco] will be considerable and will be cumulative; it will exacerbate the bad publicity on the VICEROY memorandum [a reference to a memorandum not in the documents available to us] and other more recent troubles with SNOW WHITE AND THE SEVEN DWARFS and FTC generally.
>
> 2.   Competitors will be likely to disengage from this area, not increase their *abuse* of it. And even if I am wrong, *the use of any cigarette by a movie hero advertises <u>all</u> cigarettes.* So let the competitors help advertise our brands in this way.
>
> 3.   This is a mirage. B&W gets no brand advantage in having its cigarettes stuck under a hospital mattress in a James Bond movie. The use of MARLBORO in the SUPERMAN II movie was disparagement not approval. The only thing one could say in favor of such advertising is the old Huey Long idea, I don't care what you say about me as long as you spell my name right.
>
> Accordingly, it is foolish for Brown & Williamson to continue this program both *for business and political reasons* [italic emphasis added]. {2400.02}

In addition to analyzing the value of its own product placement in movies, B&W was acutely aware of the placement of its competitors' products in films, and evidently believed that they, too, were not effectively served. For example, in a memo to N. V. Domantay, dated December 5, 1983, on the subject "Apocalypse Now—Marlboro," Coleman concludes:

1.   Martin Sheen smokes Marlboro throughout the movie.

2.   The pack is prominent at the beginning of reel #1 and #2. These shots focus on the pack for extended periods of time, particularly at the beginning of reel #2.

3.   However, the only real identification is the "red roof"—the Marlboro logo is not seen.

4.   We have heard unconfirmed estimates that PM paid $200M for the product placement in this movie.

The exposure Marlboro received from this movie is worth something but not $200M—if I had to assign a value it would be approximately $100M. This placement is not worth $200M because the actual logo is not seen, and because of the setting, they were not able to use any other product identification (i.e. billboard, cab top). This movie is a "Marlboro commercial" only to people in our industry because we know the pack and the cigarette brand even when the pack is not shown—but to an ordinary person, the pack/cigarette shots are not that intrusive. {2400.13}

Of course, Philip Morris may have had a different opinion about the value of Marlboro's appearance in this film.

On January 11, 1984, B&W met with AFP to work out termination of their agreement. The meeting is summarized in a memorandum of February 2, 1984, from Coleman to Domantay:

1.   Present at the meeting from AFP were R. Kovoloff and J. Ripslinger.

2.   AFP was told that the product placement relationship was being terminated because of a corporate policy decision.

3.   The following issues were also discussed:

a.   AFP has discussed the <u>Tempest</u> and <u>Never Say Never Again</u> with the respective producers and reached agreement on make-goods. They were told that this would violate the new corporate policy so we could not accept the offer.

b.   They will negotiate with Stallone or try to sell to someone else. Failing this, we will owe Stallone an additional $200M per agreement.

c.   As of the date of the meeting BWT products were not to be placed in any films including those we already paid for if they can be edited out.

d.   They requested payment for the invoices we have in hand, $30M and $9.7M, and a release from the two-year restriction on doing business with other tobacco companies. We agreed since the $30M is consistent with 60-day cancellation, while the $9.7M is for administration of Plitt cinema ads. [This is a reference to services AFP provided with respect to a contract between B&W and Plitt Theatres, Inc., for the running of commercial messages in theatres that Plitt operated. See {2400.23, p. 1}.]

e.   The $300M AFP received during 1983 for administering the Plitt contract was discussed. AFP's position is that the $100M ($300M less $200M payment to Plitt associate) is necessary because they will only receive $9.7M per quarter in 1984 which was initially agreed to when they were also receiving placement monies.

      . . .

4.   They were told that official written notification would be mailed at the end of the week. {2400.14, pp. 1–2}

During the period of the contract between AFP and B&W, AFP claims to have attempted to place Brown and Williamson brands in more than

150 movies or television shows and succeeded in making placements in 22 movies and one television show (table 9.6, p. 390) {2400.23, p. 10}. Significantly, product placement in the television show *The A-Team,* a program with a strong youth appeal, was paid for by the B&W advertising budget. The payment for product placement on a television show did not appear to raise any questions with those involved in the process, despite the federal law against advertising tobacco products on television. The auditors, and indeed everyone in the process, treated it in a very matter-of-fact manner.

Whatever Brown and Williamson's professed policies on advertising may have been, any advertising in theaters, particularly when an ad appears in conjunction with a movie aimed at a young audience, would reach children and teenagers. Yet, B&W stopped the theater advertising only when a public relations gaffe made its continuation too embarrassing. Similarly, product placements in the movies and on television were discontinued only when the company determined that it was not receiving sufficient value for the money being spent. There is nothing in the documents to indicate that the company was having second thoughts about the propriety of the practice.

USING MODERN MARKETING TECHNIQUES TO SELL CIGARETTES

As the public became increasingly concerned about the health dangers of smoking, the marketing of cigarettes became increasingly difficult. Thus, in addition to using the more traditional marketing methods, such as emphasizing the taste of the product and targeting various population segments, the industry attempted to develop more sophisticated marketing techniques, based on knowledge of smoking behavior; this new approach to marketing was the subject of a Smoking Behaviour–Marketing Conference held in Montreal, Quebec, from July 9 through July 12, 1984. The conference was attended by delegates from Imperial Tobacco Limited (ITL), the Canadian subsidiary of BAT, who worked in marketing or research in five countries (United States, United Kingdom, Australia, Germany, and Canada). The conference proceedings demonstrate that the tobacco companies took research about marketing at least as seriously as research about the health effects of their product.

Evidently, the purpose of the Montreal conference was to increase interaction between the marketing and research personnel at B&W and BAT, in order to devise methods of selling tobacco products in an increasingly unfavorable environment. In his opening remarks for the conference, P. J. Dunn, vice president of research and development at ITL, notes the importance of having a clearer understanding of smoking behavior:

> One way of defining smoking behaviour has been the fundamental understanding of the complete smoking process, but I feel that this definition should be enhanced to include the complete smoker process. In other words we must understand all elements which make up our customer, his wants and needs, translate these, using product, pack imagery, advertising, into some specific brand direction which inevitably will meet those needs. The basic question that begs a response is how do we provide smoker satisfaction from a lower tar base with specifically enhanced acceptability traits, and *at the same time help our consumer rationalize his decision to smoke in light of increasing external pressures.*
>
> . . . [T]he means by which this goal may be better accomplished would be if marketing and consumer research and product development techniques and methodologies are exchanged freely [emphasis added]. {1224.01, p. BW-W2-03186}

Dunn then outlines the purposes of the conference sessions:

1.   Provide a current focus and background on the existing MKTG/R&D interaction;

2.   Communicate the existing techniques and methodologies and how they are applied, looking at not only laboratory methodologies, but also case studies of identified marketing needs and R&D responses;

3.   *To look at current research and future implications as they relate to compensation, sidestream, the role of nicotine, and the role that smoking behaviour in its broadest definition has overlapped with product development and finally to look at future social pressures* specifically relating to smoking and health, biological indicators and other such topics;

4.   The last session, and probably the most critical, will look at future direction and how we as a group see our priorities and activities proceeding in order to maximize the synergy of the group [emphasis added]. {1224.01, p. BW-W2-03187}.

Topics covered at the conference included (1) discussion of a consumer survey; (2) an overview of research on human smoking behavior; (3) ITL's approach to marketing and new product development, segmentation, and models to explain brand-switching behavior; (4) marketing research methods; (5) the response of research and development to marketing needs; (6) a review of and update on the role of nicotine; and (7) social pressures, including consumer awareness of smoking and health issues. (The overview of nicotine presented is discussed in chapter 3.)

Wayne Knox, marketing director of ITL Canada, described ITL's sophisticated market assessment methodology to identify key consumer

trends on a monthly basis. After analyzing these trends, ITL developed
a "switching model" of marketing:

> Smokers don't buy products[,] they buy brands. We sell a Marketing Mix—
> Product, Package, Ads, etc. {1224.01, p. BW-W2-03245}

In other words, the product itself is only one element that contributes to
the consumer's decision to buy a particular cigarette.

The first area of discussion focused on knowledge of the consumer's
smoking behavior—specifically, his or her brand-switching behavior.
The delegates agreed that the companies needed to investigate the roles
of product, pack, imagery, and advertising in brand switching. These discussions of consumer smoking behavior clearly show that the tobacco
companies were interested in getting people to start smoking as well as
to switch brands. The tobacco companies have continued to deny that
their advertising induces people to start smoking. Nevertheless, the conference report states:

> Since our future business depends on the size of this starter population set, it
> was considered important that we know why people start to smoke and this
> may be more important than why they continue to smoke [emphasis added].
> {1224.01, p. BW-W2-03197}

Participants at the conference also discussed the significance of smoke
components, including nicotine, in relation to development and marketing of a low-retention cigarette; market segmentation; target markets; third-
party endorsements; and communication of the attributes of the product.

CONCLUSION

The sophisticated marketing, political, and public relations strategies
continued to protect B&W and the tobacco industry's interests very well
through the 1980s. Advertising and promotional techniques grew in so-
phistication, as did the industry's efforts to influence editorial decisions
and key community organizations to support the industry's position—
or at least keep the smoking and health "controversy" open. As with the
efforts surrounding scientific research, the effort was closely monitored
by lawyers, with constant attention to avoiding any statement that could
be construed as admitting that smoking causes any disease whatsoever.
At the same time, the companies were to insist that an open-minded debate on smoking and health should take place. These techniques, which
have served the tobacco industry so well, are now being applied to contest the evidence that passive, as well as active, smoking is dangerous.

TABLE 9.1 SOME ORIGINAL TEXT AND LAWYER'S
EDITORIAL COMMENTS ON THE BLACKMAN PAPER

Item	Original Text {1833.02}[1]	Lawyer's Comment {1833.01}
2	Despite a great deal of research there are no clear answers as to why people smoke. Some reasons which have been suggested are: Donald Gould in the 'New Scientist' (4.3.1976): "Cigarettes calm, they comfort, they give pleasure, they act as a kind of stockade, a visible barrier between the naked individual and a hostile and perplexing world."	Delete Donald Gould reference. The article identifies cigarettes as a drug.
3	Dr. W. S. Cain of the Yale University School of Medicine (1979 Cold Spring Harbour Conference): "Full flavour serves as a sign of effects soon to follow—such as a sense of • Relaxation • Reduced Anxiety • Power to Concentrate • Self Confidence • Social Facilitation or any of the many other positive features that smokers attribute to smoking." "Without the benefits of such features, most smokers would never establish the habit in the first place."	Delete reference to Dr. W. S. Cain. The article identifies short term and longer term pharmacological and physiological factors as important in the derivation of "habitual cigarette smoking."
4	Atsuko Chiba in the New York 'Tribune' (25.4.1983): "The prevalence of smoking in Japan, 70.1% of men and 16.2% of women, is a result of the tensions in the country, social psychologists said. Men in particular, locked in fierce competition to succeed, smoke and drink heavily as a release from stress."	Suggest reconsideration of the Chiba reference. . . . it is risky to rely on newspaper accounts for scientific information. The scientific article may equate the effects of smoking with those of heavy drinking.
5	Whatever the reason, smoking is a very stable practice: Ruth Roemer, a lawyer from the School of Public Health in Los Angeles, reviewed the legislation against smoking for the World Health Organisation. As stated in an editorial article in 'The Lancet' (24.7.1982): "A frustrating part of her review is the lack of evidence that particular laws—on advertising, selling to young people, or smoking in public or at work, for example—have had much impact."	Delete. The point made here might be said to run counter to arguments that cigarette smoking is not addictive. Thirty million people in the U.S. have quit smoking voluntarily. Cigarette excises [taxes] have dramatic impacts on consumption. Also, BAT should avoid uncritical reference to the work of Roemer, who is dedicated to anti-smoking views.

TABLE 9.1 *(continued)*

Item	Original Text {1833.02}[1]	Lawyer's Comment {1833.01}
6	From R. Doll and R. Peto—British Medical Journal (25.12.76) . . . 2. The computed annual mortality rate for heart disease in nonsmokers is some 5 times that for lung cancer in smokers. <The study and its application have been criticised and the BAT does not endorse it but discusses it here as background.>	Suggest reconsideration of the point that the annual mortality rate for heart disease in nonsmokers is greater than for lung cancer in smokers. The purpose of this statement is unclear and it emphasizes the large number of deaths due to heart disease attributed to smoking.
8	Though Professor Doll and Mr. Peto maintain that smoking is a direct cause of certain illnesses, they acknowledged in their publication that statistical association does not imply causation. Thus, apropos the published table of diseases, they stated: "To say that these conditions were related to smoking does not necessarily imply that smoking caused (or prevented) them." "The relation may have been secondary in that smoking was associated with some other factor, such as alcohol consumption or a feature of the personality, that caused the disease."	Delete Doll and Peto reference. Doll and Peto have published a table which shows "cancer of the lung" is "caused by cigarette smoking" and have concluded that "much of the excess mortality in cigarette smoking can be attributed with certainty to the habit . . ."
9	This scientific fact was supported in the July 1983 issue of the consumer magazine 'WHICH?' in an article concerned with cancer—where the following cautionary statement was made regarding epidemiology: "This kind of research does not prove that particular features of lifestyle cause cancers, but can point to possible causes. Even when these appear to be plausible in the light of what is known about how the body works, and how cancers form, further research is needed."	Delete reference to the consumer magazine. The quoted statement was made in connection with diet. The article advocates, as the first example of "the kind of thing they believe will prove to make a difference are: stopping smoking. Tobacco is a factor in about one-third of all cancers."
10	<Similarly,> Mr. R. Peto when speaking at a conference on nitrosamines and human cancer (Banbury Report No 12, 1982) <said>: " . . . this idea that you can analyse the chemistry of tobacco smoke and marijuana and predict what their human effects are going to be is completely inappropriate."	Delete reference to Peto. In the next sentence in the cited Report, Peto mentions "the carcinogenic components of tobacco smoke. . . ." Peto is convinced that the causal hypothesis is proven and, therefore, his opinions are at odds with the position of the "Controversy" section of the Draft, which is that the causal hypothesis is not proven.

TABLE 9.1 *(continued)*

Item	Original Text {1833.02}[1]	Lawyer's Comment {1833.01}
12	The following comment was made apropos lung cancer: "The maps for lung cancer indicate that excessive mortality is not limited to highly populated urban areas where cigarette smoking and air pollution are most prominent. In fact, the rates are highest along the coast of the Gulf of Mexico, particularly in Louisiana." "Further studies are needed to identify the environmental and demographic factors contributing to the increased risk of lung cancer in these predominantly rural and port areas."	Without explanation, the quotation from the cancer atlases does not stand as an anomaly. The quotation is consistent with lung cancer causation by cigarette smoking and other exposures.
14	The Epidemiological Research Unit of the Medical Research Council published in late 1983 a detailed analysis on "Trend in Cancer ~~Statistics~~ <Mortality>" in England and Wales for women and men aged 25–69 years, who were born between 1880–1950 and died between 1951–1980. For both women and men, the risk factor for a given "cohort", relative to the average for the whole period covered, varied strongly and systematically, building up to peaks in the early decades of this century and then declining. The interpretation of cohort data is complex, but it may be noted, in relation to cigarette smoking, that the 1951 cohort of women, most of whom are still alive, have already smoked about twice as many cigarettes as the 1880 cohort smoked in their entire lifetime—yet both groups have similar risk factors. For men, also, there is no direct correlation of the rise and fall of the risk factor with cigarette consumption (G. F. Todd et al, 'TRC Occasional Paper 3', 1976).	The material should be rewritten. The current version fails to distinguish between the 1983 and 1976 articles [referring to the 1983 article by the Epidemiological Research Unit of the Medical Research Council analysing the "Trend in Cancer Mortality" in England and Wales for specified groups of people, and a 1976 TRC Occasional Paper, by G. F. Todd et al., also evidently analysing cohort data], which is a problem because the 1983 article concludes that the cohort data is consistent with the causal hypothesis [that smoking causes cancer] and states that "even among young people, who have been smoking safer cigarettes, lung cancer remains a major problem."
18	More recently, Professor G. Cumming, Medical Director of the Midhurst Research Institute and a noted lung research specialist, stated on BBC Radio 4 on 12.1.1983: "What's interesting about cigarette-related diseases is that the majority of people who smoke cigarettes don't suffer ill-effects."	Suggest delete reference to Professor Cumming. In the broadcast, Cumming indicated he believed that a substantial group (perhaps 30% of smokers) "are at risk from smoking."

TABLE 9.1 *(continued)*

Item	Original Text {1833.02}[1]	Lawyer's Comment {1833.01}
	" . . . particularly some American work has shown that in cancer of the lung in smokers, this is related to another environmental cause, and the environmental cause that they have identified is the level of Vitamin A in the blood of the smoker." " . . . if the Vitamin A level is high then they don't get cancer. Their risk is the same as if they were non-smokers."	
21	Friberg and co-workers reported in 1973 ('Archives of Environmental Health', vol 27) an 11-year monitoring from 1961 to 1972 of 572 Swedish twins (both sexes). The results were: . . . Six years later in 1979 the work was reviewed in the 'Bibliography on Smoking and Health': "The findings seem to be yet another indication of the incomparability of smokers and non-smokers. The results from the twin study clearly demonstrate the importance of genetic, behavioural and psychosocial factors which have not been considered in conventional epidemiological studies. Such factors should as far as possible be included in future epidemiological research, not only in the context of smoking and health, but also in studies on other similar exposure factors that may be linked to risk factors of this type or to genetic predispositions."	Recommend delete references to Friberg and the Bibliography on Smoking and Health. Unfortunately, Friberg, Cederlof and Lundman published a monograph in 1977 which stated that "lung cancer is closely related to the amount smoked . . . ," that associations were confirmed between smoking and respiratory, cardiovascular and other symptoms of disease or ill health, that there is no doubt about a causal link between smoking and lung cancer, and that the results from the Swedish monozygotic twin studies are contrary to the constitutional hypothesis advanced by [Sir Ronald] Fisher.
26	This disease [chronic obstructive lung disease], often loosely termed 'bronchitis' <and emphysema>, is frequently cited as being causally related to smoking. It is of significance, therefore, to note the striking social class dependence for England and Wales in 1961 when, according to the 4th Report of the Royal College of Physicians, "smoking habits were fairly similar in all social classes."	Consider deleting the section dealing with COLD [chronic obstructive lung disease]. The title of the section focuses on lung cancer. The same paragraph in the fourth Report which presents the table reprinted in the Draft states "it must be emphasized that at present only the effects of tobacco are reliably known to be of substantial importance."
27	A similar result was found in earlier international comparisons of the effect of diet and smoking intervention on the incidence of coronary heart disease. As reported in "Circulation", (Volume 1, Supplement 1, 1970):	Suggest deletion of reference to work by Keys and the secondary article from the *Lancet*. In March, 1984, Keys and others published a

TABLE 9.1 *(continued)*

Item	Original Text {1833.02}[1]	Lawyer's Comment {1833.01}

"In an international cooperative study on the epidemiology of coronary heart disease, international teams examined 12,770 men aged 40 through 59 years in Finland, Greece, Italy, Japan, the Netherlands, the United States, and Yugoslavia. Strictly standardized methods and criteria were used. <Note: this is paraphrase but not a quote.> Cigarette smoking was one of the risk factors studied and it is concluded that smoking cannot be involved in the incidence and deaths from this disease."

As further reported in The Lancet (12.12.1981):

"In the seven-country study there was no significant association between coronary heart disease incidence and smoking in the different countries, and in the prospective necropsy series of the Oslo study a significant correlation between prevalence of coronary raised atherosclerotic lesions and smoking could not be shown."

study which concluded that "For coronary death, age, serum cholesterol, blood pressure, and smoking were highly significant in all regions except Japan, where coronary deaths were too few for evaluation." Keys, et al., *The Seven Countries Study: 2289 Deaths in 15 Years,* Preventive Medicine (1984), p. 141. In 1983, the Tobacco Institute published a letter which cited Keys in support of the position that cigarette smoking is not a cause of cardiovascular disease. Keys responded with a vitriolic letter complaining of "an unending stream of misrepresentations and distortions from the Tobacco Institute and the cigarette companies that attempt to persuade the public to disregard the overwhelming evidence that cigarette smoking is a major health hazard and cause of premature death."

28   ~~The largest~~ <A large> medical study ~~ever mounted~~ was completed and reported in the 'Journal of the Medical Association'. The editorial comment in 'Health Services' (15.10.1982) stated:

"A massive, $110m trial of prevention of coronary heart disease (CHD) in the United States has given disappointingly inconclusive results."

"Nearly 13,000 men at high risk of CHD were selected from 360,000 men aged between 35 and 57 who underwent health screening."

"The 13,000 men were divided into two groups. One, the 'intervention' group, was given counseling to help them stop smoking, a diet with only 10 per cent of the food intake as saturated fats, and drug treatment for raised blood pressure."

"Seven years later 265 of the men in the 'intervention' group had died, 138 of heart disease, and 260 of the control group had died, 145 of heart disease."

Reconsider. We do not have the source for the quote pertaining to the MRFIT study. At least one well-known scientist in the U.S. has studied the MRFIT data and stated his conclusion that the study failed to prove smoking was a major factor in coronary heart disease. However, comments in health related publications generally have repeated the claims by HHS that the [MRFIT] study showed smoking reduction caused a decrease in CHD incidence.

TABLE 9.1   *(continued)*

Item	Original Text {1833.02}[1]	Lawyer's Comment {1833.01}
29	Hypertension and heart disease are frequently cited as being causally related to smoking. It is interesting to note, therefore, that the time trends for hypertension in the UK closely parallel those for the US and Australia— whereas, as shown ~~above~~ <opposite>, the same does not obtain for heart disease.	Delete the material presented pertaining to hypertension. Smoking is, but hypertension is _not_, frequently cited as being causally related to heart disease.
30	In a review in the journal 'New Scientist' (23.2.1984), reference was made to the findings of Professor J. Morris of the Medical Research Council unit at the London School of Hygiene and Tropical Health: " 'Vigorously' exercising men suffered fewer heart attacks whether they were fat or lean, cigarette smokers or not, suffering from high blood pressure or not, and with or without a family history of the disease."	Suggest reconsider. . . . Is the material gratuitous? The statement [that "'vigorously' exercising men suffered fewer heart attacks whether they were fat or lean, cigarette smokers or not, and with or without a family history of disease"] is not necessarily inconsistent with smoking as a major risk factor. Our adversaries will insist that we be as careful in making any statements about health (such as the benefits, if any, of exercise) as we are about deciding whether it has been proven that cigarette smoking causes disease.
33	In 1983, the 3rd Report of the Independent Scientific Committee stated: "Carbon monoxide is suspected of having a role in their [heart disease] development but it is not clearly established that it is a factor in their causation."	Revise. The Committee also stated as a conclusion that "there are significant health grounds to require substantial reductions in carbon monoxide yields of cigarettes."
35	Many independent doctors, scientists and government/health authorities believe that the use of filters and other changes in the product have been directly responsible for the significant reduction in recent years in smoking-associated diseases (especially lung cancer) in younger age groups, in countries such as the UK, US and Finland. Certainly ~~the pioneer of smoking and health research~~ Professor R. Doll strongly believes that this is the case. At a recent Royal College of Physicians conference in Edinburgh (3.12.82), he stated regarding the drop of about 50% in lung cancer among men under 50 years of age:	Revise. The Draft can present the scientific exposition of low delivery/low risk only within a framework of an accurate description of the current status of scientific and government positions. The BAT draft mentions government and health authorities only in connection with the belief that lower delivery has been responsible for a reduction in smoking-associated disease. However, the 1983 U.S. Surgeon General's Report stated the following conclusions:

TABLE 9.1 *(continued)*

Item	Original Text {1833.02}[1]	Lawyer's Comment {1833.01}
	"This reduction can be attributed to people giving up smoking altogether, but probably even more to changing to low-tar cigarettes which, without doubt, produce less harmful effects."	Epidemiological evidence concerning reduced tar and nicotine or filter cigarettes and their effect on CHD rates is conflicting. No scientific evidence is available concerning the impact on CHD death rates of cigarettes with very low levels of tar and nicotine. Doll's conclusion that smoking causes lung cancer should be stated as well as his opinion about low delivery cigarettes. Doll's opinion about low delivery cigarettes is that they reduce the smoker's risk of lung cancer but do not reduce, and may increase, the risk of mortality from CHD. Parenthetically, any reference to Doll must be crafted carefully because he is a dedicated advocate of the causal hypothesis. . . . If the BAT article cites uncritically Doll's position on low delivery cigarettes, we must be prepared to explain why we reject his treatment of delivery levels and cohort analysis.
36	Apropos such views, an interesting comment was made by Mr. R. Peto at a Ciba Foundation meeting on preventative medicine held in London (as reported in the 'New Scientist', 19.4.1984): "Even the World Health Organisation won't advocate lowering the tar content of cigarettes. They don't want to believe that lower tar means lower death rates from lung cancer." Thus, as in virtually all areas of smoking and health, there is continuing controversy.	Revise or delete. The same article [in the *New Scientist*, April 19, 1984, regarding a comment made by Mr. R. Peto at Ciba Foundation meeting on preventive medicine in London] presents Peto's position that low-tar cigarettes could increase mortality due to heart disease and COLD [chronic obstructive lung disease]. If the Peto reference is retained, these views also should be stated in the BAT article as well as Peto's endorsement of the causal hypothesis. Why invite the reaction of an adversary when it is not necessary to an exposition of our position?

TABLE 9.1   *(continued)*

Item	Original Text {1833.02}[1]	Lawyer's Comment {1833.01}
37	AMBIENT SMOKE AND "PASSIVE SMOKING" There is a large literature on both ambient smoke and 'passive smoking'. Until recently there was little suggestion that there might be a health risk in non-smokers breathing other people's smoke. Thus: 1978. Draft Status Report of the US National Cancer Institute: "The risk of cancer of the respiratory tract, emphysema, or cardiovascular disease does not appear to be increased by passively inhaling smoke generated by others." 1979 US Surgeon General's Report "Healthy non-smokers exposed to cigarette smoke have little or no physiological response to the smoke, and what response does occur may be due to psychological factors." 1979 Chairman of the American Heart Association Task Force on the Environment and Cardiovascular Disease "Studies indicate that non-smokers have negligible levels of carboxyhemoglobin under good conditions of ventilation, and with no ventilation have acceptably low levels." 1978 C. Hugod, K. Hawkins and P. Astrup <'International Archive of Occupational and Environmental Health, 42'> "It is pointed out that in spite of an often considerable subjective discomfort, exposing non-smokers to tobacco smoke under realistic conditions will not cause inhalation of such amounts of the components of tobacco smoke traditionally considered harmful, that a lasting, adverse health effect in otherwise healthy, grown up individuals seems probable."	Revise and reconsider. The purpose of the quotes with 1978 and 1979 dates is not clear. The authors made the statements <u>after</u> suggestions had been publicized that smoking caused disease in nonsmokers, not before such suggestions as implied by the introductory text. All four of the quotes are outdated and the U.S. NCI and Surgeon General have substantially changed their positions from these quotes.
38	—the Japanese as a race are very different from the Western world in terms of living environment and social cultures. —smoking ~~habits~~ <patterns of wives> were determined only at the beginning of the period —the majority of the cancers (17 out of 23 in a sample) were not of the type most commonly found in ~~lung cancer~~ <smokers> —the two-fold increased risk in wives of heavier smokers is similar to that found by Dr. Hirayama for women actively smoking about 5 cigarettes a day—whilst their heavy smoking husbands averaged only about 8 cigarettes a day at home.	The first listed "criticism" of the Hirayama article must be deleted. The statement that perhaps only Japanese nonsmokers get lung cancer from cigarette smoke is little comfort to the Japanese.

TABLE 9.1 *(continued)*

Item	Original Text {1833.02}[1]	Lawyer's Comment {1833.01}
40	~~Dr.~~ <Mr.> L. Garfinkel, <Munchener Medizinische Wochenschrift, 1981> "Passive smoking may be a political matter, but it is not a main issue in terms of health policy."	Delete. Dr. Garfinkle has published a letter in the *New York Times* (June 5, 1984) which protests R. J. Reynolds' use of the passage quoted in the Draft and states: It is irresponsible of Reynolds to attempt to create a false sense of security about the potential dangers of passive smoking, especially at a time when incriminating evidence continues to accumulate.

[1]Handwritten inserts by lawyer indicated in "< >" and deletions indicated as ~~strikeouts~~.

TABLE 9.2   TOBACCO INSTITUTE, 1987 BUDGET: CONTRIBUTIONS TO NATIONAL ORGANIZATIONS

	1986 Budget	1986 Estimated	1987 Budget
National headquarters			
American Legislative Exchange Council (ALEC)	$7,500	$10,000	$12,000
American Society Legislative Clerks & Secretaries (ASLC&S)	$1,500	$1,500	$1,500
Council of State Governments (CSG)			
CSG Annual Meeting	$4,000	$4,000	$4,000
Corp. Associates Program (national)	$2,500	$1,500	$1,500
Eastern Regional CSG	$2,000	—	$2,000
Southern Regional CSG	$2,000	$2,000	$2,000
Midwest Regional CSG	$2,000	$2,000	$2,000
Western Regional CSG	$2,000	$2,000	$2,000
CSG Committee Hearings	$2,000	$2,000	$2,000
National Assoc. of Attorneys General (NAAG)	$2,000	—	—
National Assoc. of Counties (NACO)	$3,000	$2,000	$2,000
National Assoc. of Latino Elected Officials (NALEO)	$1,000	$1,000	$1,000
National Assoc. of State Depts. of Agriculture (NASDA)	$500	$600	$500
Southern Assoc. of State Depts. of Agriculture (SASDA)	$300	$300	$300
National Black Caucus of State Legislators (NBCSL), prorated among national & state Black Caucuses in AL/CT/FL/GA/LA/MA/MD/ NY/SC/TX	$7,000	$6,000	$7,000
National Center for Initiative Review (NCIR)	$5,000	—	$5,000

TABLE 9.2   *(continued)*

	1986 Budget	1986 Estimated	1987 Budget
National Conference of State Legislatures (NCSL)			
Foundation for State Legislatures	$2,500	$2,500	$2,500
Annual Meeting	$5,000	$5,000	$5,000
NCSL—State/Federal Assembly	$2,000	$2,000	$2,000
NCSL—Assembly Legislature	$2,000	$2,000	$2,000
NCSL Committee Meetings	$1,000	$2,000	$2,000
Regional Governors' Assoc.			
Northeast Governors' Assoc.	$2,000	$2,000	$2,000
Midwestern Governors' Assoc.	$2,000	$2,000	$2,000
Southern Governors' Assoc.	$2,000	$2,000	$2,000
Western Governors' Assoc.	$2,000	$2,000	$2,000
NGA Annual Meeting	—	$2,500	$2,500
National League of Cities (NLC)	$1,500	$1,500	$1,500
National Legislative Services & Securities (NLSS)	$1,000	$1,000	$1,000
National Order of Women Legislators (NOWL)	$1,000	—	—
Public Affairs Council (PAC)	$500	$500	$500
State Governmental Affairs Council (SGAC)	$2,500	$2,500	$2,500
State Legislative Leaders Foundation (SLLF)	$10,000	$10,000	$10,000
US Conference of Mayors (USCM)	$1,500	$1,500	$1,500
Allies/Coalitions			
Amusement and Music Operators Assoc. (AMOA)	$4,000	$5,000	$5,000
National Assoc. of Convenience Stores (NACS)	$2,000	—	—
National Assoc. of Neighbors (NAN)	$2,000	$2,000	$2,000
National Licensed Beverage Assoc. (NLBA) (prorated among state chapters)	$4,000	$3,000	$3,000
Women Involved in Farm Economics (WIFE)	$1,500	$2,000	$2,000
State/local festivals in tobacco producing states	$2,000	$2,000	$2,000
Contingency (special events and meeting expenses)	$20,000	$15,000	$15,000
Totals	$118,300	$104,900	$114,800

SOURCE: Cost Center, State Activities Division, Headquarters No. 1401, Account 7520 {2229.01, pp. 9056–9057}.

TABLE 9.3 THEATRE CHAINS FOR "KOOL JAZZ" ADVERTISEMENT, 1984

Theaters	Screens	Yearly Attendance
United Artist	937	75,000,000
Gulf State Theatres	139	7,500,000
FLW Theatres	23	2,100,000
Universal Amusement	8	530,000
Theatres West	7	575,000
Cineplex Theatres	67	3,900,000
Kent Theatres	33	2,800,000
LAM Theatres	15	1,000,000
Davis Theatres	6	432,000
Martin Theatres	421	20,800,000
AMC Theatres	712	55,000,000
Georgia Theatres	100	5,600,000
Fairlane Litchfield	135	12,000,000
Santikos Theatres	65	5,000,000
Mann Theatres	275	27,000,000
General Cinema	1,054	100,000,000
Cobb Theatres	188	15,700,000
Total	4,185	334,937,000
Currently Screening	1,235	93,837,000

SOURCE: {2400.06}.

TABLE 9.4 AUDITOR REPORT ON B&W PAYMENTS TO ASSOCIATED FILM PROMOTION (AFP) FOR SPECIAL MOTION PICTURE PLACEMENTS

Date	Movie	Amount
8/81 & 3/82	Tempest[1]	$70,000
4/82	Shaker Run	5,000
4/82	Blue Skies Again	7,500
7/82	Smokey & Bandit III	10,000
8/82	Never Say Never Again	20,000
1/83	Harry & Son	100,000
3/83	Tank	25,000
3/83	Where the Boys Are	100,000
4/83	Killing Ground	50,000
6/83 & 8/83	Sylvester Stallone (5 movies)[2,3,4]	300,000
Total		$687,500

[1]B&W was to receive a bonus placement in Traces for this payment.
[2]Not yet released.
[3]B&W owes AFP an additional $200,000 for the Sylvester Stallone movies.
[4]It is our [B&W's auditors] understanding that the Marketing Department is pursuing the possibility of having AFP obtain life and disability insurance on Mr. Stallone in order to protect B&W's position in the matter. We [the auditors] support this as an additional control measure.

SOURCE: {2400.23, p. 2}.

TABLE 9.5   AFP PAYMENTS FOR B&W PRODUCT
PLACEMENTS, AS REPORTED IN B&W AUDIT, 1983

Movie	AFP Check Payable[1]	Amount	Description[2]
Never Say Never Again	Arta Diamond	$ 7,170	Jewelry for Sean Connery
	Robinsons	5,545	" " " "
	Fisher Corp.	2,782	Television for Production Mgr.
	Robert Kovoloff	4,000	Mr. Kovoloff stated that he would rather not say what this payment was for.
	Bally Aladdin Castle	1,248	Pac Man Machine for Property Master
	Total AFP Payments	$ 20,745	
	B&W Payment	$ 20,000	
Harry & Son	Pan Am. Air Travel	$ 50,000[3]	
	Henry Kaye	9,850	Jewelry for Property Master
	Auto Stiegler	42,307	Car for Paul Newman
	Edward & Sons	1,185	Jewelry—Mr. Kovoloff could not remember who this was for.
	Total AFP Payments	$103,342	
	B&W Payment	$100,000	
Tank	David Levy	$ 13,000	Payment to Assistant Producer
	Beverly Hills Camera Shop	1,132	Camera for Property Manager
	La Brea Dodge	5,535	Car for Crowd Drawing[4]
	Lorimar Production	5,000	Prize for Crowd Drawing[4]
	Total AFP Payments	$24,667	
	B&W Payment	$25,000	
Where the Boys Are	Henry Kaye Jewelers	$ 7,500	Watch for producer
	Coral Cadillac	31,063	Car for producer
	Martin Cadillac	16,762	Car for assistant producer
	Robert Kovoloff	6,000	Cash for production coordinator
	Joe Amega & Co.	25,000	Jewelry for producer
	Beverly Hills Camera	10,552	Camera for production coordinator
	Total AFP Payments	$ 96,877	
	B&W Payment	$100,000	
Killing Ground	Cash	$ 10,030	Cash for production coordinator
	Evans, Inc.	6,500	Jewelry for Producer
	Auto Stiegler	22,047	Car for Clint Eastwood
	Auto Diamond	4,452	Jewelry for Producer
	Phil Adams	5,988	Payment for Property Master
	Total AFP Payments	$49,017	
	B&W Payment	$50,000	

TABLE 9.5 *(continued)*

Movie	AFP Check Payable[1]	Amount	Description[2]
Sylvester Stallone Movies	Tom Saccio	$ 2,000	Payment to Property Master
	Falconer Jewelry	24,200	Jewelry for S. Stallone
	Cash	8,000	Cash for Producer
	Autistic Children's Foundation	25,000	Contribution
	Wenpe Jewelry	7,290	Watch for S. Stallone
	Sub-total	66,490	
	American Saddlebred	80,000[5]	
	Stallone Automobile	97,000[6]	
	Total AFP Payments	$243,490[7]	
	B&W Payments	$300,000	

[1] We [Brown and Williamson auditors] examined canceled checks for all items . . . of this exhibit with the exception of the AFP/Pan Am agreement ($50,000) and the AFP/Stallone American Saddlebred agreement ($80,000).

[2] Per conversations with Mr. Kovoloff and Mr. Ripslinger, we made <u>no attempt to verify</u> the accuracy of this information. Because of the nature of these payments, the actual distribution of these payments (money and/or merchandise) <u>could</u> have been different.

[3] Agreement between AFP and Pan Am where Pan Am will provide $50,000 worth of travel free to the production company of "Harry & Son" in return for AFP providing movie placement services for Pan Am. We examined a copy of the contract. (There is no check.)

[4] Prizes are offered to the public by the production company on location in order to draw people for a crowd scene.

[5] Sale of horse owned by Mr. Kovoloff to Mr. Stallone (no check involved). We examined a copy of the sales agreement.

[6] Mr. Kovoloff informed us that he has ordered a Stallone automobile for Mr. Stallone. No payment has been made yet.

[7] Mr. Stallone has yet to give payment instructions on the remainder of the money.

SOURCE: {2404.04, pp. 2–4}. Emphasis in original.

TABLE 9.6   FILMS AND TELEVISION PROGRAMS
WITH B&W PRODUCT PLACEMENTS,
AS REPORTED IN B&W AUDIT, 1983

Movies

1. Cheaper to Keep Her	12. Making Love
2. Honky Tonk Freeway	13. Sharkey's Machine
3. Nine to Five	14. The Entity
4. Wacko	15. Jinxed
5. Night People (All Night Long)	16. First Blood
6. Body Heat	17. Love Child
7. Body & Soul	18. Blue Skies Again
8. All the Marbles	19. Star Chamber
9. Kill & Kill Again	20. Private School
10. Two for the Price of One	21. Summertime
11. Only When I Laugh	22. Savannah Smiles

Television Show

The A-Team

SOURCE: {2400.23, p. 10}.

REFERENCES

1. Taylor P. *The Smoke Ring: Tobacco, Money, and Multi-national Politics*. New York: Pantheon Books, 1984.

2. Garfinkel L. Time trends in lung cancer mortality among nonsmokers and a note on passive smoking. *J Natl Cancer Inst* 1981;66(6):1061–1066.

3. Garfinkel L, Auerbach O, Joubert L. Involuntary smoking and lung cancer: A case-control study. *J Natl Cancer Inst* 1985;75:463–469.

4. Bero L, Galbraith A, Rennie D. Sponsored symposia on environmental tobacco smoke. *JAMA* 1994;271:612–617.

5. Pollay RW. *A Scientific Smoke Screen: A Documentary History of Public Relations Efforts for and by the Tobacco Industry Research Council (TIRC), 1954–1958*. Vancouver, Canada: History of Advertising Archives, 1990. Tobacco Industry Promotion Series.

6. USDHHS. *The Health Consequences of Smoking: Cancer. A Report of the Surgeon General*. US Department of Health and Human Services, Public Health Service, Office on Smoking and Health, 1982. DHHS Publication No. (PHS) 82–50179.

7. Levin M. Tobacco pitchman agrees stars did not receive gifts. *Los Angeles Times* 1994 June 14:1.

8. Hazan A, Lipton H, Glantz S. Popular films do not reflect current tobacco use. *Am J Pub Health* 1994;84:998–1000.

CHAPTER 10

Environmental Tobacco Smoke and the Nonsmokers' Rights Movement

Strategic objectives [of sidestream smoke research] remain as follows: 1. Develop cigarettes with reduced sidestream yields and/or reduced odour and irritation. 2. Conduct research to anticipate and refute claims about the health effects of passive smoking.

Summary of BAT research activities, 1984
{1181.12, p. 2}

INTRODUCTION

During the 1970s, as the scientific evidence of the dangers of environmental tobacco smoke (ETS) was beginning to accumulate, a grassroots movement for nonsmokers' rights emerged (1). When it became evident that tobacco smoke can harm nonsmokers who inhale it passively, the public became less tolerant of smoking in public places and the workplace, and restrictions on smoking began to be implemented, by both government and private businesses. Although the mainstream health establishment was slow to appreciate the significance of the passive smoking issue, the tobacco industry was quick to recognize the need to counter this emerging shift in social attitudes toward smoking, particularly smoking in the workplace, and mobilized its public relations and political resources to deal with the potential threat. It used scientists, who were funded through the Council for Tobacco Research (CTR) special projects and special accounts (see chapter 8), to oppose restrictions on smoking in public places and workplaces, and it organized to fight ballot measures for clean indoor air in California and elsewhere.

The smoke that cigarette smokers draw into their lungs is "mainstream" smoke, while the smoke that comes off the burning tip of a cigarette is "sidestream" smoke. Sidestream smoke actually contains higher concentrations of many toxic chemicals than mainstream smoke (2), because sidestream smoke is not filtered and because cigarettes burn at a lower temperature when they are smoldering, leading to a less complete, dirtier combustion. The air pollution resulting from sidestream and extracted mainstream smoke is called secondhand smoke or environmental tobacco smoke, and people who breathe this smoke are known as passive smokers or involuntary smokers. Research conducted in the 1970s showed that children exposed to ETS have higher rates of respiratory diseases (2). In 1981 several published studies showed that nonsmoking women married to smokers have a higher risk of dying from lung cancer than nonsmoking women married to nonsmokers (3–5). This work was widely reported in the press, and provided the first strong evidence that passive smoking causes fatal diseases such as lung cancer. Research on ETS rapidly accumulated during the 1980s, and in 1986 major consensus reports by the National Academy of Sciences' National Research Council (6) and the Surgeon General (7) confirmed the evidence that ETS endangers children and causes lung cancer in adults. In 1992 the Environmental Protection Agency listed environmental tobacco smoke as a Class A (known human) carcinogen and a major source of respiratory problems in children (2). Subsequent studies have shown that exposure to ETS also increases the risk of heart disease (8–11).

In 1978 the Roper Organization conducted a confidential study for the Tobacco Institute on the attitudes of the public toward smoking (12). This report, which was obtained by the Federal Trade Commission and subsequently made public, stated:

> The original Surgeon General's report, followed by the first "hazard" warning on cigarette packages, the subsequent "danger" warning on cigarette packages, the removal of cigarette advertising from television and the inclusion of the danger warning in cigarette advertising, were all "blows" of sorts for the tobacco industry. They were, however, blows that the cigarette industry could successfully weather because they were all directed against the smoker himself.
>
> The anti-smoking forces' latest tack, however—on the passive smoking issue—is another matter. What the smoker does to himself may be his business, but what the smoker does to the non-smoker is quite a different matter. . . . six out of ten believe that smoking is hazardous to the nonsmoker's health, up sharply over the last four years. More than two-thirds of non-smokers believe it; nearly half of all smokers believe it.
>
> *This we see as the most dangerous development yet to the viability of the tobacco industry that has yet occurred* [emphasis added]. (p. 6)

The Roper report recommended that the industry engage in research to discredit the evidence that passive smoking is dangerous to nonsmokers.

The strategic and long run antidote to the passive smoking issue is, as we see it, developing and widely publicizing clear-cut, credible, medical evidence that passive smoking is not harmful to the non-smoker's health [emphasis added]. (p. 7)

The documents indicate that the tobacco industry followed this advice.

EARLY RECOGNITION OF THE PASSIVE SMOKING ISSUE

The tobacco industry's early awareness of the importance of the passive smoking issue is reflected in a March 15, 1973, document that summarizes the results of a literature review on issues related to smoking and health {2114.02}. It specifically notes that passive smoking is a growing issue of concern to the industry because of the negative impact that increased regulation will have on the social acceptability of smoking:

4. *Increasing emphasis is being given to the smoking habits of employees and the whole question of occupational exposure.* One anticipated result can be the increased attention of government and organized labor to the personal smoking habits of employees.

5. The popular claims that heart and lung disease are closely associated with community air pollution are being extended to include passive smoking, often to the degree that industrial smokestacks and vehicular emissions are ignored. In many instances, cigarette smoking is taking the rap for environmental pollution.

6. *More and more, smoking is being pictured as socially unacceptable.* The goal seems to be the involvement of others—non-smokers, children, etc.—in addition to health and government organizations. The main thrust of these zealots seems to be that "smoking is not a personal right because it hurts others; that smoking harms non-smoking adults, children, and even the yet unborn" [emphasis added]. {2114.02}

This document reflects themes that the tobacco industry has used for over two decades when dealing with secondhand smoke: it has argued that cigarette smoke is "taking the rap" for environmental pollution and that people concerned about secondhand smoke are "zealots."

In contrast to the tobacco industry's claims, the scientific and medical communities are well aware that environmental toxins such as radon and asbestos are hazardous to health. However, they also are aware of the large body of scientific evidence indicating that exposure to environmental tobacco smoke can cause disease as well (2, 6, 7). Interestingly, the tobacco industry also appears to have recognized that it would have very few natural allies in its effort to alleviate concern over passive smoking:

Many major U.S. industries are quite willing to let cigarettes take the full rap (government control, anti-pollution forces) and the tobacco industry can expect little help or sympathy from fellow manufacturers. {2114.02, p. 2}

Tobacco industry lawyers also became interested in the passive smoking issue at an early stage. In 1978 William Shinn, an attorney at Shook, Hardy, and Bacon, wrote a memo discussing various scientific activities, particularly the activities of Dr. Gary Huber {1910.05}, then director of the Kentucky Tobacco and Health Research Institute. As discussed in chapter 8, the institute, a state program funded through cigarette taxes, claimed to be independent but actually worked closely with tobacco industry lawyers on occasion. In addition, Dr. Huber was a consultant for Shook, Hardy, and Bacon (table 8.1). Shinn's memo states that Huber will be conducting a two-hour presentation at an American Thoracic Society/American Lung Association meeting, and that he might include a section on passive smoking in his presentation {1910.05}. In addition, Shinn states:

> Dr. Huber has mentioned from time to time the possibility of engaging in "passive smoking" research. . . . He is also curious as to what factors may contribute to the strong feelings of certain anti-smokers with respect to the smoking of others. {1910.05}

The attorneys' interest in secondhand smoke has not waned over the years. On September 13, 1984, Donald K. Hoel, a lawyer at Shook, Hardy, and Bacon, wrote a letter to attorneys at B&W in which he discussed tentative arrangements for a meeting of the "Public Smoking Advisory Group" at the Tobacco Institute. The purpose of the meeting was to discuss possible research on "normally encountered" tobacco smoke {1832.02}. (Some of the research sponsored by tobacco industry lawyers is discussed later in this chapter.)

RESEARCH AND PRODUCT DEVELOPMENT RESPONSE TO THE ETS ISSUE

As discussed in chapters 3, 4, and 7, BAT held annual research conferences so that its subsidiaries from around the world could share their research findings and agree on the research agenda for the following year. BAT research was carried out at facilities operated by the individual companies, and also through a joint research program headquartered at the Group Research and Development Centre (GR&DC) in Southampton, England. Most of the research on environmental tobacco smoke appears to have been conducted in Southampton.

DUCK KEY RESEARCH CONFERENCE, 1974

During the early 1970s concern over ETS was focused on its irritating effects. For example, the minutes from a meeting of the Biological Testing Committee that was held in Southampton on January 27, 1970, note that research technicians have been complaining about irritation caused by sidestream smoke from one of the cigarettes under evaluation:

> Dr. [S. J.] Green [of BAT R&D] drew attention to the additional point . . . that the operators of the smoking machines at Battelle [which was conducting research for Project Janus at the time] have complained about the odour/irritating nature of the sidestream smoke from the cigarette containing 100% I-308. {1164.04, p. 3}

Minutes from later meetings indicate that most BAT scientists did not take these complaints seriously at first. At the 1974 research conference in Duck Key, Florida, Dr. Green proposed that irritation caused by sidestream smoke should be evaluated in all new products. His colleagues, however, reacted without enthusiasm. The conclusions and recommendations from the Duck Key conference state:

> 16.   It was suggested by Dr. Green that now that we have an objective sensory difference test for assessing irritation of sidestream smoke, we might write in to all new product developments a constraint in the specification in this respect. *This suggestion had a cool reception and most members felt that passive smoking was relatively unimportant.* It was agreed to note disagreement on this subject [emphasis added]. {1125.01, p. 4}

Just one year later, however, BAT scientists began to pay more attention to the irritating and potentially dangerous effects of ETS.

MERANO RESEARCH CONFERENCE, 1975

At the BAT research conference held in Merano, Italy, in April 1975, BAT scientists discussed passive smoking at length. Participants agreed that research into the irritating effects of sidestream smoke should be undertaken. The minutes from the meeting state:

> 12.   Passive smoking was discussed and reviewed in detail. *It is considered that this is an important area and interest in it is unlikely to recede.* The meeting felt that the work on sidestream irritation at Southampton was a useful contribution to a part of the whole problem. R & D Southampton were asked to extent [*sic*] their studies to cover a wider range of cigarettes and chemical constituents in the sidestream. *It is desirable to be in a position to anticipate the identification of new sidestream constituents which may be considered harmful to non smokers* [emphasis added]. {1173.01, p. 3}

BAT's scientists made this statement nearly a decade before the general scientific community had recognized ETS as a serious threat to public health.

BIOLOGICAL RESEARCH MEETING, SOUTHAMPTON, 1976

By the mid-1970s the scientific community had begun to identify toxic substances such as carbon monoxide (13, 14) and N-nitrosamines (15, 16) in sidestream smoke. In addition, Carl Becker, a researcher at Cornell University, had published a series of studies on glycoproteins in tobacco smoke (17–19). Glycoproteins are a class of proteins that often induce allergic reactions. Becker's first study showed that glycoprotein isolated from tobacco could produce allergic reactions in some individuals (17). His report caught the attention of BAT researchers, who discussed his findings at a biological research meeting held on October 14, 1976, in Southampton. The minutes of the meeting note that BAT scientists at Southampton had repeated Becker's experiments and had confirmed that glycoprotein is present in mainstream smoke. The researchers agreed that the studies should be repeated for sidestream smoke.

> The work in GR&DC . . . has shown that glycoproteins with characteristics similar to those found by [Carl] Becker and Stedman are present in tobacco leaf and in saline extracts of mainstream smoke. It was agreed that there was no intention to examine the biological effects of such materials and there was no necessity to examine condensate. Nevertheless, SJG [Dr. S. J. Green, of BAT R&D] considered that it was important to know whether or not these materials were present in sidestream smoke.
>
> It was concluded that the project should be extended to an examination of sidestream smoke and to the examination of one or two other tobacco types including experimentally de-proteinated tobacco. {1164.17, p. 11}

By the next year's meeting, BAT researchers announced that they had found glycoproteins in sidestream smoke as well.

BIOLOGICAL RESEARCH MEETING, CHELWOOD, 1977

Becker published a second study on tobacco glycoproteins in 1977 (18). This study showed that glycoproteins from tobacco increase the formation of clots in human blood, and he concluded that tobacco glycoproteins "may be important to the pathogenesis of cardiovascular and pulmonary diseases associated with cigarette smoking" (18). Becker's findings were reported in the *New York Times* (20).

Ironically, Becker's second study had been funded by CTR. As mentioned in chapter 8, publication of his results had prompted correspondence between Robert Hockett, the scientific director of CTR, and Addison Yeaman, president of CTR {1910.01}. Hockett stated in his memo that he was unhappy with Becker's publication and that he had attempted, but failed, to have acknowledgment of CTR funding deleted from the publication.

While CTR was attempting to distance itself from Becker's findings, tobacco industry lawyers and scientists took his findings very seriously. A letter from Timothy M. Finnegan, an attorney at Jacob and Medinger, to William W. Shinn, an attorney for Shook, Hardy, and Bacon, notes that the lawyers have hired a scientist to repeat Becker's experiments.

> As a result of Dr. Carl Becker's report of a glycoprotein in tobacco leaf, tobacco smoke condensate and tobacco smoke, Dr. [John] Salvaggio and his colleagues have undertaken an analysis of these compounds for the presence of glycoproteins. {1910.06}

Dr. Salvaggio received $283,777 from 1976 to 1981 to conduct a CTR special project on the physical, chemical, and immuno-chemical properties of components present in tobacco smoke (table 8.1).

Scientists at BAT also repeated Becker's experiments and replicated his results. They adopted a defensive posture, however, regarding the implications of their research. The minutes from a biological research meeting held on November 27, 1977, in Chelwood note:

> RB [R. Binns of BAT GR&DC] explained that, whereas Becker's findings in relation to the presence of glycoproteins in mainstream and sidestream smoke had been confirmed, this did not mean that we agreed with his interpretation of their effects on man. {1164.24}

Although Binns was hesitant to concur with Becker's conclusions, the researchers at the Chelwood meeting agreed that the presence of glycoproteins in sidestream smoke was an important problem. They recommended that it should be addressed on an industry-wide basis through the Tobacco Research Council (TRC) in the United Kingdom {1164.23; 1164.24}.

> SJG [Dr. S. J. Green of BAT R&D] proposed that the glycoproteins question is an industry problem and should be pursued by TRC. This was accepted. {1164.23}

The documents and our review of the literature do not indicate whether the health effects of glycoproteins were ever studied by the TRC. The role, if any, that glycoproteins play in the mechanisms underlying tobacco-related disease also is not known precisely. It is noteworthy, however, that BAT had confirmed the presence of a potentially dangerous substance in sidestream smoke as early as 1977.

SYDNEY RESEARCH CONFERENCE, 1978

The research conference held in Sydney, Australia, in March 1978 marked two major shifts in BAT's research policy toward environmental tobacco smoke. First, the emphasis shifted from glycoproteins to nitrosamines. Second, BAT executives began to realize that the passive smoking issue represented a potential new commercial opportunity for the company.

Nitrosamines are potent carcinogens. Tobacco contains several types of tobacco-specific N-nitrosamines (TSNA), most of which are by-products of nicotine formed during the curing, fermentation, aging, and burning of tobacco (21, 22). TSNA cause a variety of cancers—most notably lung cancer—in laboratory animals, and most researchers today believe that they are one of the primary causes of many tobacco-induced cancers in humans (21–23).

BAT was actively engaged in measuring levels of nitrosamines in both mainstream and sidestream smoke by the late 1970s. Notes from BAT's Sydney conference explain BAT's concern over nitrosamines in ETS:

> It is clear that in many countries there is concern over the level of nitrosamines in foodstuffs. This explains in part the sensitivity to the presence of nitrosamines in tobacco smoke and, perhaps particularly, the levels in sidestream smoke. The latter is a potential threat to the currently held view by many authorities that passive smoking does not constitute a direct hazard. {1174.01}

Minutes from later conferences indicate that research on nitrosamines in both mainstream and sidestream tobacco smoke grew in importance at BAT throughout the 1980s. Unfortunately, the conference reports in the documents rarely include the results of these studies, but only indicate that research was ongoing.

While BAT scientists acknowledged that nitrosamines in sidestream smoke could present a problem for the industry, they also began to realize during the late 1970s that the passive smoking issue could be used to their advantage. The report from the 1978 Sydney conference indicates a growing awareness that BAT could capitalize on the growing anti-smoking sentiment by developing a new cigarette with less irritating side-stream smoke. The notes from the meeting state:

> 21. ... A worthwhile aim is to modify the quality of sidestream smoke, and it should be remembered that governments can produce markets by endorsing a particular aspect of the cigarette, e.g., charcoal filters. {1174.01, p. 3}

Throughout the 1980s BAT's research on environmental tobacco smoke was focused on measuring nitrosamine levels and on developing a new low-sidestream cigarette.

UK RESEARCH CONFERENCES, 1979

The tobacco industry was concerned that government agencies would use the nitrosamine issue to impose further regulations on tobacco products. BAT group scientists discussed this concern at an R&D policy conference held in the United Kingdom on February 10 to 14, 1979. The notes from the conference, prepared by Dr. S. J. Green of BAT R&D, indicate that BAT executives agreed that they should attempt to establish "safe level" thresholds for nitrosamines:

> The likely increase in pressure in this area from the anti-smoking lobby was noted. In the absence of threshold figures (e.g. safe levels for nitrosamines) any measured number could harm the Industry. Consideration should be given to the possibility of establishing thresholds. It was agreed that on nitrosamines some sighting shots should be aimed on both ambient air and sidestream smoke. {1175.03, p. 4}

The implication here is that the industry would attempt to show that nitrosamine levels in all cigarettes were below the "safe level," thus preventing government regulation of cigarettes based on their nitrosamine content. On the other hand, the industry realized that any mention of a "measured number" could be dangerous because it would be an explicit admission that tobacco smoke contains hazardous substances.

An R&D conference held later in 1979 in London confirmed the growing realization of the importance of the passive smoking issue. The notes from the meeting, prepared by Dr. L. C. F. Blackman of BAT R&D, state:

> 18. <u>SIDESTREAM</u>
> *Concern for the passive smoker was regarded as likely to become a key issue in the future and the GR&DC programme was regarded as of importance—both for defensive and offensive (i.e., possible commercial advantage) purposes* [emphasis added]. {1176.02, p. 9}

SEA ISLAND RESEARCH CONFERENCE, 1980

By 1980 BAT's researchers were trying to develop a cigarette with low sidestream smoke emission. The direction of the research was discussed at a research conference held in Sea Island, Georgia, on September 15 to 18, 1980. Notes from the conference, prepared by Dr. L. C. F. Blackman of BAT, state:

SIDESTREAM

20.   There was strong support for research into the generation and control of sidestream smoke. Factors investigated should include the role of pH on sidestream nicotine and aroma. Research into the attitude of smokers and non-smokers to substantial reduction or elimination of sidestream smoke should be established.

21.   Effort should be directed to developing a smoking article with greatly reduced tobacco content to reduce the material available for generation of sidestream. {1177.01, p. 4}

In addition, the notes from the meeting indicated that the BAT Group continued to support research on nitrosamines in sidestream smoke.

19.   The research into the source and mechanism of formation of nitrosamines in both sidestream and mainstream should be continued with urgency. {1177.01, p. 4}

The entry suggests that the researchers had already isolated nitrosamines in sidestream and mainstream smoke, because the purpose of the research was to determine their source and formation. Thus, BAT may have again confirmed in its own laboratories that ETS contains dangerous substances.

While BAT's scientists were quietly conducting research on sidestream smoke, the general scientific community was becoming increasingly aware that passive smoking could cause a variety of diseases, including lung cancer. In 1981 a large epidemiological study on the relationship between passive smoking and lung cancer was published by Dr. Takeshi Hirayama (3). The study showed that nonsmoking women married to smokers were more likely to develop lung cancer than nonsmoking women married to nonsmokers. The Hirayama study received a great deal of publicity and, as we will discuss later in this chapter, was criticized vehemently by the tobacco industry. Nonetheless, shortly after the publication of Hirayama's paper, BAT began to study the "biological activity" of sidestream smoke. As discussed in chapter 4, the tobacco industry uses the term "biological activity" as a euphemism for carcinogenicity and other adverse health effects.

PICHLARN RESEARCH CONFERENCE, 1981

The issue of environmental tobacco smoke grew in importance at BAT throughout the 1980s. A document describing BAT's proposed research program for 1982–84, which was prepared after a research conference in Pichlarn, Austria, in August 1981, states:

> The broadly based Programme [on sidestream smoke] was approved. Particular points were:

> - It was agreed that GR&DC should continue short-term testing (inhalation, Ames [test for mutagenicity] etc) to get a better understanding of the relative specific activity of sidestream and mainstream smoke. This should form a basis for a future decision as to the need, or otherwise, for more extensive biological testing (eg, mouse-skin painting) of sidestream smoke. {1178.01, p. 6}

The fact that BAT was studying the "specific activity" of sidestream smoke indicates that BAT was concerned about studies suggesting that ETS is carcinogenic and that it was attempting to measure the carcinogenicity of ETS in laboratory tests.

The proposed 1982–84 research program also contains a reference to a study of sidestream smoke emissions using different cigarette papers:

> - Information on inorganic fibres thought to be available in Canada from prior use in cigar wrapper should be evaluated with respect to the current cigarette sidestream project. {1178.01, p. 6}

As discussed below, one of BAT's primary techniques for minimizing sidestream smoke was to use new cigarette papers.

MONTEBELLO RESEARCH CONFERENCE, 1982

The summary of BAT's 1982 research conference, held in Montebello, Canada, notes that the bulk of the conference was devoted to discussing topics of major importance to the group {1179.01}. One of the five topics discussed was environmental tobacco smoke. The summary of the meeting reflects the growing awareness that the passive smoking issue represented an opportunity for new product development. Under the topic of environmental tobacco smoke, the summary states:

> 14.   The strong growth of medical, scientific and media concern and comment in this area was acknowledged. The subject is extremely complex and it is essential to keep separate in our thinking:
> (a)   health issues
> (b)   social issues
> (c)   new commercial product opportunities.

(a) and (b) represent constraints on the tobacco industry as a whole, but within them lies the opportunity for commercial exploitation (c). {1179.01, p. 6}

The next item in the summary is very vague. It appears to suggest that BAT had determined that sidestream smoke had different biological effects than mainstream smoke, but also that BAT may have found a way to reduce the toxicity of sidestream smoke:

> 15. Sidestream has long been known to be different chemically from mainstream, but only very recently have there been signs from GR&DC inhalation studies that *the biological activity of sidestream may also be significantly different from mainstream.*
>
> *An early design of reduced sidestream product developed at GR&DC has recently been screened* [emphasis added]. {1179.01, p. 6}

Sidestream smoke contains higher levels of toxic substances—such as carbon monoxide, benzo(a)pyrene, and nitrosamines—than mainstream smoke (24). The item above confirms that BAT's inhalation experiments had shown that sidestream smoke is "biologically active" and that researchers were actively seeking designs that reduced sidestream emissions.

The summary of the 1982 Montebello conference also mentions a paper written by Dr. Ian Ayres of BAT GR&DC, which apparently was presented or discussed at the conference:

> The personal paper by Dr Ian Ayres was regarded as a useful contribution in that it highlighted our need for better knowledge and understanding of the key chemical and biological aspects of environmental smoke. Much further thought is clearly required but specifically it was recommended that:
>
> (a) We must get hard data both to help counter anti-smoking attacks, and to support the design of future products. . . .
>
> (b) *We should keep within BAT:*
>
>> i) *animal results on sidestream activity*
>>
>> ii) *thoughts on the biological activity of sidestream*
>>
>> iii) research findings on the consumer annoyance aspects of environmental smoke—since these have potential commercial value.
>
> (c) Dr. Ayres' paper should be discussed in confidence with Peter Lee [a British statistician and tobacco industry consultant] and Francis Roe [another British scientist and tobacco industry consultant] with the aim of guiding the research under (i).
>
> It was also recommended that BAT should be prepared to share on an industry basis the development of techniques for monitoring chemicals in environmental smoke [emphasis added]. {1179.01, pp. 7–8}

This item demonstrates that BAT was attempting to develop a sophisticated understanding of the health effects of passive smoking and the public's attitude toward environmental tobacco smoke. BAT planned to use some of its data to "counter anti-smoking attacks," while data supporting the evidence that ETS is dangerous would be withheld from the public. This is the same strategy that the tobacco industry has employed regarding active smoking.

REVIEW OF BAT RESEARCH PROGRAM, 1983

In May 1983 BAT conducted an extensive review of its group research at Southampton. BAT's research operations at that time were divided into fifteen work areas: Biological, Filters, Nitrosamines, Future Technologies, Combustion, Sidestream, Human Smoking/Smoke Aerosol, Psychology and Sensory Testing, Smoke Taste and Flavour Improvement, Leaf and Biotechnology, Tobacco Processing, Tobacco Expansion, Novel Cigarette Making Technology, Process Control and Physical Test Method Development, and Chemical Test Method Development and Analytical Projects. The review of BAT's research program summarizes the activities in each of these work areas {1180.17}.

Work on environmental tobacco smoke was being carried out in several of the work areas. For example, the review notes that 20 percent of the work in the Biological area was related to the evaluation of sidestream smoke. In the Nitrosamine work area, "the importance was emphasized of . . . Work on both mainstream <u>and</u> sidestream [emphasis in original]" {1180.17}. In addition, one of the projects in the Combustion work area was related to "The mechanism by which magnesium oxide filler in the cigarette paper reduces *visible* sidestream" [emphasis added] {1180.17}.

In the Sidestream work area, BAT's research effort was directed at designing a low-sidestream cigarette, primarily by developing new types of cigarette paper that would release less irritating or smaller volumes of sidestream smoke.

> The general thrust of the work on sidestream is to design and evaluate cigarettes with reduced emission of sidestream smoke. This will also include the generation of data on the build-up of smoke in confined areas and the effect of this on occupants and furnishings. The project areas are:—
>
> (a)   The development of analytical techniques for measuring sidestream smoke constituents.
>
> (b)   Development of new cigarette paper for sidestream reduction using alternative fillers and additives. Work to improve existing papers is also included.

(c)   The development of low sidestream cigarettes using cigarette papers described under (b) and currently available papers.

(d)   The evaluation of the effects of low sidestream products on ambient smoke in rooms. This involves bringing into operation soon of a suitably designed room. {1180.17}

This research was aimed primarily at reducing the visibility and irritation of sidestream smoke. The review does not mention any attempts to study the health effects of sidestream smoke released from these new products. Evidently, BAT's first inclination was to develop a "health-image" cigarette to respond to public concern over ETS, just as it had initially responded to concern over active smoking by introducing filter cigarettes (see chapter 2).

BAT's 1983 review of its work program also mentions several other projects related to environmental tobacco smoke. For example, "Interest was expressed in determining the extent to which the level of visible sidestream smoke influences subjects [sic] irritation response" {1180.17}. In addition, a smoking machine was being built that would collect both mainstream and sidestream smoke from the same cigarette; and the range of sidestream analysis was being expanded to include more vapor phase components, such as carbon monoxide and nitrogen oxide. Taken together, these projects indicate that BAT's scientists were making a sophisticated evaluation of the chemical, social, and biological aspects of environmental tobacco smoke. The primary focus of its program, however, was on producing a new cigarette with reduced sidestream smoke emissions.

Following this review of the research program, BAT subsidiaries were asked to provide priority rankings for each research project {1180.18}. The projects were rated on a scale of 1 to 3, with 1 having the highest priority. The documents include the rankings provided by the major countries in the BAT group—Australia, Brazil, Canada, Germany, and the United States—along with the average score that each project received. Virtually all the projects related to environmental tobacco smoke, described above, were given a priority of 1 by most of the delegates {1180.18}.

BROAD OBJECTIVES OF BAT'S RESEARCH PROGRAM, CIRCA 1983

BAT's primary objective in conducting research on environmental tobacco smoke was to develop a new cigarette that produced less sidestream smoke. However, by the end of 1983 BAT had added a second primary objective to its ETS research program: to gather scientific data to refute the evidence that passive smoking is dangerous to health. This shift is shown in a document titled "Broad Objectives of the Group R&D Programme" {1180.14}. This document contains a series of tables describing eleven areas of research, corresponding loosely, but not exactly, to the work areas mentioned above. BAT's research on environmental tobacco smoke was considered both "defensive and offensive" in nature and was given a priority of 1. The main objectives of the program in this area were to "find ways of reducing the nuisance aspects of sidestream" and to "obtain scientific data to refute the alleged health risks of sidestream smoke" {1180.14} (see table 10.1, p. 433).

A document written by W. D. E. Irwin of BAT GR&DC and titled "Sidestream Research" confirms that BAT's main priorities for ETS research during the mid-1980s were to develop a low-sidestream cigarette and to conduct defensive research. This document appears to have been written in mid-1983, possibly in anticipation of BAT's research conference in Rio de Janeiro. It begins:

> The B.C.A.C. [BAT Chairman's Advisory Committee] *confirmed two requirements:*
>
> 1. *Develop cigarettes with reduced sidestream emissions and/or reduced perceived smell and irritation.*
> 2. *Conduct research to anticipate and refute claims about the health effects of passive smoking* [emphasis added]. {1180.24}

Again, it is noteworthy that BAT appeared more concerned with the irritative aspect of smoke than with whether passive smoking is dangerous to health. Its interest in health appeared to be limited to refuting any claims made by others about the effects of exposure to ETS.

Irwin then notes that a joint GR&DC/Marketing/Public Affairs Sidestream Working Party has been formed to coordinate BAT's effort to develop and market a low-sidestream product.

> The Working Party will propose a programme of gradual reductions in sidestream emission levels as well as developing products taking maximum reductions. The former would be a safeguard to any future debate, *but would not be communicated to the consumer at present* [emphasis added]. {1180.24}

BAT appears to have been planning to make cigarettes with a range of sidestream emissions that would leave it free either to reduce sidestream smoke gradually, without informing the customer, or to introduce a radically new product if it were deemed marketable.

Irwin also summarizes BAT's research on cigarette papers that would reduce ETS emissions. Two types of papers were being evaluated: slow-burning papers and "sidestream filtration papers." However, the sidestream filtration papers did not appear to work well; two of them failed to reduce fresh sidestream irritation and smell {1180.24}.

RIO DE JANEIRO RESEARCH CONFERENCE, 1983

At BAT's 1983 conference in Rio, the biological activity (i.e., carcinogenicity) of sidestream smoke was addressed as a major issue. The meeting summary states:

> 5.   The programme of work set up in response to the BCAC directive was supported—but *it was stressed that the programme should consider the reduction of specific biological activity, as well as the reduction of visible smoke irritation and unpleasant odour.* It should also consider the more general question of ambient smoke [emphasis added]. {1180.07, p. 5}

This statement suggests that BAT's scientists believed sidestream smoke could be biologically active, that is, carcinogenic. In addition, it implies that they were hoping to create a new product with less carcinogenic sidestream smoke, just as they had initially hoped to create a "safe" cigarette for active smokers.

The summary of this conference also refers to several contracts being negotiated to develop special cigarette papers that would reduce sidestream smoke emissions. The use of slow-burning cigarette paper could serve a dual purpose: reducing sidestream emissions and creating a self-extinguishing cigarette, which would be less likely to set accidental fires (see chapter 7) {1180.07, p. 5}. In addition, the participants agreed that defensive research should continue:

> The analysis of ambient smoke was regarded as a priority need—to provide firm data to counter misleading statements in the literature and the media. {1180.07, p. 23}

The increasing emphasis that BAT placed on ETS research during the early 1980s is indicated in a document that provides projected resource allocations for 1984 {1180.16}. In 1983, 4.1 "graduate years" and 4.7 "assistant years" were allocated for ETS research (7.6 percent and 5.2 percent, respectively, of BAT's budget); in 1984 these values had increased by roughly 60 percent to 6.5 graduate years and 6.7 assistant years

(12.5 percent and 8.2 percent, respectively). The revenue expenditure for 1984 was estimated at 318,000 pounds for the sidestream research group {1180.16}.

SOUTHAMPTON RESEARCH CONFERENCE, 1984

BAT's 1984 research conference, held in Southampton, included lengthy discussions of BAT's research activities related to environmental tobacco smoke and to the psychology of smoking. In addition, several other technical conferences held earlier in the year were summarized. The main objectives of BAT's ETS research program remained unchanged from the previous year: to "Develop cigarettes with reduced sidestream yields and/or reduced odour and irritation" and to "Conduct research to anticipate and refute claims about the health effects of passive smoking" {1181.12}. As in previous years, the first objective was being addressed by attempting to reduce sidestream emissions through changes in cigarette composition and construction. This research was being coordinated with efforts to maintain satisfactory mainstream deliveries, taste, and ash characteristics {1181.12}. There was also an attempt to develop an alternative cigarette paper. Consumer tests had shown that a noticeable reduction in visible sidestream smoke could be achieved with "a 50% reduction in the rate of sidestream PMWNF [perhaps, particulate matter] emission" {1181.12}. For example, the paper company Ecusta had conducted consumer tests of a magnesium oxide–filled cigarette paper, but the ash and taste properties of this cigarette were judged unsatisfactory. BAT had next turned to Papeteries de Mauduit (PDM), which was testing cigarette papers with a combination of 8 percent potassium citrate additive and 11 percent magnesium oxide. This product performed fairly well in terms of taste but did not result in a large enough reduction of ETS emissions. PDM was currently testing papers with higher percentages of potassium citrate or magnesium oxide {1181.12}.

BAT was also measuring the buildup and decay of ambient smoke under carefully controlled conditions. In addition, it was monitoring levels of smoke in public places such as bars. Tests of human uptake of various smoke components as well as tests for odor and irritation were also being performed {1181.12}.

Turning to BAT's secondary objective of conducting defensive research, the 1984 conference summary notes that evidence related to the "alleged" health effects of passive smoking could be classified as:

1.   Claims based on smoke component concentrations in rooms.

2.   Claims based on measuring body uptake of various smoke components.

3.   Clinical studies, such as lung function measurements of non smoking subjects exposed to tobacco smoke over a period of time.

4.   Epidemiological studies, e.g. claiming increased lung cancer risk for non-smoking wives of smoking husbands. {1181.12}

The report noted that the rate of publication on ETS, particularly clinical and epidemiological studies, was continuing to grow. However, BAT's research effort was restricted to measurements of smoke components and body uptake.

> [C]linical and epidemiological testing of the effects of ambient smoke are not part of the GR&DC programme [emphasis added]. {1181.12}

Also discussed at the 1984 meeting was BAT's research on the psychology of smoking. The group's strategic objective was threefold:

> a)   To research means of measuring consumer needs, attitudes and motivations, and develop models to relate these to product development and marketing activity.
>
> b)   To research means of optimising communication of product features to the consumer, particularly in the context of restricted advertising.
>
> c)   To interface Product Applications and Research group collaborative activity with the development and application of novel product testing methodology and psychophysical models. {1181.12}

Among the projects undertaken in this area was a study of whether nonsmokers' reactions to environmental tobacco smoke might be affected more by the actions of smokers than by the smoke itself.

> It has been hypothesised that the smoker, rather than the cigarette smoke, plays a key role in determining non smoker reaction to sidestream smoke. An alternative to modifying the cigarette may therefore be to encourage more "acceptable" behavior by the smoker. {1181.12}

BAT's preliminary results suggested that this hypothesis was correct. Studies were planned for 1985 that would further characterize nonsmokers' reactions to ETS. Specifically, BAT planned to study how nonsmokers react to the smoker's manner, the degree to which the nonsmoker perceives control over the passive smoking situation, and the effect of same-sex and different-sex pairs of smokers and nonsmokers {1181.12}. This and similar work may have contributed to current tobacco industry activities to create a "smokers' rights" movement and to provide social support for smokers (25, 26).

BAT's 1984 R&D conference report also contains summaries of several smaller technical exchange meetings that had been held earlier that year. Environmental tobacco smoke was discussed at several of these smaller conferences. For example, at a biological conference held in Southampton, BAT researchers confirmed their commitment to studying the health effects of the sidestream smoke produced by any new products.

> It was thought prudent to ensure that the Company could show *no adverse effects on sidestream toxicity* for a product designed to have a lower *visible* sidestream [emphasis added]. {1181.06}

This statement raises the question of whether the additives and other modifications to the paper and tobacco rod used to reduce visible sidestream smoke may have increased overall toxicity of the smoke.

Southampton also sponsored a "structured creativity" conference in June 1984. The conference was essentially a brainstorming session to discuss the feasibility of developing a variety of new products. One of the products discussed was the "low sidestream/ameliorated aroma product." The purpose of this product was:

> *To pre-empt potential volume decline from smokers under pressure in social and work environments* by providing them with an offer which combines re-assurance in social smoking with taste and satisfaction [emphasis added]. {1181.10}

This statement indicates that the motivation behind BAT's effort to develop a low-sidestream cigarette was profit rather than public health. The goal was to keep smokers smoking even though acceptance of smoking in public places was declining. The conference attendees rated this project as having "large market potential, high behavioral validation (evidence of need) but potentially high associated risks to the business" {1181.10}.

After the 1984 research conference in Southampton, BAT circulated a document titled "Proposed Revisions to the Group R&D Programme" {1181.13}. Few revisions were proposed for the work on ETS. However, in the section on "Novel Cigarette Technology," the research that had been carried out that year on low-sidestream cigarettes is described as promising.

> Initially promising work using a food extruder, at the Food Research Institute, Norwich, produced highly expanded tobacco materials with low density and reasonable smoke character. Lower CO [carbon monoxide]/tar ratio and sidestream smoke levels were recorded in prototype products. Significant effort will be allocated to this activity during 1985–86. {1181.13}

Another study described as promising had to do with the effect of changing cigarette combustion/pyrolysis temperature profiles by the use of thermal conductors. The result was reduced carbon monoxide and tar levels.

> Unexpected observations of reduced CO/tar ratios, especially in sidestream smoke, have encouraged a wider investigation of products employing the principle, as it is thought that there may be accompanying changes in specific activity. {1181.13}

These items suggest that BAT was meeting with some success in its efforts to reduce the carcinogenicity of sidestream smoke.

The reports from BAT's annual research conferences demonstrate that BAT's internal research efforts supported the conclusion that environmental tobacco smoke is dangerous to health. BAT had shown in its own laboratories that sidestream smoke contains toxic substances, such as nitrosamines, and that sidestream smoke was "biologically active," and therefore potentially carcinogenic. Publicly, however, BAT and the other tobacco companies have denied that ETS is dangerous.

PUBLIC ATTACKS AND PRIVATE ACCEPTANCE OF ETS RESEARCH

One of the techniques used by the tobacco industry to counter the evidence that passive smoking is dangerous is to fund scientific research specifically designed to "refute claims about the health effects of passive smoking" {1181.12}. The industry also has funded special projects related to ETS through CTR. As discussed in chapter 8, CTR special projects were funded at the request of tobacco industry lawyers, and their purpose was to generate data that could be used on the tobacco industry's behalf.

USING CTR SPECIAL PROJECTS TO EXONERATE SECONDHAND SMOKE

In 1981 Patrick Sirridge, an attorney at Shook, Hardy, and Bacon, wrote a letter to a group of tobacco industry lawyers known as the Committee of Counsel recommending funding for a revised proposal that had been submitted by Dr. Theodor D. Sterling {2026.01}. The purpose of Sterling's project was to study sick building syndrome. (Sick building syndrome refers to buildings in which a substantial proportion of occupants experience symptoms such as headaches or eye irritation when inside the building. Sick building syndrome has become increasingly common since the 1970s, when new buildings were built without windows that opened and in which air was recirculated to conserve energy. Outgassing of building materials, carpeting, and furnishings and accumulation of bacteria and other contaminants can contribute to sick building syndrome, as can tobacco smoke.) In his letter Sirridge notes that "Dr. Sterling has incorporated into the current proposal plans for collection of data on substances [other than tobacco smoke] present in buildings." In Dr. Sterling's previous work on sick building syndrome, Sirridge points out, "[s]moking was considered and found not to be a problem." Dr. Sterling's request of $207,913 for eighteen months was recommended for funding.

> It is our opinion that this study could be useful with respect to the controversial issue of restriction of smoking in the workplace. {2026.01}

As discussed in detail in chapter 8, Sterling has regularly appeared on behalf of the tobacco industry at scientific meetings and legislative and administrative hearings as an independent scientist who believes that the risks associated with passive smoking are being overstated by health authorities. The documents indicate that Sterling has received more than $6 million in special project funding from 1971 to 1990 (table 8.1).

Another special project related to ETS was conducted by ACVA Atlantic, Inc. ACVA Atlantic was awarded $13,800 in 1985 to conduct a special project on air quality in the home. The proposal for the project stated:

> Results of such a study . . . could demonstrate that environmental tobacco smoke has a relatively insignificant effect on indoor air quality. {2041.03}

The methodology for the study is described as follows:

> Twelve homes will be selected in three discrete areas of the country giving a total of 36 homes, *the selection will be by the Tobacco Institute* who will provide the names, addresses, phone numbers and contact at each of the homes chosen to ACVA [emphasis added]. {2041.04}

ACVA Atlantic, which later changed its name to Healthy Buildings International (HBI), characterizes itself as an independent firm that specializes in monitoring indoor air quality and in diagnosing causes of sick building syndrome. However, it is highly unusual for an "independent" company to allow an organization such as the Tobacco Institute, which clearly has a strong interest in the outcome of the study, to select the sites for its study.

To our knowledge, the ACVA Atlantic study has never been published, and the tobacco industry has never used the data for any purpose. However, a study conducted by ACVA Atlantic's successor, HBI, has been cited extensively by the tobacco industry. This study—which was funded by the Center for Indoor Air Research (CIAR), a tobacco industry–sponsored organization similar to CTR (27)—was published in a peer-reviewed journal. Its authors measured levels of ETS in typical office buildings and concluded that "with good ventilation, acceptable air quality can be maintained with moderate amounts of smoking" (28). A congressional inquiry subsequently found, however, that more than 25 percent of the data from the HBI study was falsified (27, 29, 30). For example, employees of HBI who conducted the study stated that they had been instructed to put their measuring devices in lobbies and other open areas, in order to keep ETS readings as low as possible (31, exhibit 2). In addition, HBI employees stated that their data collection sheets were routinely altered, so that the levels of ETS recorded were lower than those that had actually been measured (31, exhibit 2). An independent analysis of HBI's data concluded that there were "many unexplained anomalies, raising serious questions about the integrity of [the] data" (27, exhibit 10). A reanalysis of HBI's data revealed that, in areas where moderate smoking occurred, "the impact of ETS on indoor air quality is 40-fold greater than HBI asserts publicly" (27, exhibit 10).

Gray Robertson, the president of HBI, and other HBI employees have testified on at least 129 occasions before local, state, and federal government agencies regarding various proposals to ban smoking in public places (27, exhibit 9). Their standard statement is that, according to their studies, moderate levels of smoking can be tolerated with adequate ventilation (27, 33). In many cases they did not acknowledge tobacco industry support (31, 32).

ANALYZING LONDON'S SMOKE-FREE UNDERGROUND TRAINS

A decision by the London Underground to end smoking in 1984 reflected the accelerating trend toward smoke-free environments that was beginning in the mid-to-late 1980s. One of the B&W documents is a report titled "An Investigation of the Atmosphere in London Underground Trains" {1181.04}, which was part of the papers for the 1984 research conference. Neither the author nor the audience is identified in the report, but it appears to have been part of an effort to gather data to demonstrate that ETS is not an important source of indoor air pollution. The report notes that smoking was ended on all Underground trains for a one-year trial period beginning July 9, 1984, and that a study was conducted to measure the air quality before and after ending smoking. Before smoking was ended, levels of nicotine and particulates were higher in the smoking cars than in the nonsmoking cars. However, all levels were below the industrial safety limits.

> Before the total ban on smoking was introduced, smoking compartments contained on average five times the concentration of nicotine and four times the concentration of airborne particles as compared to non-smoking carriages. However, the concentration of nicotine (c. 30 μg/m^3) and particulates (c. 0.7 mg/m^3) found in the smoking areas are similar to those that are likely to be encountered in typical offices and public houses, and are far below recommended industrial limits for safe exposure (500 μg/m^3 for nicotine). {1181.04}

One month after smoking had been ended, nicotine levels were lower than they had been in both smoking and nonsmoking cars. These results suggest that some smoke had been leaking into the nonsmoking cars. Moreover, there had been significantly elevated levels of air pollution when smoking was present, and these levels were reduced by ending smoking. The report, however, does not comment on either of these findings. Instead, it reiterates that levels of nicotine and particulates measured did not exceed recommended exposure levels.

INTERESTING DEVELOPMENTS IN THE HIRAYAMA MATTER

Another technique that the tobacco industry has used to create a controversy surrounding the passive smoking issue is to attack published research on ETS. The documents show that, in at least one case, the industry has even criticized research that some of its own consultants acknowledged was valid.

In 1981 Takeshi Hirayama published a major study indicating that lung cancer could be caused by passive smoking as well as active smoking (3). The study, which was published in the *British Medical Journal,* received international attention. The tobacco industry responded by launching a public relations campaign to discredit Hirayama's work. The Tobacco Institute hired Nathan Mantel, a well-known epidemiologist, to critique the study, and it then cited Mantel's criticisms in a press release that was widely reported (34). The institute also reprinted several critical news articles as full-page advertisements in newspapers and magazines (35) (figure 10.1). Several months after the original publication of Hirayama's study, the *British Medical Journal* responded to the public attacks against Hirayama's work by reopening correspondence on his study. In particular, the editors stated that they were taking the "exceptional step" of publishing letters that had not been sent to *BMJ,* including

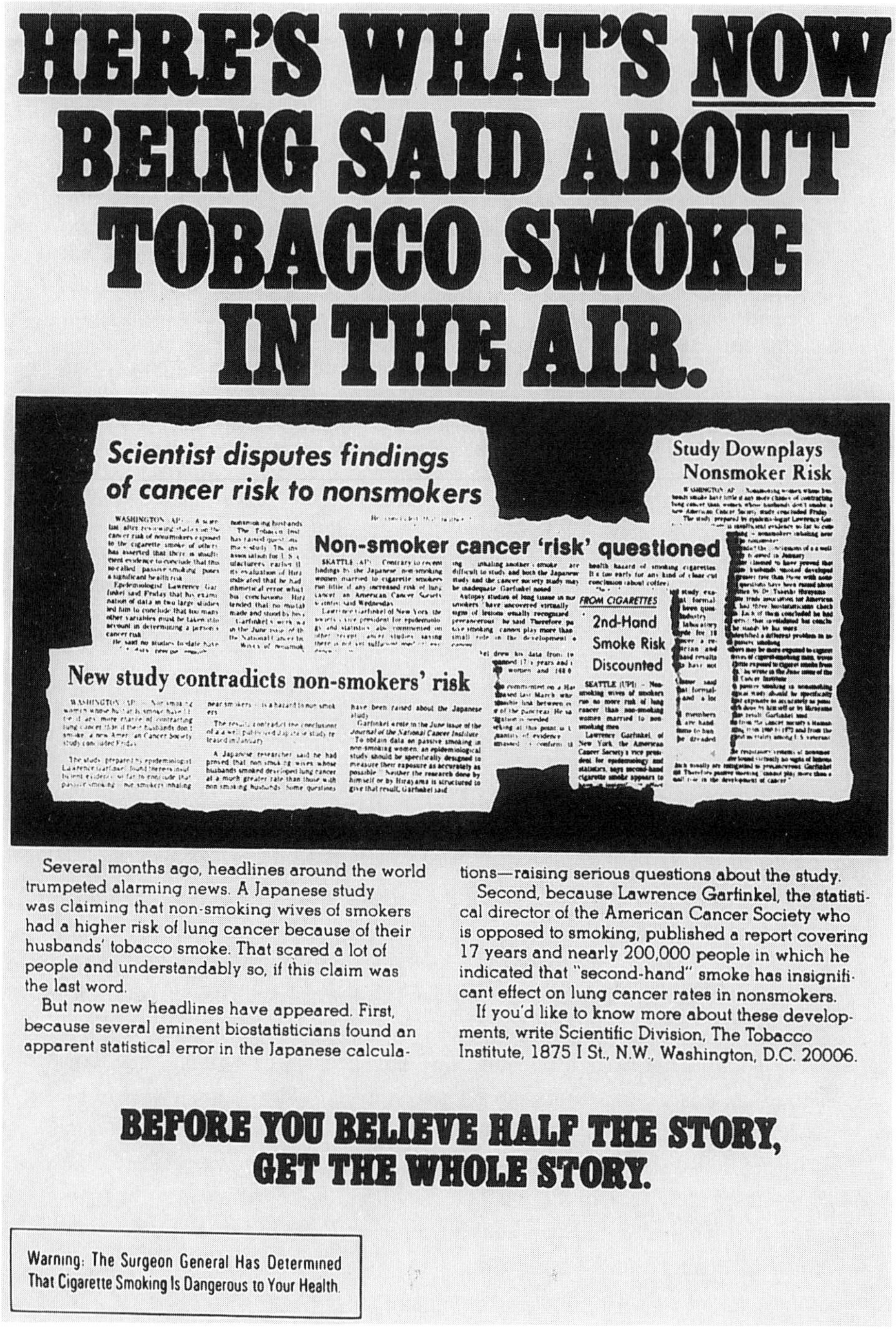

FIGURE 10.1. The Tobacco Institute ran this advertisement in newspapers and magazines all over the United States shortly after publication, in 1981, of the first scientific paper linking environmental tobacco smoke with lung cancer in nonsmokers.

Mantel's original report to the Tobacco Institute, to allow Hirayama to respond publicly to the criticisms of his work (33).

The documents show that, although the tobacco industry was publicly attacking Hirayama's paper, several of its own experts were privately admitting that his conclusions were valid. On July 24, 1981, J. K. Wells, B&W corporate counsel, wrote a memo to Ernest Pepples, B&W's vice president of law {1825.01}. The memo summarized a telephone conversation between Pepples and Tim Finnegan, an attorney with the firm of Jacob, Medinger, and Finnegan, regarding "Interesting Developments on the Hirayama Matter."

> Dr. Adlkofer, who is the Scientific Director of the German Verband [the German equivalent of CTR, see chapter 2], has committed himself to the position that Lee [presumably Peter Lee, a British statistician and tobacco industry consultant] and Hirayama are correct and Mantel and TI [Tobacco Institute] are wrong. Adlkofer called Frank Colby at Reynolds [R. J. Reynolds Tobacco Co.] and said that Germany has received new data from Japan which confirms the Hirayama work. Adlkofer and Lee and another German associate were all asked to review Hirayama's work and did not find the error picked up by Kastenbaum [a statistician at the Tobacco Institute]. *They believe Hirayama is a good scientist and that his nonsmoking wives publication was correct.* Adlkofer invited Tsokos [affiliation unknown] and Kastenbaum to Germany to view the new data, although they would not be allowed to work with it or make copies. The proposal added that after the session in Germany Tsokos, Kastenbaum, and apparently Adlkofer would proceed to Japan to visit Hirayama. Adlkofer had previously proposed four research projects to examine the Hirayama work to be done by the research arm of the Verband. At a meeting of the board of the research arm of July 15 Adlkofer was asked how he could continue to support the projects if Hirayama's work was dead. *He replied with a strong statement that Hirayama was correct, that the TI knew it and that TI published its statement about Hirayama knowing that the work was correct.* Mr. von Specht [affiliation unknown] is reported to have cut Adlkofer short. Subsequently Adlkofer told Colby that unidentified authors would publish in an unnamed publication an article claiming that Hirayama was correct and that TI published its statement while privately acknowledging Hirayama's correctness. Within a few days Adlkofer called again to say that the article was off.
>
> . . .
>
> No comment is needed on the proposal to have Kastenbaum and Tsokos visit Germany to review the Hirayama data unless you believe the visit should take place. [Horace] Kornegay [of the Tobacco Institute] gave a forceful veto of the program and as of this point there is no dissent [emphasis added]. {1825.01}

The threatened letter from Adlkofer never materialized, and the industry and its consultants have maintained a unified public position that

Hirayama's study was flawed and that the health dangers of passive smoking have not been proven. Since then, Philip Morris and R. J. Reynolds have both run a series of full-page advertisements criticizing the U.S. Environmental Protection Agency's risk assessment of environmental tobacco smoke (2) (see figures 5.2 and 5.3). The Tobacco Institute has also continued to criticize Hirayama's paper and its use by regulatory bodies such as the Environmental Protection Agency and the Occupational Health and Safety Administration (35, 36). The scientific community, however, widely regards Hirayama's work as a landmark study on the health effects of ETS, and his findings have been confirmed by several other studies showing a link between passive smoking and lung cancer (37).

This episode indicates that the tobacco industry is not committed to learning and disseminating the truth about the health effects of its products. Rather, it has consistently attempted to discredit research even when its own scientists have admitted that the research results are valid. Just as the industry has continued to deny that active smoking has been proven dangerous to health, it continues to deny that the case is proven against passive smoking.

STATE AND LOCAL EFFORTS TO REGULATE PUBLIC SMOKING

As discussed in chapter 7, during the 1960s and 1970s the tobacco industry lobbied to pass legislation limiting the federal government's authority to regulate tobacco products and preempting state and local actions aimed at protecting smokers. This legislation was ineffective, however, against government regulations designed to protect *nonsmokers*. During the 1970s the nonsmokers' rights movement emerged at the state and local levels (1). The goal of the movement was to protect nonsmokers from the effects of tobacco smoke by restricting smoking in public places.

In 1975 Minnesota became the first state to pass a Clean Indoor Air Law, which (by 1990s standards) mildly restricted where people could smoke. Tobacco control activists in California then attempted to convince the California Legislature to pass a similar bill. After failing in the Legislature, the activists (including one author of this book, Peter Hanauer) succeeded in passing a strong (for the time) nonsmokers' rights law in Berkeley. They then attempted to pass a stronger law statewide by placing it on the ballot as an initiative measure in 1978. California ballot initiatives are proposed laws that are placed on the ballot for a direct vote by the people after petitions have been collected with the signatures of a sufficient number of registered voters. The tobacco industry defeated the initiative known as Proposition 5, as well as a similar initiative, known as Proposition 10, in 1980. The documents describe in detail how the tobacco industry worked behind the scenes to defeat these initiatives, which had initially enjoyed wide public support. The description of the industry's successful strategy provides important insights—still relevant today—into how these campaigns are waged.

CALIFORNIA'S PROPOSITION 5 (1978)

Proposition 5, the California Clean Indoor Air Act of 1978, was the first attempt in the nation to pass a statewide clean indoor air law through the initiative process. Proposition 5 would have required smoking and no-smoking sections in workplaces, public places, and restaurants. The initiative petitions were circulated in late 1977 and early 1978, and the initiative was voted on in the November 1978 election. Brown and Williamson, working with the other tobacco companies, played a major role in defeating Proposition 5. In fact, the tobacco companies financed the effort to defeat Proposition 5 in direct proportion to their market shares of the California market (1).

The tobacco industry recognized the importance of the Proposition 5 campaign early in the initiative process. Since (as shown by its own polling) the industry knew that it had virtually no public credibility, it decided to act through a nominally independent campaign committee known as Californians for Common Sense (CCS). Even though CCS was created and controlled by the tobacco companies through a closely coordinated effort, it attempted to minimize and, in some respects, even hide its industry connections. The industry wanted the public to believe that CCS was a group of concerned California citizens.

Ernest Pepples wrote a detailed analysis of the industry's strategy for defeating Proposition 5 in a report dated January 11, 1979. Pepples's report summarizes the campaign from the industry's point of view and provides important insights into the organization and structure of the industry's campaign as well as the strategies employed.

> Two decisions made in 1977 account for the victory that was achieved on November 7, 1978:
>
> (1) The commitment by five major cigarette manufacturers to participate in a program of early planning and research.
>
> (2) The commitment by these companies to provide early and adequate financing for the project.

The foregoing decisions were made before the terms of Proposition 5 were
even known or concepts to combat it had been developed. Because of the early
start a California Action Plan was presented to the chief executive officers
within three weeks of the time the sponsors filed their "Clean Indoor Air Act"
initiative and its provisions became known for the first time. That Action Plan
became the basic blue print of the campaign concepts, strategy, organization
and tactics for the entire campaign to defeat Proposition 5. The Tobacco Institute made Jack Kelly a full time employee—he had been the paid executive
of California's tobacco distributors group—to devote all his efforts to the
campaign [emphasis added]. {2302.05, p. 1}

The tobacco companies' sponsorship of the CCS campaign is indicated
by a memo dated February 15, 1978, from Pepples to the managers of
B&W's major cigarette brands. Pepples stated that the industry had formed
a campaign committee called Californians for Common Sense, Inc., to run
the campaign against Proposition 5, and asked the brand managers to
give him the names of any people they knew in California who could be
recruited to participate in the campaign {2301.01}. This active role of the
tobacco companies contrasts sharply with the industry's public position
during the campaign: that Proposition 5 was a local California matter
and that Californians for Common Sense was a campaign organization
established by local citizens as a free-standing, autonomous organization. The tobacco industry's approach contrasted sharply with that of
national voluntary health organizations, which did, in fact, stand back
and treat Proposition 5 as a local California matter.

Pepples's "Campaign Report" continues:

The first step was to form a California-based campaign organization, Californians for Common Sense.
    The concept: A broad based citizen membership, operating under the bi-
partisan co-chairmanship of prominent and respected Californians who had
no past or present connection with the tobacco industry. That the proponents
would attack the presence of tobacco money in the campaign was obvious.
The answer was a non-tobacco organization with leadership so prestigious
and membership so broad that its composition clearly belied the charge that
only the tobacco companies opposed Proposition 5. {2302.5, pp. 1–2}

Although the tobacco industry sought local people to appear on behalf
of the campaign, control rested firmly with the tobacco companies. In
addition, in contrast to most initiative campaigns, the nominal local leaders were not required to contribute their own money or raise money. Like
all campaigns involving the tobacco industry since then, more than 99
percent of the money came from the industry itself (1).

The industry conducted benchmark surveys in December 1977 and January 1978 which showed that the "vote no" side was a staggering underdog: California voters favored smoking restrictions by 68 percent to 24 percent {2302.05, p. 2}. Overcoming this significant voter deficit was the essence of the industry's (ultimately) successful plan. Indeed, the tobacco industry started its research well before the initiative had even qualified for the ballot; Pepples's "Campaign Report" states:

> The first Tarrance data [from the tobacco industry's pollster V. Lance Tarrance and Associates of Houston, Texas] came in *June 1977*. It showed that more than 82% of the electorate approved the idea of a new state law requiring smoking and nonsmoking sections in public places.
>
> . . .
>
> *The same survey showed that the California voters' perception of the tobacco industry's credibility was very low.* It removed all doubts that this campaign had to be a [*sic*] California-grounded, with the Tobacco Institute as far in the background as possible and with tobacco industry involvement limited to financial contributions to a California citizens committee [emphasis added]. {2302.05, p. 10}

As soon as Californians for Common Sense was established, the tobacco industry began an active campaign for securing local endorsement, with particular emphasis on union leadership.

> Perhaps the most significant achievement during this period was the amazing sign-up of California labor leaders first as individuals and later with official anti–Proposition 5 positions by their trade union organizations. Brown & Williamson's labor relations group, especially C. H. Teague and C. R. Baumgardner and Wilson Wyatt in Corporate Affairs, encouraged the TWIU [Tobacco Workers International Union] and other labor organizations to get in touch with labor officials in California on behalf of the NO-On-5 position. Lorillard and Philip Morris were similarly active in rounding up labor support. {2302.05, p. 3}

Having the union leadership on their side proved to be of tremendous benefit to the tobacco industry, not only because it gave the campaign an air of legitimacy but also because the union's connections in Democratic party politics were useful in neutralizing efforts to get prominent politicians to support the initiative. In particular, then-governor Jerry Brown was persuaded to take a neutral position on the initiative through the efforts of people in the union movement {2302.05}. The tobacco industry also used the industry's mailing lists of customers to provide direct mail access to smokers in the state {2302.05}. This technique was expanded in later years as part of the effort to develop the smokers' rights movement (25).

The tobacco industry knew that, since it had very low public credibility, identification of the industry with the No-on-5 campaign would hurt it. Thus, it established several important guiding principles to keep its profile as low as possible. In his description of how the tobacco industry defeated Proposition 5, Pepples lists these guiding principles:

> All campaign functions would be operated through the citizens committee, Californians for Common Sense.
>
> Tobacco company visibility would be confined to financial contributions to CCS. There would be no attempt to disclaim or discount the amount of tobacco contribution.
>
> Tobacco company personnel would not make campaign appearances, occupy campaign positions or make public statements relative to the campaign.
>
> No campaign events, programs or advertising would be directed to college campuses, specifically, or to youth in general. {2302.05, p. 8}

Although Pepples says that "there would be no attempt to disclaim or discount the amount of tobacco contribution," the tobacco industry kept a low profile during the campaign and campaign spokesmen denied the industry's role until campaign disclosure statements proved that the industry was financing the campaign. On one occasion CCS issued a press release that misstated the amount of tobacco industry contributions to the campaign by leaving out approximately $270,000 of in-kind campaign contributions (38, 39).

The documents make it clear, however, that the tobacco companies maintained tight control of CCS activities from behind the scenes. Pepples's "Campaign Report" notes,

> Extreme caution was exercised in preparation of the publicity. *Company legal counsel approved all releases prior to dispatch* [emphasis added]. {2302.05, p. 17}

In addition, high-level tobacco industry officials maintained contact with CCS throughout the campaign:

> A group of 5 tobacco company representatives consisting of Jim Dowdell who was succeeded by Charles Tucker from RJR, Ed Grefe from Philip Morris, Arthur Stevens from Lorillard, Joe Greer from Liggett & Myers and Ernest Pepples from B&W kept in constant contact with the operation of CCS. Visits were made at least once a month by the group to the CCS headquarters in both San Francisco and Los Angeles. Also frequent telephone conferences were held between Woodward & McDowell [the firm hired to manage the campaign] and the five company people. During the final month of the cam-

paign, almost daily conferences were held by telephone including Woodward
& McDowell and Jack Kelly together with Lance Tarrance [the pollster] in
Houston conferring with the five company representatives. Occasionally it
was necessary for the five company people to meet to iron out differences. At
one point, for example, Reynolds insisted on launching a campaign to deal
affirmatively with the nonsmoker issue in newspaper advertising. This was a
clear deviation from the California Action Plan as originally submitted to the
company CEO's. The RJR proposal was contrary to the advice of the professional campaign advisors who had been employed in California. RJR finally retreated from its insistence on a separate campaign.

> . . .

> As a rule, however, the injection of company views into the operation of
> the campaign was kept to a minimum, *while at all times retaining in the com-*
> *panies complete control over legal approval both as to advertising copy and*
> *general operation of the campaign* [emphasis added]. {2302.05 pp. 27–29}

Despite the tight control of the campaign by the tobacco industry, the
public face of the campaign was very different. CCS sought to present
opposition to Proposition 5 as a purely local matter involving prominent
local opposition:

> Public attention was focused on the three carefully chosen and prestigious co-
> chairmen of the Californians for Common Sense campaign:
>
> John F. Henning, Secretary Treasurer of the California Labor Federa-
> tion (AFL-CIO), a University of California regent, former U.S. Under-
> secretary of Labor, former U.S. Ambassador to New Zealand and an ac-
> tive and prominent Democrat (a nonsmoker).
>
> Houston I. Flournoy, Vice President Governmental Affairs, University
> of Southern California, former California State Controller, former mem-
> ber of the Legislature. In 1974, Republican candidate for governor (a
> heavy smoker).
>
> Katherine D. Dunlap, President of the California Council for Environ-
> mental and Economic Balance, Director of the Metropolitan Water Dis-
> trict of Southern California, a prominent civic leader and conservationist
> (a nonsmoker). {2302.05, pp. 13–14}

The campaign that the tobacco industry ran against Proposition 5 was
to become the industry's classic three-phase approach to tobacco control measures, whether at the local or state level, which is still in use today. Pepples continues:

> (1)   First phase program was to redefine the enemy. The enemy CCS selected
> is the foe of every voter. He passes stupid laws, wastes billions of taxpayer
> dollars, contributes nothing useful, dreams up useless initiatives. He is ubiq-
> uitous and he is obnoxious. Who is he? To take a small liberty with the im-
> perishable wisdom of Pogo "We has met the enemy, and they is <u>They</u>" Phase
> one: "<u>They're at it again!</u>"

(2)   Phase two sharpened the picture of the enemy, defined him more narrowly, crowded him into a small territory. It introduced the thought that this
kind of regulation is dangerously precedent setting. Voters were reminded
that freedom dies a bit at a time. If they regulate smoking now, what will they
regulate next? Freedom of assembly? Freedom of speech? Phase two: "What
will they regulate next?"

(3)   Third phase asked for the order. Voters had moved to our side in grati-
fying numbers but there still were many who hadn't taken the last step. They
were no longer sure that Proposition 5 was right; but still hadn't decided to
vote against it. Question, yes; conviction, no. Objective was to convert the
doubt to a No vote. It is, of course, better to show than tell—better to demonstrate than argue. CCS showed its conviction and confidence by offering to
send voters a copy of the initiative. CCS made the voter a part of the progress
[sic], suggested they read it for themselves—read the fine print—then decide.
This not only made our point, it suggested inferentially that the other side
had something to hide and CCS didn't. Phase three: "Read the fine print"
[emphasis in original]. {2302.05 pp. 33–34}

Pepples's discussion of the industry's strategy of equating the "right"
to smoke with the constitutionally guaranteed rights of assembly and
free speech is particularly ironic, given statements he had made in a memorandum only five months earlier that there is no constitutionally protected "right" to smoke and that regulating smoking is a legitimate government activity {2201.01, pp. 3–4} (see chapter 7).

The tobacco industry made the cost of implementing the initiative—
primarily the posting of signs and the expenses of enforcement—a piv-
otal issue in the campaign. The supporters of Proposition 5 had obtained
a copy of an industry-funded poll showing that there was a direct relationship between this cost and the percentage of people who would vote
against the measure. Specifically, the poll indicated that a majority of voters would vote "no" if the costs were to exceed $60 million (1). A con-
sulting firm hired by the tobacco industry, San Francisco–based Economic
Research Associates, produced a study concluding that implementation
of the initiative would cost $63 million. The proponents of the initiative,
who had also obtained a copy of the calculations used to reach this conclusion, discovered an arithmetic error in the calculations that, when corrected, reduced the actual projected cost to only a few thousand dollars.
Although the proponents attempted to publicize the error to undercut the
industry's cost claims, as Pepples noted, the industry successfully shifted
the debate into terms favorable to itself {2302.05}.

The tobacco industry's polling showed that the issues of health in general and secondhand smoke in particular were dangerous ones for the

industry. It therefore worked very hard to steer the campaign away from these questions and was largely successful at doing so.

> The Tarrance [polling firm] tracking showed that it was not necessary to change our game plan; the health issue and the nonsmoker issue had not become dominant. Indeed the best issue for the Yes side was not health, despite the strong propaganda push by ACS and the lung and heart associations. Only 25% of those favoring the Yes position cited Health as their reason for voting Yes. The best issue for the Yes side was Smoke Bothers (50%). Tobacco smoke is seen by persons in the Smoke Bothers category as a nuisance and as an annoying invasion of their "life space". {2302.05, p. 36}

At the same time, the industry realized that the health effects of passive smoking might be introduced as an issue:

> Lance Tarrance's organization kept a close watch on the effect of the pro-5 advertising. If other people's smoke became a dominant issue in the closing days of the campaign, we had an alternate ad campaign which was prepared and kept in the can in case it was needed. It had been tested in Madison, Wisconsin. It was based on work done by BBD&O [Batten, Barton, Durstine, and Osborne, an advertising firm with long-standing tobacco accounts]. The testing at Madison showed no perceptible improvement in attitudes about "other people's smoke," but it seemed to be bombproof. {2302.05, p. 35}

These advertisements were never needed.

Nevertheless, the industry did make use of a number of physicians to contest the evidence that passive smoking is a cause of disease.

> Also we furnished witnesses such as Dr. Cosentino, who appeared before a legislative hearing that had been stimulated by the proponents of Proposition 5. Also Dr. Albert H. Niden was prevailed on to write a piece for the *Los Angeles Times* opinion page. It appeared on Sunday, October 29, 1978 in opposition to a similar article by Dr. Luther L. Terry [former Surgeon General; responsible for first report on smoking and health]. Niden's comment was simply "little is known about the effects, if any, of ambient tobacco smoke on people suffering from lung disease." In short the nonsmoker issue has not been conclusively decided. What little is available does not support the claims by the anti-cigarette lobby. This was in direct contradiction to the wild statements by Luther Terry. {2302.05, pp. 35–36}

At the time, in radio debates with one of the authors (Glantz), Dr. Cosentino denied that he had any financial involvement with the tobacco industry and stated that his testimony was based on his views as a libertarian and physician concerned about the misrepresentation of science. The documents show that he was paid an estimated $2,500 for "preparation of statement re: public smoking" by the tobacco industry through its special accounts, although the date of payment is not specified (table 8.1). Similarly, Dr. Niden was paid on several occasions (the documents show no dates) through the industry's special accounts to prepare testimony on smoking-related issues. Niden's quote is typical of the way in which the tobacco industry spokesmen muddied the issue by carefully constructing restrictive clauses: he stated that little was known about the effects of ETS "on people suffering from lung disease," implying that lung disease was the only disorder associated with exposure to ETS. He did not mention what was known about the effects of ETS on other diseases or the implications of the weight of scientific evidence when examined as a whole.

Pepples's "Campaign Report" also notes the weaknesses of the pro–Proposition 5 campaign:

> The reaction of the proponents was belligerent. They falsely accused Californians for Common Sense of deceit and misrepresentation. They challenged the accuracy of the cost estimates—with a variety of conflicting versions of their own. Their unfounded accusations influenced some broadcast station managers to remove certain of our spots. Most of them did so temporarily. Once the backup material supporting the claims was presented, the spots were allowed to resume. In presenting the backup for our claims, CCS took the opportunity to point out that the stations were offering free time for ACS and lung association PSA's [public service announcements] which were clearly pro-Proposition 5. As a result, several stations declined to continue running the PSA's until after November 7.
>
> But most importantly the proponents abandoned their own battleground and came to fight on the battleground staked out by CCS.
>
> The attacks by the opposition were troublesome and presented many concerns and additional work burdens on the campaign management and its legal defenses. They were major problems but in most cases they were overcome.
>
> As troublesome as these battles were it meant that the proponents of Proposition 5 were now on CCS' turf arguing about the amount of costs, the degree of infringement, the technicalities of arrests and fines and trying to explain away such ridiculous inconsistencies as the Proposition's exemption of rock concerts and the smoking prohibition it would impose during jazz concerts in the same auditorium. {2302.05, pp. 5–6}

Pepples also notes that the tobacco industry had considered the long term as well as the short term when it planned the campaign.

> On another occasion, Woodward & McDowell [the political campaign management firm that ran the day-to-day operations of the No-on-5 campaign] very much wanted to carry a theme in the advertising which was a parody on the legislature. The opinion surveys indicated that the voters currently hold the legislature in very low esteem. The proponents had begun to respond to

our original message that this was a bad law, poorly drafted. They conceded that it had some flaws but said not to worry, the legislature will take care of any flaw by amendment. Woodward & McDowell, therefore, urged a direct attack on the legislature to take advantage of the negative voter attitudes toward the legislature and to crowd the proponents into a corner. *The companies differed in their reaction but after internal discussion, it was agreed that the tobacco industry must live with the California legislature for years to come and should not damage its relations by supporting advertising which made fun of the legislature* [emphasis added]. {2302.05, p. 28}

This caution proved to be a wise move, since the California Legislature consistently supported the tobacco industry on a wide range of issues in succeeding years (40, 41).

Although the tobacco industry won the battle over the Proposition 5 campaign, Pepples notes in his report that the industry has not necessarily won the war:

Indeed the findings of the post-election survey indicate that a majority of California voters would still approve smoking regulations that they consider reasonable.

After election surveys show that 71% of the electorate say they would support "some regulation" of smoking in public places. Those who would stand for "no restrictions" numbered only 26%. Those numbers are not greatly different from the early 68–24 reading taken in 1977 and in January 1976. {2302.05, p. 40}

The report points to the need for a more active role in the Legislature to protect the tobacco industry's interests:

In California there has been little legislative equity of the type available to the tobacco industry. Strong personal relationships with legislators developed over the years by the companies were beneficial but should be reinforced more realistically in California and in other states where the industry may face problems. {2302.05, p. 41}

Passive smoking, Pepples realizes, is an ongoing issue that requires addressing, albeit carefully:

In the post-election survey 72% of the voters agreed with the belief that secondhand smoke is "hazardous" to nonsmokers; only 16% disagreed.

A measurement of the voting citizens who believe that secondhand smoke can "cause disease" in nonsmokers continues to be discouraging:

Agree 49%

Disagree 31%

Not Sure 21%

Perhaps the industry should consider a program of public education in hope of shifting this ratio of misconception.

Any program, however, must be cautiously designed and should be tested in selected markets before being applied nationally. The lesson of California is that such a program must never be part of—or coincide with—an election campaign in which smoking regulation is an issue. *Credibility will be diminished or destroyed in a competitive atmosphere of a political campaign* [emphasis added]. {2302.05, p. 42}

The fact that the tobacco industry viewed Proposition 5 as a potentially serious economic threat is underscored in a letter sent from Pepples to Jack S. Swaab of BAT on January 23, 1979 {2302.01}. Pepples notes that he is sending Swaab a copy of his report on the Proposition 5 campaign in response to Swaab's request.

We ask that you maintain the strictest sort of confidence for this report because it does contain our battle plan. {2302.01, p. 1}

Pepples clearly recognized that the financial stakes for the tobacco industry were very high in the Proposition 5 campaign. In the letter he attempts to quantify the effects of the initiative and to justify the expenses the industry paid to defeat it:

Although it is obviously conjectural to try to quantify the results of [B&W'S] expenditures [of over $1 million to defeat Proposition 5], we have looked at it from several points of view. . . .

If it is assumed that the passage of Proposition 5 would have caused a decline in volume of just one cigarette per California smoker per day, the chart attached to this letter shows the industry would have suffered an after tax loss equal to $5.9 million in the first year. On that basis, it can be said that the industry [which spent $6.6 million to defeat the proposition] will recover its "investment" over a period of one year. If it is assumed that the passage of Proposition 5 would have caused a decline of 2 cigarettes per day per smoker, then the industry can expect to recover the $5.9 million expense in only 6 months.

California represents about 10% of the population of the United States or 20 million people. *California is regarded as a trendsetter and theoretically if Proposition 5 had passed it would have had an impact on sales elsewhere in the United States.*

. . .

A University of California study reported that the volume decline from the passage of Proposition 5 in California would be in the 15–20% range due to inconvenience. At 15% the annual incremental after-tax loss by the industry would be $24.6 million, and at 20% it would be $32.4 million. The 15–20% range translates into 4–6 fewer cigarettes per day per California smoker. In the 4–6 range, the payback period is less than three months. Limited strictly to the cigarette market in California, if Proposition 5 had resulted in a decline of 1–6 cigarettes, the industry can be said to recover its costs for preventing that loss within 1–12 months' time [emphasis added]. {2302.01, pp. 2–3}

Ironically, the University of California report used by Brown and Williamson for its analysis was written by Stanton Glantz, one of the authors of this book, as part of material prepared to analyze the potential costs and benefits of Proposition 5. While the health community may have been slow to recognize the economic impact of smoking restrictions, the tobacco industry was acutely aware of how much even a small decline in smoking would affect its profits.

The Proposition 5 campaign also provided evidence that smokers could be motivated to vote for the industry's political and economic interests. At the beginning of the campaign, before the tobacco industry's massive advertising campaign, most smokers supported the initiative. However, the tobacco industry was successful in its attempt to sway them. In his letter to Swaab, Pepples observes:

> Close to 90% of the smokers who voted on Proposition 5 voted against its enactment. They stood up against a restriction on their smoking pleasure. The opinion sampling indicates that *smokers were in fact quite enthusiastic in support of the position of Californians for Common Sense* [that Proposition 5 represented unnecessary government intrusion].
>
> This contrasts with the pre-campaign mood which even among a majority of smokers was solidly in favor of restricting public smoking. Verbatims [comments?] from the early public opinion surveys had the *smokers saying that Proposition 5 might help them quit or cut back and for that reason, at that early point in time, they expected to vote for it.*
>
> As the campaign progressed and as these smokers heard the messages which Californians for Common Sense put on radio and television, the attitudes of the smokers toward the right to smoke in public underwent a favorable change. Verbatims from focus groups held toward the end of the campaign demonstrated that smokers became much less defensive in the sessions and would actually pull out their packages of cigarettes and proudly display them on the conference table. *The health issue was never addressed in the "Vote NO" messages; they raised instead the basic economic and freedom issues. It is possible to theorize, therefore, that in addition to avoiding a negative sales impact from the legislative restrictions which Proposition 5 would have represented, the industry may have achieved a positive effect among smokers in support of their custom of smoking* [emphasis added]. {2302.01, pp. 2–3}

Since that time, the tobacco industry has continued to use this strategy, not only to oppose local and state clean indoor air laws but also in its attacks on the efforts of the federal Occupational Safety and Health

Administration to regulate passive smoking in the workplace and the Food and Drug Administration to regulate cigarettes and smokeless tobacco products as drug delivery devices.

The Proposition 5 campaign was only the first in a large number of initiative and referendum measures throughout the country, most notably in California, Colorado, and Florida, in which the tobacco industry became intimately involved. Just as in the Proposition 5 campaign, the industry usually formed local campaign committees with names designed to mask industry involvement. For example, in an effort to defeat a ballot measure in Dade County, Florida, the industry formed an organization named "Floridians Against Increased Regulation," or "FAIR" for short.

Tobacco industry executives appear to have expected that initiatives similar to Proposition 5 would be proposed in other localities. A memo from B. D. Cummins [affiliation unknown] to a group of tobacco industry lawyers and executives, dated August 24, 1979, suggests that money be set aside for voter referendums (a term sometimes used synonymously with "initiatives"):

> [A]n amount of $500,000 should be budgeted for "Smoking Voter Referendum" and included in General Corporate as a separate line item. This is budgeted for any state or city referendums on smoking that may come up in 1980. {1503.12}

It is possible that the tobacco companies were already aware that tobacco control activists were planning to sponsor another initiative to restrict smoking in California, Proposition 10.

CALIFORNIA'S PROPOSITION 10 (1980)

In 1980 the same people who had sponsored Proposition 5 made a second attempt to pass a statewide initiative to restrict smoking in workplaces, public places, and restaurants. This initiative was known as Proposition 10. While the documents do not contain the same kind of detailed analysis of the Proposition 10 campaign as the Proposition 5 campaign, one interesting document illustrates how the industry approaches scientific research implicating secondhand smoke as a cause of disease in nonsmokers.

In 1980, when Proposition 10 was before the voters, an important paper on the health effects of secondhand smoke, by James R. White and Herman F. Froeb (42), was published in the *New England Journal of*

Medicine. The paper demonstrated that nonsmokers working in smoky offices have pulmonary function similar to that of light smokers. This study represented the first medical evidence that workplace exposure to secondhand smoke could impair lung function in otherwise healthy non-smoking adults. On October 7, 1980, Californians Against Regulatory Excess (CARE), the tobacco industry's organization that ran the campaign against Proposition 10, issued a statement to the press criticizing the White and Froeb paper.

> This publication of White and Froeb has aroused new activity by the proponents of legislation and regulation aimed at restricting smoking in public places. This activity has occurred despite the many defects in the study and widespread criticism of the study by members of the medical and scientific communities. {2303.02}

The CARE statement drew heavily on an editorial comment by Claude Lenfant and Barbara Liu of the National Heart, Lung and Blood Institute that had accompanied the White and Froeb publication in the *New England Journal of Medicine*. The editorial (43) had stated:

> [T]he evidence that passive smoking in a general environment has health effects remains sparse, incomplete, and sometimes unconvincing. Yet the dearth of scientific data has not prevented this issue from becoming the focus of major debates that have resulted in national and local legislative actions. These actions, in turn, have reinforced the endless conflict between the rights of smokers and those of nonsmokers. {2303.02, p. 2}

The CARE press release then asserts that many authorities have criticized the study:

> Much criticism and many doubts about the study methods utilized and conclusions reached by White and Froeb have been voiced in letters to the *New England Journal of Medicine*. {2303.02, p. 3}

The authors of the criticisms included Franz Adlkofer, Gary Huber, Allan P. Freedman, Domingo Aviado, Michael Halberstam, and George E. Schafer (a former Surgeon General of the Air Force and a self-identified consultant to the Tobacco Institute). As table 8.1 shows, Huber and Aviado received funding through the industry's special projects division. Aviado was paid $85,000 for a CTR special project from 1977 to 1978 and also received $675,500 as a consultant through Special Account 4 from 1981 to 1990. Huber received "computer and staff expenses" through a Shook, Hardy, and Bacon consultancy. Except for Schafer, none of this information was disclosed at the time. Adlkofer works at the German

Verband, which conducts activities similar to the Tobacco Institute and the Council for Tobacco Research.

CARE's press release also directs ad hominem attacks against White, suggesting that White's research was biased because he had volunteered to work in favor of the Proposition 5 and 10 campaigns.

> White's extreme anti-smoking statements reveal his bias against smoking. ("When children are playing ball in the Little League, smoking parents should not be allowed within 50 yards of them.")
>
>   Dr. White, besides his involvement on the pro-Proposition 5 campaign in 1978, is a member of the Campaign Support Committee of Californians for Smoking & No Smoking Sections (the pro-Proposition 10 people) and appeared with Paul Loveday, the campaign chairman, at the news conference announcing the initiative drive. This "political" involvement may affect the objectivity necessary in science. {2303.02, pp. 11–12}

CARE's statement also included general comments from Dr. Hiram T. Langston, Duncan Hutcheon, Edwin R. Fisher, Suzanne Knoebel, and John Salvaggio criticizing the evidence that passive smoking is dangerous. All these individuals received money through the industry's special accounts (table 8.1).

Attacks on the White and Froeb study were not limited to the California campaign. A memo dated July 24, 1981, from J. K. Wells, B&W corporate counsel, to Ernest Pepples notes that a letter criticizing White has been sent to a member of Congress:

> [Dr. Michael] Liebowitz has sent Congressman [Charlie] Rose [D-NC] an extensive and hardhitting letter very critical of James White. It is not clear whether the letter can be used by the industry in the present posture of the situation. {1825.01}

"The situation" might refer to a National Academy of Sciences report (44), completed for the EPA, urging increased restrictions on smoking in public buildings.

Proposition 10 was defeated in 1980. Nevertheless, the tobacco industry realized that the issue of secondhand smoke was here to stay. Five years later, in 1985, the "B&W Public Issues Environment" memorandum views the growth of smoking restrictions as a threat to the industry and predicts that smokers will probably support these restrictions.

> *Large numbers of local governments will adopt smoking restrictions which require segregation of smokers in indoor areas with public access and government office buildings.* A substantial number of restrictions will apply to

office areas and a growing number will apply to factories. A minority of the restrictions will virtually prohibit smoking, with the severity and incidence of restrictions varying by geographical region. The trend of private businesses to adopt smoking restrictions and cessation programs for employees will accelerate. The Federal government will adopt tight smoking restrictions for its offices. The insurance industry will broaden the application of nonsmoker discounts, which will appear as a feature of health care plans. *Few smokers will complain about these events and the press will continue to publish assessments that smoking restrictions are seen by all parties concerned as working well* [emphasis added]. {2228.02, p. 3}

To put this memorandum in perspective, in November 1983 the tobacco industry had just suffered its first defeat in a ballot measure when the voters in San Francisco approved Proposition P, a referendum that ratified a city ordinance requiring employers to provide smoke-free areas for nonsmoking employees in office workplaces (45). The victory was accomplished despite an expenditure of $1,250,000 by the tobacco industry, including a sizable contribution from Brown and Williamson, which set a new national record for a local ballot measure. The success of Proposition P encouraged people throughout the country to work for legislation to protect nonsmokers from second-hand smoke and literally opened the door to the passage of hundreds of local laws regulating public smoking. Pepples therefore had good reason to predict that "large numbers of local governments will adopt smoking restrictions." Many of Pepples's other predictions have also since materialized. Nevertheless, the tobacco industry has continued to oppose controls on smoking in the workplace and public places with increasing intensity.

THE NEW JERSEY SANITARY CODE

The documents provide a small glimpse of one tobacco industry effort in New Jersey to oppose the regulation of public smoking. When the Public Health Council of New Jersey planned hearings in October 1977 to amend the New Jersey sanitary code to restrict smoking, Brown and Williamson and the other tobacco companies, both directly and through the Tobacco Institute, organized to oppose this proposal, and worked to mobilize local groups, such as the Restaurant and Tavern Association and law enforcement associations {2300.01}. As a result of their efforts, the Public Health Council was shorn of its rule-making authority in this area, and within a few years the Legislature passed a series of weak laws with strong preemption language that prevented localities and other jurisdictions from taking action to protect nonsmokers.

CONCLUSION

Privately, B&W and BAT have conducted internal research on environmental tobacco smoke, most of which has supported the conclusion that ETS is dangerous to health. The reports from BAT's annual research conferences show that BAT has identified harmful substances in sidestream smoke, including glycoproteins and tobacco-specific N-nitrosamines. In addition, the reports imply that sidestream smoke was "biologically active," and therefore potentially carcinogenic, in BAT's laboratory tests. BAT researchers were working throughout the 1980s to develop a new cigarette that would emit less sidestream smoke.

In contrast, the documents also show that, in their public pronouncements, B&W, BAT, and the tobacco industry in general have actively sought to mislead the public about the dangers of passive smoking. BAT's conference reports state that BAT and B&W were engaged in research to "refute the evidence" that passive smoking is dangerous. In addition, US tobacco companies jointly funded "special projects" related to ETS. In at least one case, data from a special project were apparently falsified to make passive smoking appear less harmful than it actually is. Also, according to its conference reports, BAT had a policy of "no disclosure" regarding internal research on the health effects of ETS. The tobacco industry has also publicly attacked scientific research on ETS in order to "create a controversy" over the evidence that passive smoking is dangerous. In at least one case, it publicly attacked research that its own consultants had privately acknowledged was valid.

Finally, the tobacco industry has actively sought to block efforts to minimize the exposure of nonsmokers to tobacco smoke. Although the industry states publicly that it is motivated by a dedication to freedom of choice, its true motivation is maintenance of profits.

Taken together, the documents demonstrate that the tobacco industry's strategy regarding passive smoking has been virtually identical to its strategy regarding active smoking. It has privately conducted internal research, which has largely supported the evidence that passive smoking is dangerous to health, while it has publicly denied that the dangers have been proven.

TABLE 10.1 BROAD OBJECTIVES OF THE GROUP R&D PROGRAMME: SIDESTREAM RESEARCH

Main Objective	Comment	Work Area	Projects
(a) To find ways of reducing the nuisance aspects of sidestream (visibility/smell/irritation).	*Defensive and Offensive* *CAC Priority 1* While attacks on sidestream smoke represent a considerable threat to the industry, success could lead to new marketing opportunities.	05 Combustion	07 Studies of the formation of sidestream—both experimental and computer models.
	Consumer reaction to perception of 'passive' smoking is important.	06 Sidestream	01 Development of analytic methods and facilities for sample evaluation. 02 Testing and development of papers and additives that reduce sidestream emissions. 03 Development of prototype products. 04 Study of ambient smoke in rooms.
		08 Psychology and Sensory Testing	01(a) Smoker reaction. 03(a) Sensory evaluation.
		09 Smoke Taste and Flavour Improvement	07 Inclusion of flavour in sidestream smoke.
		13 Novel Cigarette Making Technology	01 Novel products.
		15 Chemical Test Method Development	02(d) Analysis of constituents.
(b) To obtain scientific data to refute the alleged health risks of sidestream smoke.	Here we are concerned not only with the (small) quantity of smoke inhaled by non-smokers, but also with the biological activity of the smoke components in sidestream.	03 Nitrosamines	03 Ambient monitoring. 02 Nitrosamines in smoke.
		06 Sidestream	04 Study of ambient smoke in rooms.

SOURCE: [1180.14, pp. 03649–03650]. Emphasis in original.

REFERENCES

1. Taylor P. *The Smoke Ring: Tobacco, Money, and Multi-national Politics*. New York: Pantheon Books, 1984.
2. USEPA. *Respiratory Health Effects of Passive Smoking: Lung Cancer and Other Disorders*. Indoor Air Division, Office of Atmospheric and Indoor Programs, Office of Air and Radiation, US Environmental Protection Agency, 1992. EPA/600/6-90/006F.
3. Hirayama T. Non-smoking wives of heavy smokers have a higher risk of lung cancer: A study from Japan. *Brit Med J* 1981;282(6259):183–185.
4. Trichopoulos D, Kalandidi A, Sparros L, MacMahon B. Lung cancer and passive smoking. *Int J Cancer* 1981;27:1–4.
5. Garfinkel L. Time trends in lung cancer mortality among nonsmokers and a note on passive smoking. *J Natl Cancer Inst* 1981;66(6):1061–1066.
6. National Research Council Committee on Passive Smoking. *Environmental Tobacco Smoke: Measuring Exposures and Assessing Health Effects*. Washington, DC: National Academy Press, 1986.
7. USDHHS. *The Health Consequences of Involuntary Smoking: A Report of the Surgeon General*. US Department of Health and Human Services, Public Health Service, Centers for Disease Control, 1986. DHHS Publication No. (CDC) 87-8398.
8. Glantz, S, Parmley W. Passive smoking and heart disease. *Circulation* 1991;83:1–12.
9. Taylor A, Johnson D, Kazemi H. Environmental tobacco smoke and cardiovascular disease. A position paper from the Council on Cardiopulmonary and Critical Care, American Heart Association. *Circulation* 1992;86:1–4.
10. Gidding S, Morgan W, Perry C, et al. Active and passive tobacco exposure: A serious pediatric health problem. A statement from the Committee on Atherosclerosis and Hypertension in Children, Council on Cardiovascular Disease in the Young, American Heart Association. *Circulation* 1994;90:2582–2590.
11. Glantz S, Parmley W. Passive smoking and heart disease: Mechanisms and risks. *JAMA* 1995;273:1047–1053.
12. Roper Organization. *A Study of Public Attitudes toward Cigarette Smoking and the Tobacco Industry in 1978*. Vol. 1. Roper Organization, 1978.
13. Russell M, Cole P, Brown E. Absorption by non-smokers of carbon monoxide from room air polluted by tobacco smoke. *Lancet* 1973;1(803):576–579.
14. Cuddeback J, Donovan J, Burg W. Occupational aspects of passive smoking. *Am Industr Hyg Assoc J* 1976;37(5):263–267.
15. Brunnemann K, Yu L, Hoffman D. Assessment of carcinogenic volatile N-nitrosamines in tobacco and in mainstream and sidestream smoke from cigarettes. *Cancer Res* 1977;37(9):3218–3222.
16. Brunnemann K, Hoffman D. Chemical studies on tobacco smoke LIX. Analysis of volatile nitrosamines in tobacco smoke and polluted indoor environments. *IARC Sci Publ* 1978;19:343–356.
17. Becker C, Dubin T, Wiedemann H. Hypersensitivity to tobacco antigen. *Proc Natl Acad Sci* 1976;73(5):1712–1716.
18. Becker C, Dubin T. Activation of factor XII by tobacco glycoprotein. *J Exp Med* 1977;146:457–467.
19. Becker C, Levi R, Zavecz J. Induction of IgE antibodies isolated from tobacco leaves and from cigarette smoke condensate. *Am J Pathol* 1979;96(1):249–255.
20. Altman L. Tobacco protein viewed as link to heart disease. *New York Times* 1977 September 18:29.
21. Hoffman D, Brunnemann K, Adams J, Hecht S. Formation and analysis of N-nitrosamines in tobacco products and their endogenous formation in consumers. *IARC Sci Publ* 1984;57:743–762.

22. Hoffmann, D, Brunnemann K, Prokopczyk B, Djordjevic M. Tobacco-specific N-nitrosamines and Areca-derived N-nitrosamines: Chemistry, biochemistry, carcinogenicity, and relevance to humans. *J Toxicol Environ Health* 1994;41:1–51.

23. Tobacco-specific N-nitrosamines (TSNA): Papers presented at the 15th International Cancer Congress in Hamburg, Germany, August 1990. *Crit Rev Toxicol* 1991;21(4): 235–313.

24. Guerin M, Jenkins R, Tomkins B. *The Chemistry of Environmental Tobacco Smoke: Composition and Measurement.* Ann Arbor, MI: Lewis Publishers, 1992.

25. Samuels B, Glantz S. The politics of local tobacco control. *JAMA* 1991;226: 2110–2117.

26. Cardador TM, Hazan AR, Glantz SA. Tobacco industry smokers' rights publications: A content analysis. *Am J Pub Health* 1995;85:1212–1217.

27. Barnes DE, Bero LA. Industry-funded research and conflict of interest: An analysis of research sponsored by the tobacco industry through the Center for Indoor Air Research. *J Health Politics Policy Law* 1995; in press.

28. Turner S, Cyr L, Gross A. The measurement of environmental tobacco smoke in 585 office environments. *Environ Int* 1992;18(1):19–28.

29. Levy D. Smoking data tampered with, researchers say. *USA Today* 1994 Nov 2:D1.

30. Tobacco firms called data fakers. *San Francisco Chronicle* 1994 December 21:A3.

31. Subcommittee on Health and the Environment. *Environmental Tobacco Smoke Investigation: Exhibits.* Subcommittee on Health and the Environment, Committee on Energy and Commerce, U.S. House of Representative, 1994.

32. Levin M. Who's behind the building doctor? *The Nation* 1993 August 9/16:168–171.

33. Levy D. Struggling to clear the air on tobacco. *USA Today* 1994 October 12:A1.

34. Editor. Correspondence: Non-smoking wives of heavy smokers have a higher risk of lung cancer. *Brit Med J* 1981;283:914–917.

35. Glantz S. Tobacco industry response to the scientific evidence on passive smoking. In *Proceedings of the Fifth World Conference on Tobacco and Health, 1983* (pp. 287–292). Winnipeg: Canadian Council on Smoking and Health, 1983.

36. Glantz S, Parmley W. Dissent: Passive smoking causes heart disease and lung cancer. *J Clin Epidemiol* 1992;45(8):815–819.

37. Fontham E, Correa P, Reynolds P, et al. Environmental tobacco smoke and lung cancer in nonsmoking women: A multicenter study. *JAMA* 1994;271(22):1752–1759.

38. Burns, J. Millions given to defeat Prop. 5. *San Francisco Chronicle* 1978 October 3:8.

39. Campaign Finance Statement filed by Californians for Common Sense, September 30, 1978.

40. Traynor M, Begay M, Glantz S. New tobacco industry strategies to prevent local tobacco control. *JAMA* 1993;270:479–486.

41. Glantz S, Begay M. Tobacco industry campaign contributions are affecting tobacco policymaking in California. *JAMA* 1994;272:1176–1183.

42. White J, Froeb H. Small airways and dysfunction in nonsmokers exposed chronically to tobacco smoke. *N Engl J Med* 1980;302:720–723.

43. Lenfant C, Liu B. (Passive) smokers versus (voluntary) smokers (editorial). *N Engl J Med* 1980;302:742.

44. National Research Council. *The Airliner Cabin Environment: Air Quality and Safety.* Washington DC: National Academy Press, 1986.

45. Hanauer P. Proposition P: Anatomy of a nonsmokers' rights ordinance. *NY State J Med* 1985;85:369–374.

CHAPTER 11

Where Do We Go from Here?

The industry has retreated behind impossible demands for
"scientific proof" whereas such proof has never been required
as a basis for action in the legal and political fields.

> *Dr. S. J. Green, head of BAT research and*
> *development and a member of the BAT board,*
> *1976 {2231.08, p.1}*

The Brown and Williamson documents reveal that the tobacco industry
has been amazingly successful in protecting its ability to market an addictive product that kills its customers in epidemic numbers. In 1989 tobacco killed 420,000 smokers and 53,000 nonsmokers in the United
States alone (figure 11.1). This toll dwarfs the 20,000 deaths from illegal drugs and 40,000 deaths from AIDS. Nevertheless, at a time when
the government spends billions fighting illegal drugs and AIDS, it has yet
to mount a serious effort to control tobacco (figure 11.2).

This situation is, however, changing. In recent years there has been a
flowering of grass-roots efforts to pass clean indoor air laws, which—as
the tobacco industry feared when it successfully opposed California's
Proposition 5 in 1978—are undermining the social acceptability of
smoking and helping smokers stop. In addition, since 1987 the people
of three states—California, Massachusetts, and Arizona—have ignored
multimillion-dollar tobacco industry campaigns and enacted, by voter
initiative, tobacco tax increases tied to aggressive (and effective) tobacco
control programs. Starting in 1994 several states mounted legal action
to recover the hundreds of millions of dollars the tobacco industry costs
taxpayers in medical costs, and the private bar is organizing a new wave
of products liability lawsuits against the industry. At the federal level, in
1992 the Environmental Protection Agency firmly established that tobacco smoke is air pollution, and in 1995 the Occupational Safety and
Health Administration and the Food and Drug Administration started
regulatory action on tobacco smoke as a workplace toxin and nicotine
as an addictive drug, respectively.

US Deaths in 1989

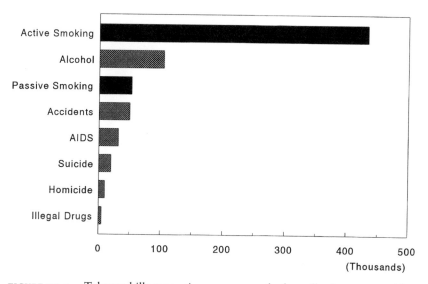

FIGURE 11.1. Tobacco kills many times more people than all other preventable causes of death. Active smoking is the leading preventable cause of death, and passive smoking is the third leading preventable cause of death (1). From S. Glantz, *Tobacco: Biology and Politics*. Waco, TX: HealthEdCo, 1992.

As promising as these efforts are, the tobacco industry is well practiced, resourceful, and highly motivated to mount a vigorous defense. The documents discussed in this book give the first clear view into the sophisticated knowledge the industry had developed—years before the general scientific community—about nicotine pharmacology and the health dangers of smoking. Moreover, they illuminate how, despite the crushing scientific evidence against tobacco, the industry has successfully mustered legal, political, and public relations talent to deny and obfuscate the science. In this effort the industry has been assisted by a small group of scientists—both inside and outside the industry—who served the industry's economic, political, and legal needs.

The role of lawyers in selecting research projects and methodologies and controlling the dissemination of results is, perhaps, the most important insight offered by the documents. The industry's increasing reliance on lawyers to manage research reveals an industry policy toward research that was adversarial and elevated advocacy over objectivity. By putting lawyers in charge of scientific research, the tobacco companies

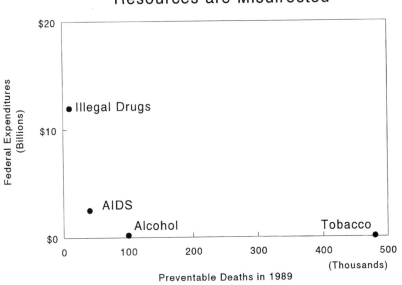

US Deaths versus Federal Expenditures
Resources are Misdirected

FIGURE 11.2. Despite causing many more deaths than illegal drugs, AIDS, or other preventable causes of death, tobacco control receives relatively little attention by the federal government (2). From S. Glantz, Actual causes of death in the United States, *JAMA* 1994;271:660.

effectively adopted a research policy that had nothing to do with finding out and disseminating the truth about the health effects of tobacco or with sponsoring truly independent research on that subject. It had everything to do with protecting the political and legal position of the industry and protecting its profits.

Lawyers were involved in decisions about what research to do and how to do it. For example, industry lawyers played a key decision-making role in the design of experiments related to cancer, such as the investigation of the additive Chemosol, which was thought to reduce the carcinogenicity of cigarette smoke. Initially, lawyer rationales favored serious research into the causation and addiction hypotheses. As the results clearly demonstrated that tobacco causes cancer and other diseases, enthusiasm for such research waned among lawyers. They seemed afraid that in-house or sponsored research would either directly confirm that smoking is addictive and causes disease or provide indirect confirmation by, for example, using methodologies that the tobacco companies would prefer to claim were unreliable. Ultimately, the lawyers made active efforts to stop research that might turn "sour," even if that research had scientific merit. Lawyers also designed elaborate procedures to prevent BAT research results from becoming "known" to B&W, so that B&W could continue to claim that it did not accept the causation and addiction hypotheses.

The tobacco companies appear to have used lawyers as part of a conscious effort to contain the dissemination of scientific information that might be adverse to the companies' economic and legal interests. Most of the documents reflecting lawyer participation in managing research were explicitly marked "confidential" or subject to attorney-client or work-product privilege. This practice had the effect of concealing the extent of lawyer participation in managing research, contrary to the industry's assurances that its support of scientific work was disinterested and subject to peer review procedures by objective scientists. It also enabled the industry to use a confidential conduit for funds provided to nominally independent outside scientists, and it enabled the industry to suppress adverse results by cloaking the work in attorney-client privilege or work-product privilege.

Finally, the documents suggest that in some instances the companies relied on lawyers to keep research results away from the United States if they had been produced by industry scientists and confirmed the causation and addiction hypotheses. The documents reveal instances in which lawyers were involved in removing documents labeled "deadwood" from company files and actually recommended that adverse data be destroyed. Such conduct is inconsistent with the companies' professed interest in the scientific truth about smoking and disease.

Just as the attitudes and roles of the lawyers evolved over the thirty years spanned in the documents, so did the roles of the scientists. In the 1960s they had frank discussions about nicotine addiction and the carcinogenic nature of cigarette smoke, and they tried to develop a cigarette that would deliver an acceptable dose of nicotine but would avoid the cancer risks caused by smoking. The scientists also focused on specific compounds, such as polycyclic aromatic hydrocarbons and phenols, as the bad actors in cigarette smoke. Their work was almost entirely scientific in nature, and there was little mention of marketing considerations.

By the late 1970s the adverse health consequences of smoking had been conceded, although efforts to make a less "biologically active" cigarette were continuing. Specifically, the scientists were trying to measure and remove or neutralize potent carcinogens, such as nitrosamines, as well as other toxins, including hydrogen cyanide and carbon monoxide, from cigarettes. This work caused real problems for the lawyers, who were worried about what to do with the more "biologically active" products. Sophisticated research continued in the areas of nicotine pharmacology and the effects of nicotine on the central nervous system. Sidestream smoke began to emerge as an issue in the early 1970s, and by the early 1980s considerable research was being conducted in this area—for instance, research related to perceptions of smoking by nonsmokers and smokers as well as research on how to make a cigarette with less visible sidestream smoke.

By the 1980s the scientists' subservience to the lawyers was complete. Before they proceeded to work in potential areas of investigation, they would check with the lawyers. The use of scientific approaches to marketing also became much more prominent.

In vigorously pursuing the development of a "safe" cigarette while at the same time continuing to market cigarettes that they knew were dangerous, cigarette company executives could say to themselves and their boards that they were doing the very best they could to do the right thing. Was this true? After all, the products they were selling and profiting from continued to cause illness and death in an enormous number of their best customers year after year after year. The January 1954 "Frank Statement" advertisement declared that the health of its customers was the industry's "paramount concern," rising above every other aspect of the business (figure 2.1). But if health really was their primary concern, the only ethical course for B&W and BAT (and, presumably, the rest of the tobacco industry)—given the scientific data available to them in the mid-1960s—would have been to withdraw their products from the market until safe ones could be reintroduced. Likewise, they would have disclosed—not withheld—their scientific results on nicotine addiction and tobacco smoke carcinogenicity to the Surgeon General's Advisory Committee in 1963.

The same dynamic continues today. In 1994 R. J. Reynolds announced a novel product called Eclipse, which, according to newspaper accounts, delivers a nicotine aerosol to the smoker together with lower levels of other toxins than cigarettes deliver in their smoke. This product, like Reynolds's Premier in the 1980s, was based on the same general technology as was developed in BAT's Project Ariel, which, in turn, grew out of research into making cigarettes safe that had been pursued in a conscientious manner by BAT in the 1960s. Does R. J. Reynolds plan to withdraw Camel, Winston, and Salem cigarettes and replace them with Eclipse? Not at all. If the industry can make a substantially less dangerous product, why does it not cease marketing the more dangerous ones that are presently being sold?

While the tobacco industry has earned the bulk of the credit—or blame—for successfully continuing to market its products over the last forty years, the role of the health and scientific community also bears comment. In 1963, the year before the original Surgeon General's report was published, there was genuine panic in the industry. The tobacco companies' executives feared that the health community would use the 1964 Surgeon General's report to force decisive government action to curb the industry. Unfortunately for public health, the feared decisive action by the health community never materialized, and the industry was allowed time to regroup and mount the effective campaign reflected in the documents. While the health community has become more active in tobacco control in recent years, it still does not devote the resources—either financial or institutional—required to achieve effective control over tobacco. The industry's efforts to create "controversy" continue to work to this day.

The documents reveal that the tobacco industry effectively manipulated the terms of debate in the scientific and legal communities in a way that led to an obsessive concern about "causality," to the exclusion of common sense. In 1976 Dr. S. J. Green, head of BAT research and development and a member of the board, wrote a thoughtful essay entitled "Cigarette Smoking and Causal Relationships," which addresses this point:

> The public position of the tobacco companies with respect to causal explanations of the association of cigarette smoking and diseases is dominated by legal considerations. In the ultimate companies wish to be able to dispute that a particular product was the cause of injury to a particular person. By repudiation of a causal role for cigarette smoking in general they hope to avoid liability in particular cases. This domination by legal consideration thus leads the industry into a public rejection in total of any causal relationship between smoking and disease and puts the industry in a peculiar position with respect to product safety discussions, safety evaluations, collaborative research, etc. Companies are actively seeking to make products acceptable as safer while denying strenuously the need to do so. To many the industry appears intransigent and irresponsible. The problem of causality has been inflated to enormous proportions. *The industry has retreated behind impossible demands for "scientific proof" whereas such proof has never been required as a basis for*

action in the legal and political fields. Indeed if the doctrine were widely adopted the results would be disastrous. I believe that with a better understanding of the nature of causality it is plain that while epidemiological evidence does indicate a cause for concern and action it cannot form a basis on which to claim damage for injury to a specific individual [emphasis added]. {2231.08, p. 1}

Green concludes with an opinion that makes the very point upon which state lawsuits seeking recovery of medical care costs are based:

> In summary, for social policy purposes it is sensible and totally relevant to use the experimental evidence pertaining to large groups and also to select the simplest hypothesis. *It may therefore be concluded that for certain groups of people smoking causes the incidence of certain diseases to be higher than it would otherwise be* [emphasis added]. {2231.08, p. 4}

It remains to be seen whether the medical, public health, legal, and political systems will muster the courage and resources to act on this fact and hold the tobacco companies accountable for the havoc their products cause.

In the meantime, every day 3,000 American children will become addicted to nicotine, and another 1,300 smokers and nonsmokers will die.

REFERENCES

1. Glantz S. *Tobacco: Biology and Politics.* Waco, TX: HealthEdCo, 1992.
2. Glantz S. Actual causes of death in the United States (letter). *JAMA* 1994;271:660.

Statements by
Brown and Williamson

Portions of chapters 1, 5, 7, 8, and 10 of this book appeared as articles in the July 19, 1995, issue of the *Journal of the American Medical Association*.[1-5] In response to a request from *JAMA* for comment on the substance of our articles,[6] Brown and Williamson issued the following statement:

June 8, 1995

BROWN AND WILLIAMSON TOBACCO CORP.
STATEMENT TO JOURNAL OF THE AMERICAN
MEDICAL ASSOCIATION

We believe there is a right way and a wrong way to deal with these documents. We refuse to be drawn into media hysteria over these stolen, attorney-client privileged documents. Despite this, it is obvious that B&W and other companies will continue to be "tried in the media" in advance of any proper forum to address these issues. Dr. Glantz has admitted cooperating with plaintiffs' attorneys and we seriously question his objectivity in addressing these issues.

It is important to remember that similar documents have been addressed in courts of law before—rather than in the news media—and juries did not buy these allegations.

Documents stolen by a person who is "out to get the company" should not be portrayed as presenting the whole story. Lifting single phrases or sentences from 30-year-old documents and using that information to distort and misrepresent B&W's position on a number of issues is clearly what is occurring.

B&W has done, and will continue to do, nothing to waive any privilege or confidentiality associated with these documents and we are taking every step necessary to preserve those rights.

We continue to believe that nicotine is not addictive because over 40 million Americans have quit smoking, 90 percent of them without any help at all. . . .

On July 12, 1995, after release of the *JAMA* papers to the media, Brown and Williamson issued the following statement:

TO BUSINESS AND MEDICAL EDITORS:
BROWN & WILLIAMSON'S STATEMENT
REGARDING AMA ARTICLE

LOUISVILLE, Ky., July 12/PRNewswire/—Brown & Williamson today issued the following statement regarding the American Medical Association's planned publication of tobacco-related JAMA articles on July 13:

The American Medical Association's planned publication of articles relating to Brown & Williamson's stolen documents is little more than a cherry-picking exercise designed to advance its stated mission to eliminate smoking.

The AMA admitted that despite its so-called scientific review, the documents addressed in the JAMA articles "could be subject to a form of selection bias." In addition, the release said that the "documents do not provide a complete picture." In fact, the AMA also stated its motive for publishing the articles. According to its own news release, "the AMA maintains an unequivocal stance against tobacco" and added later that its mission was to "force the removal of this scourge from our nation. . . ." Clearly, the JAMA articles do not represent independent scientific review.

The bottom line is that the AMA's approach to selectively present company documents advances only one agenda—that of the anti-tobacco establishment, including the plaintiffs' bar, which is involved in extensive litigation against tobacco companies. Brown & Williamson would hope to achieve a fair hearing in the court of public opinion. However, based on continued one-sided presentation of the issues, the company will continue to rely on the legal system, where the facts are presented in an impartial manner and decided by impartial juries.

The subjects addressed in JAMA, including passive smoking, lawyer involvement and nicotine, represent a rehashing of allegations previously reported at length by the news media and discussed in testimony before Congress. In addition, similar allegations have been made in previous product liability litigation, and when the full facts are presented, juries consistently have found in favor of tobacco companies.

Among the issues addressed in the JAMA articles:

Passive smoking: The AMA claims company research concluded that so-called passive smoking "is harmful to health." In fact, the University of California at San Francisco documents do not even include environmental tobacco smoke (ETS) research studies. There is nothing in the reported documents which changes Brown & Williamson's view that ETS has not been established as harmful to health.

Lawyer involvement: Even the AMA admits to its readers that "lawyers by nature are asked to evaluate proposed courses of action in terms of their legal risks." Since tobacco companies have been involved in product liability litigation for decades, it is even more "natural" that attorneys be involved in defending the company's position. Brown & Williamson's lawyers have conducted themselves appropriately.

Nicotine addiction: Scientists have yet to agree on a definition or precise set of circumstances that distinguishes a state of "addiction" from "habit" or "enjoyment." In that context, as B&W stated a year ago, when many of these same documents were attacked in Congress, none of these documents established that nicotine is addictive. The fact that 40 million people have quit smoking by themselves flies in the face of the "addiction label."

REFERENCES

1. Glantz SA, Barnes DE, Bero L, Hanauer P, Slade J. Looking through a keyhole at the tobacco industry: The Brown and Williamson documents. *JAMA* 1995;274:219–224.

2. Slade J, Bero L, Hanauer P, Barnes DE, Glantz SA. Nicotine and addiction: The Brown and Williamson documents. *JAMA* 1995;274:225–233.

3. Hanauer P, Slade J, Barnes DE, Bero L, Glantz SA. Lawyer control of internal scientific research to avoid products liability lawsuits: The Brown and Williamson documents. *JAMA* 1995;274:234–240.

4. Bero L, Barnes DE, Hanauer P, Slade J, Glantz SA. Lawyer control of the tobacco industry's external research program: The Brown and Williamson documents. *JAMA* 1995;274:241–247.

5. Barnes DE, Hanauer P, Slade J, Bero LA, Glantz SA. Environmental tobacco smoke: The Brown and Williamson documents. *JAMA* 1995;274:248–253.

6. Graham T. The Brown and Williamson documents: The company's response. *JAMA* 1995;274:254–255.

List of Available Documents

This list describes the documents that were used to write this book. Much of the material we originally received was disorganized and fragmentary. We started our analysis by attempting to match up fragments of different documents and then to assemble related documents in files. Several documents appear more than once in the document set, sometimes from different sources, with different marginal comments, or as complete and incomplete copies. While we have attempted to delete frank duplicates, there is some repetition of material. (Some of the duplicate copies differ slightly in terms of marginalia, Bates numbers, or source.) The numbering system is generally by topic and date. The bracketed descriptions are supplied by the authors.

Copies of the actual documents are deposited in the Archives and Special Collections Department of the library at the University of California, San Francisco, where they are available to the public. They are also available over the Internet at World Wide Web address http://www.library.ucsf.edu/tobacco. The library also has a CD-ROM version of the documents for sale.

LISTS (1000 SERIES)

1000.01. Master Summary for B&W Subjective Document Review. 1989.

1001.01. Definitions for the Brown and Williamson Subjective Coding Taxonomy. 1988.

1002.01. Document Control Project. 19??

1002.02. B&W Subjective Coding. 19??

1002.03. Brown and Williamson Texas Document Review. 1988.

1003.01. BATUS, B&W Industries, BATI, BATCO & Affiliates Personnel. Draft, March 17, 1989.

1003.02. Brown and Williamson Personnel. Draft, November 30, 1988.

1004.01. Advertising/Marketing Glossary. 1989.

1005.01. Chronology of Projects. 1988.

1005.02. Chronology of Projects by Name/No. 1988.

1006.01. Chronology of Brown and Williamson Smoking and Health Research. 1988.

1007.01. [Partial chronology of tobacco-related political, scientific, and media events between 1962 and 1968.] 19??

1008.01. [Briefing on history of B&W public relations activities.] 19??
1009.01. Ex-Employees of B&W (or Still Employed) Available for Trial or Deposition Significant to Witness—Local Addresses. 19??
1010.01. B&W Corporate Organizational Chart. 19??
1011.01. [People involved with Special Account 4; incomplete.] 1986.
1012.01. Personnel/Affiliation [of Tobacco Institute or Council for Tobacco Research]. As of May 27, 1988.
1013.01. Tobacco Industry Companies, Committees, and Organizations. As of May 6, 1988.
1013.02. Tobacco Industry Companies, Committees, and Organizations. 1988.
1014.01. [Organizations of interest to tobacco industry.] List, 19??
1015.01. Code Names for B&W New Products. 1988.
1016.01. Creighton A. Re: Summary for Week Ending November 18, 1988. To All Subjective Coders, 1988.
1017.01. Law Firms & Individual Attorneys for Coding for Attorney/Client Privilege. 1989.
1018.01. RD&E [abbreviations]. 19??
1019.01. Benner R. Re: Brown & Williamson Tobacco Corp. Subjective Coding Project—Cardiovascular Disease. Memo to All Subjective Coders, February 24, 1988.

HEALTH AND MEDICAL SCIENCE (1100 SERIES)

1100.01. RD 14 Smoke Group Program for Coming 12–16 Week Period. Southampton: Research & Development Establishment [R&DE], British American Tobacco Co. Ltd [BATCO], 1957.
1101.01. Farr W. Re: F & R—3. Experiment Foreign Body. Letter to T. Wade, April 8, 1959.
1102.01. McCormick A. Smoking and Health: Policy on Research. Minutes of Southampton Research Conference, 1962.
1102.02. Ellis C. The Importance of Phenols to the Health Question and Their Possible Elimination from Cigarette Smoke. Opening remarks at Southampton Research Conference, 1962.
1103.01. Wade T. Re: Report of Sir Charles Ellis to Mr. Dobson, January 3, 1964. Memo to E. Finch, January 10, 1964.
1103.02. Ellis C. [Proposing a research program to reduce cigarette toxicity through filtration.] Memo to Richard Dobson, January 3, 1964.
1104.01. Reid W. Some Aspects of the Chemistry and Biology of Tobacco Smoke. 1964.
1105.01. Griffith R. Report to Executive Committee [of a site visit to TRC Harrogate research laboratory in UK]. 1965.
1106.01. Griffith R. [Expressing concern about effects of releasing Harrogate results on public opinion and government action.] Memo to E. Finch, J. Crume, and A. Yeaman, July 19, 1965.
1107.01. *Feasibility Studies on Tissue Tests—Second Progress Report.* Southampton: R&DE, BAT. 1966. RD.434-R.
1108.01. Salerno J. Benchwork Research & Development Meeting. Minutes, December 13, 1966.
1109.01. Current Chemistry Research at Southampton. 1967.
1110.01. Griffith R. [Importance of benzpyrene versus other PAH's in Project Janus.] Memo to E. Finch, August 8, 1967.
1111.01. Sanford R. Re: Recommendation. Memo to J. Burgard, November 14, 1968.
1112.01. Green S. Research Conference Held at Hilton Head Island, S.C. Minutes, September 24, 1968.

1128.01. Massey S. *A-Chloroethers in Cigarette Smoke: Assessment Based on a Review of the Literature.* Southampton: GR&DC, BAT, 1976. RD.1378 Restricted.

1129.01. Scherbak M, Smith T. *Use of the Nitromethane Fraction Index (NMFI) as an Indicator of Biological Activity of Smoke.* Montreal: Imperial Tobacco Limited, Research & Development Division, 1977. 151.

1130.01. Browne C. [Transmitting analytical report on vapor phase analysis of tobacco smoke for selected brands.] Letter to J. Wall, Celanese Fibers Corp., January 11, 1978.

1130.02. Celenase Fibers Corp. *Gas Phase Analysis of Commercial Brands.* Celanese Fibers Corp., 1978. CLB-78-09.

1131.01. Frank M. Re: Oven Moisture vs. Nine-Day Sulfuric Acid Moisture. Memo to D. Strubel, May 10, 1978.

1132.01. Sanford R. [Avoid "dangerous" research.] Letter to A. Heard, August 18, 1980.

1133.01. [Report on the Toxicology of Eugenol.] July 20, 1982.

1134.01. Sachleben L. Re: Cadmium Changes in Stem via Lab Process/537. Memo, March 23, 1983.

1135.01. Massey E, Few G. *Tobacco Smoke Mutagenicity: The Influence of Nitrogenous Compounds. Status Report.* Southampton: GR&DC, 1983.

1136.01. Kohnhorst E. Re: Your Letter to Tom Whitehair of Feb. 19, 1985. Letter to J. Kellagher, April 26, 1985.

1137.01. Wells J. Re: BAT Science. Memo to E. Pepples, February 17, 1986.

1138.01. [Fragment of report on Project Janus.] Frankfurt: Battelle Institute, 19??

1138.02. Karbe E, Kiendl J, Königsmann G, Kramer H, Preuss W, Schmidt I, Wilkes E. *Carcinogenicity of Smoke Condensate to Mouse Skin: Experiment B1.* Frankfurt: Battelle Institute, 1973. [partial copy of {1155.01}]

1138.03. Kiendi J, Königsmann G, Kramer H. *Long-Term Skin Painting Experiment: General Report on Project "JANUS."* Frankfurt: Battelle Institute, 1970.

1138.04. Willes NE. *A Survey of the Janus Mouse Skin–Painting Experiments.* Southampton: R&DE, BAT, 1971. RD.773-R.

1138.05. Evelyn S. *Project Janus: Annual Report, 1970–71.* Southampton: BAT, 1971.

1139.01. Tobacco Institute. [Proposed response to press inquiries anticipated upon release of the Dontenwill study.] Memo, 19??

1140.01. *Sodium and Potassium Chlorates.* 19??

1140.02. *The Biological Activity of Smoke from Hallmark Cigarettes.* 19??

1141.01. [A discussion of CO uptake in lungs and tissues; incomplete document.] 19??

1142.01. Research Conference Held at Kronberg, 2nd–6th June 1969. Minutes, June 2, 1969.

1143.01. Fisher P, Newton R. *Janus Airferm Sample Anaerobic Yeast Fermentation.* Louisville: Research & Development Department, B&W, 1968? 68-12R.

1144.01. Ayres C. *Biological Testing: Short-Term Hyperplasia Test.* Southampton: BAT, 1966. B-1.

1145.01. Hofmann A. *Further Results of Work Aimed at the Development of a Goblet Cell Test.* Frankfurt: Battelle Institute, 1969. B-14.

1146.01. Horsewell H. *Evaluation of filters containing water capsules submitted for project Janus.* Southampton: R&DE, BAT, 1970. L.318-R.

1146.02. Duplicate of {1146.01}.

1147.01. Visit to Battelle Institute, 19th–22nd May, 1970.

1148.01. Partial copy of {1149.01}.

1149.01. Wilkes E. *A Survey of the Janus Mouse Skin-Painting Experiments.* Southampton: R&DE, BAT, 1971. RD.773-R.

1150.01. Chakraborty B, Thornton R. *Analysis of Janus Condensate Solutions.* Southampton: R&DE, BAT, 1971. RD.808-R.

1151.01. Kennedy J. Project Janus Status Report. Memo to J. Burgard, I. Hughes, R. Sanford, and J. Esterle, September 30, 1971.

1152.01. Karbe E, Schwaier A. *Investigation of the Mutagenic Effect of Inhaled Smoke from Two Cigarettes (B8-1, B8-3) on Mice Using the Dominant Lethal Method.* Southampton: GR&DC, BAT, 1972.

1152.02. Duplicate of {1152.01}.

1153.01. Kennedy J. Project Janus Status Report. Memo to J. Burgard, I. Hughes, R. Sanford, and J. Esterle, October 3, 1972.

1154.01. Karbe E. *The Promotion Activity of Tobacco Smoke Condensates to Mouse Skin: Cigarettes B 9-2, B 9-3, B 9-4, and B 9-5.* Southampton: GR&DC, BAT, 1972.

1155.01. Karbe E, Kiendl J, Königsmann G, Kramer H, Preuss W, Schmidt I, Wilkes E. *Carcinogenicity of Smoke Condensate to Mouse Skin, Experiment B1.* Frankfurt: Battelle Institute, 1973.

1156.01. Karbe E, Kiendl J, Königsmann G, Kramer H, Preuss W, Schmidt I, Wilkes E. *Carcinogenicity of Smoke Condensate to Mouse Skin, Experiment B3.* Frankfurt: Battelle Institute, 1974.

1157.01. Karbe E, Kiendl J, Königsmann G, Kramer H, Preuss W, Schmidt I, Wilkes E. *Carcinogenicity of Smoke Condensate to Mouse Skin, Experiment B4.* Frankfurt: Battelle Institute, 1974.

1158.01. Gwiebner S, Langbein D. *Analysis of Progressive Lesions: Programme Description/System Definition for Janus/Optim/Tranra Programme.* Frankfurt: Battelle Institute, 1976.

1159.01. Karbe E, Preuss W, Wilkes E. *The Promotion Activity of Tobacco Smoke Condensate to Mouse Skin, Dose Dependence and Interaction of Dmba B9/1 and B9/6 Condensates.* Frankfurt: Battelle Institute, 1977. BF-F-63.051-3/B9.

1160.01. Wilkes E. *A Statistical Analysis of the Incidence of Tumour-Bearing Animals in Janus Promotion Study B30/31.* Southampton: GR&DC, BAT, 1977. RD.1517 Restricted.

1161.01. Wilkes E. *A Comparison of the Tumorigenic Activities of Janus Condensates Bo, B2 and B4.* Southampton: GR&DC, BAT, 1977. RD.1537 Restricted.

1162.01. Karbe E, Kiendl J, Königsmann G, Preuss W, Schmidt I, Chudzinski R, Wilkes E. *Carcinogenicity of Smoke Condensate to Mouse Skin, Experiment B11.* Frankfurt: Battelle Institute, 1978. BF-F-63.051-5/B11.

1163.01. Ayres C. *Long-Term Skin-Painting Experiments—Progress Report: July 1967.* Southampton: BAT, 1967. B-8.

1163.02. Ayres C. *Project Janus Annual Report.* BAT, 1969.

1163.03. Ayres C. *Quarterly Report: April–June 1969, Project Janus.* BAT, 1969.

1163.04. Ayres C. *Project Janus Quarterly Report: July–September 1969.* BAT, 1969.

1163.05. Ayres C. *Project Janus Quarterly Report: October–December 1969.* BAT, 1970.

1163.06. Evelyn S. *Project Janus Annual Report 1969–1970.* BAT, 1970.

1163.07. Ayres C. *Project Janus Quarterly Report: January–March 1970.* BAT, 1970.

1163.08. Evelyn S. *Project Janus Quarterly Report: April–August 1970.* BAT, 1970.

1163.09. Evelyn S. *Project Janus Quarterly Report: September–December 1970.* BAT, 1971.

1163.10. Evelyn S. *Project Janus Annual Report 1970–71.* BAT, 1971.

1163.11. [Report from Project Janus dealing with high-dose anomaly occurring in mouse skin–painting experiments.] 19??

1163.12. Evelyn S. *Project Janus Progress Report: January–April 1971.* BAT, 1971.

1163.13. Evelyn S. *Project Janus Progress Report: May–August 1971.* BAT, 1971.

1163.14. Evelyn S. *Project Janus Progress Report: September–December 1971.* BAT, 1971.

1163.15. Evelyn S. *Project Janus Progress Report: January–April 1972.* BAT, 1972.

1164.01. Minutes of Biological Testing Committee Meeting Held in Millbank 8th July, 1968. Minutes to C. Ellis, S. Green, D. Felton, D. Wood, C. Ayres, L. Laporte, R. Griffith, H. Sottorf, W. Fordyce, and R. Sanford, July 16, 1968.

1164.02. Minutes of the Biological Testing Committee [meeting]. Minutes, October 28, 1968.

1164.03. Green SJ. Minutes of 16th Biological Testing Committee Meeting Held in R.&D.E., Southampton, 13 June 1969. Minutes, June 25, 1969.

1164.04. Minutes of 17th Biological Testing Committee Meeting Held in R.&D.E., Southampton, 27th January 1970. Minutes to C. Ellis, S. Green, D. Felton, C. Ayres, D. Wood, L. Laporte, J. Burgard, F. Seehofer, and W. Fordyce, January 27, 1970.

1164.05. Minutes of 18th Biological Testing Committee Meeting Held in R.&D.E. Southampton, 5th May 1970. Minutes to C. Ellis, S. Green, D. Felton, C. Ayres, D. Wood, S. Evelyn, L. Laporte, I. Hughes, F. Seehofer, W. Fordyce, and H. Bentley, May 5, 1970.

1164.06. Duplicate of {1164.05}.

1164.07. Minutes of 19th Biological Testing Committee Meeting Held in Millbank, 8th February, 1971. Minutes to C. Ellis, S. Green, F. Haslam, C. Ayres, D. Felton, S. Evelyn, I. Hughes, R. Wade, and F. Seehofer, February 17, 1971.

1164.08. Minutes of 2nd Biological Research Committee Meeting, Southampton, 11th May 1972. Minutes, May 18, 1972.

1164.09. Evelyn S. Biological Research Meeting, Minutes of the Meeting Held in Southampton on 22nd May, 1974. Minutes to S. Green, I. Hughes, R. Gibb, F. Seehofer, R. Nicholls, D. Felton, F. Haslam, C. Ayres, and R. Binns, May 30, 1974.

1164.10. Evelyn S. Minutes of the Biological Research Meeting Held on 8th October. Minutes to S. Green, I. Hughes, R. Gibb, F. Seehofer, R. Nicholls, D. Felton, F. Haslam, C. Ayres, S. Evelyn, and R. Binns, October 28, 1975.

1164.11. Partial duplicate of {1164.10}.

1164.12. Duplicate of {1164.10}.

1164.13. Duplicate of {1164.10}.

1164.14. Duplicate of {1164.10}.

1164.15. Evelyn S. Biological Research Meeting, Minutes of the Meeting Held in Southampton on 13th July, 1976. Minutes to S. Green, I. Hughes, R. Gibb, F. Seehofer, R. Nicholls, D. Felton, C. Ayres, S. Evelyn, and R. Binns, July 16, 1976.

1164.16. Duplicate of {1164.15}.

1164.17. Evelyn S. Biological Research Meeting, Group Research and Development Centre, Southampton, Thursday, 14th October, 1976. Minutes to S. Green, I. Hughes, R. Wade, F. Seehofer, R. Nicholls, D. Felton, C. Ayres, S. Evelyn, and R. Binns, October 25, 1976.

1164.18. Duplicate of {1164.17}.

1164.19. Duplicate of {1164.17}.

1164.20. Duplicate of {1164.17}.

1164.21. Duplicate of {1164.17}.

1164.22. No document at this number.

1164.23. Esterle J. Biological Research Meeting—Chelwood, Sunday, November 27, 1977, J. G. Esterle's Notes. Minutes to I. Hughes, R. Sanford, and C. Rosene, December 13, 1977.

1164.24. Duplicate of {1164.23}.

1164.25. Duplicate of {1164.23}.

1164.26. Thornton R. Biological Meeting Held at Gr&Dc, 19–20 May 1983. Minutes, July 27, 1983.

1165.01. BAT: R&D Conference, Montreal. Proceedings—Tuesday, October 24, 1967. Minutes, 1967.

1165.02. BAT: R&D Conference, Montreal. Proceedings—Wednesday, October 25, 1967. Minutes, 1967.

1165.03. BAT: R&D Conference, Montreal. Proceedings—Thursday, October 26, 1967. Minutes, 1967.

1166.01. [Illegible slides that appear to be from a presentation on filters.]

1167.01. McCormick AD (chairman). Smoking and Health: Policy on Research, Research Conference, Southampton, 1962.

1168.01. Green S. Research Conference Held at Hilton Head Island, S.C., 24th–30th September, 1968. Minutes, January 27, 1969.

1168.02. Green S. Research Conference Held at Hilton Head Island, S.C., 24th–30th September, 1968. Minutes, October 14, 1968.

1169.01. Green S. Research Conference Held at Kronberg, 2nd–6th June, 1969. Minutes, June 23, 1969.

1170.01. Summary & Conclusions: BAT Group Research Conference, November 9th–13th, 1970, St. Adele, Quebec. 1970.

1171.01. Group R&D Conference—Chelwood 1972. Minutes, 1972.

1171.02. Green S. Group R&D Conference—Chelwood 1972 (October 14th–19th). Minutes, November 1, 1972.

1171.03. Green S. Group R&D Conference—Chelwood 1972 (October 14th–19th). Minutes, November 1, 1972.

1171.04. The Changing Emphasis in Industrial R&D. March 2, 1972.

1171.05. Drummond J. *Survey on the use of Crop Chemicals on Tobacco.* 1972.

1172.01. Duplicate of {1125.01}.

1172.02. Green S. Notes on the Group Research & Development Conference at Duck Key, Florida, 12th–18th January, 1974. Minutes, January 28, 1974.

1173.01. Green S. Notes on Group R&D Conference Held in Merano, N. Italy, 2nd to 8th April 1975. Minutes, April 16, 1975.

1174.01. Green S. Notes on Group Research & Development Conference Sydney, March 1978. Minutes, April 6, 1978.

1175.01. Reynolds M. Notes from Group R&D Conference, Part I, February 5–9, 1979. Minutes, 1979.

1175.02. Duplicate of {1175.01}.

1175.03. Green S. Notes on the R. & D. Policy Conference 1979. Minutes, March 1, 1979.

1176.01. Preliminary Minutes of Group Research Conference, London, October 30–November 1, 1979. Minutes, 1979.

1176.02. Blackman L. Notes on the R&D Conference 29th October–1st November, 1979, London. Minutes, November 7, 1979.

1177.01. Blackman L. Research Conference 15th–18th September 1980, Sea Island, Ga. Minutes, October 2, 1980.

1178.01. Blackman L. Research Conference, Pichlarn, Austria, 24–28 August 1981. Minutes, 1981.

1179.01. Blackman L. Research Conference, Montebello, Canada, 30th August–3rd September 1982. Minutes, September 10, 1982.

1179.02. Ayres, C. [Information growing out of Montebello Research Conference.] Letter to E. Kohnhorst, F. Seehofer, R. Nicholls, C. Desiqueira, and P. Dunn, February 9, 1984.

1180.01. Denton P. [Arranging visit to B&W in Louisville.] Letter to R. Sanford, July 22, 1983.

1180.02. No document at this number.

1180.03. Wiethaup W, Schneider W. Research Conference 1983, Brasil.

1180.04. Companhia de Cigarros Souza Cruz. Research Conference 1983, Rio de Janeiro, Tobacco Processing Research Programme.

1180.05. Blackman L. Research Conference—Brazil, 22–26 August, 1983. Letter to E. Kohnhorst, July 13, 1983.

1180.06. Wiethaup W. Lowering Tobacco Weight: Supporting Methods. 1983.

1180.07. Blackman L. Research Conference Rio de Janeiro, Brazil, 22–26 August 1983. Minutes [final], October 13, 1983.

1180.08. R&D Conference 1983 Rio de Janeiro, Brazil [agenda]. BAT, 1983.

1180.09. Blackman L. Research Conference Rio de Janeiro, Brazil, 22–26 August 1983. Minutes [draft], September 9, 1983.

1180.10. Research Conference Brazil 1983. BAT, 1983.

1180.11. Blackman L. Research Conference—Brazil, August 1983. Memo to C. Ayres, P. Denton, P. Dunn, M. Hardwick, A. Heard, E. Kohnhorst, R. Nicholls, E. Rittershaus, R. Sanford, F. Seehofer, and C. Desiqueira, August 15, 1983.

1180.12. Group Research & Development [from Rio R&DE Conference]. BAT, 1983.

1180.13. RA5 Topic—Nicotine [handwritten notes]. Notes, 1983.

1180.14. Broad Objectives of the Group R&D Programme. BAT, 1983.

1180.15. Group Research & Development Centre Organization Chart. 1983.

1180.16. Research Conference, Brazil, August 1983, Summary of Forecasted Resource Allocation. 1983.

1180.17. Wilson T. May Review of GR&DC Work Programme. BAT, 1983.

1180.18. GR&DC Research Programme Priority Ratings. BAT, 1983.

1180.19. [Handwritten notes on flavorings.] Notes, 1983.

1180.20. *Research Conference—Brazil, August 1983, Agenda.* BAT, 1983.

1180.21. [Handwritten notes on Ames test.] Notes, 1983?

1180.22. Thornton R. Project Rio: Status and Discussion, Note: July 1983. BAT, 1983.

1180.23. Massey E. Vitamin A and Cancer: Explanatory Notes. BAT, 1983.

1180.24. Irvin W. Sidestream Research. BAT, 1983.

1180.25. Hedge R. GR&DC Programme on the Effect of Tobacco Processing on Tobacco Chemistry and Smoke Flavour. BAT, 1983.

1180.26. Hook R. Effects of Tobacco Processing on Cigarette Physical Properties. BAT, 1983.

1180.27. Ayres C. Smoking Behaviour. BAT, 1983.

1180.28. Ferris R. The Significance of Smoking in Everyday Life. BAT, 1983.

1180.29. Read G. Proposed Modifications to the New Work Programme to Evaluate the Pharmacological Properties of Eugenol. BAT, 19??

1181.01. Research Conference United Kingdom 1984 [cover page]. BAT, 1984.

1181.02. Ayres C. Addendum [to Research Conference, United Kingdom, 1984]. BAT, 1984.

1181.03. Heat Is On to Ban "Sidestream" Smoke. *IPCS-Bulletin,* July 1, 1984.

1181.04. An Investigation of the Atmosphere in London Underground Trains. 1984?

1181.05. Research Conference United Kingdom, 1984, Contents and Meeting Agenda. R&DE, BAT, 1984.

1181.06. Biological Conference, Southampton, 9th–11th April, 1984. R&DE, BAT, 1984.

1181.07. Nicotine Conference, Southampton, 6th–8th June, 1984. R&DE, BAT, 1984.

1181.08. Smoking Behavior/Marketing Conference, Montreal, 9th–12th July, 1984. R&DE, BAT, 1984.

1181.09. Flavorists Workshop II, Louisville, 7th–9th November, 1983. R&DE, BAT, 1983.

1181.10. Structured Creativity Conference, Southampton, 25th–28th June, 1984. R&DE, BAT, 1984.

1192.02. Green S. *Smoking, Associated Diseases and Causality.* 19??

1192.03. Transcript of Note by Dr. S. J. Green. 19??

1193.01. Walker D, Jackson M. *A Study on the Tumour Promoting Activity of Tobacco Smoke Condensates Applied to Mouse Skin: Cigarettes B13/1–8.* Report prepared for British-American Tobacco Co. by Wickham Research Laboratories, 1976. BA41.

NICOTINE (1200 SERIES)

1200.01. Haselbach C, Libert O. A Tentative Hypothesis on Nicotine Addiction. London: BAT, 1963.

1200.02. Ellis C. [Regarding nicotine addiction and Project Hippo.] Letter to A. Yeaman, June 28, 1963.

1200.03. [Fragment of report on external research on health effects of smoking and nicotine.] Memo, 19??

1200.04. Johnson RR. Comments on Nicotine. 19??

1200.05. Johnson R, Yeaman A. Implications of Battelle Hippo I & II and the Griffith Filter. Minutes, 1963.

1200.06. Wade T. [Re: *The Fate of Nicotine in the Body*]. Memo to E. Finch, July 31, 1963.

1200.07. Finch E. [Acknowledging receipt of *The Fate of Nicotine in the Body.*] Letter to C. Ellis, July 31, 1963.

1200.08. [Fragment of document on marketing and political issues, including addiction.] Memo, 1973?

1200.09. No document at this number.

1200.10. Note for Mr. Cutchins [regarding beneficial effects of nicotine]. Memo to W. Cutchins from A. D. McCormick, June 19, 1963.

1200.11. Yeaman A. [Regrets that Todd sent copies of Battelle reports to Tobacco Industry Research Committee (TIRC).] Letter to A. McCormick, June 28, 1963.

1200.12. Yeaman A. [Cable regarding disclosure of research on nicotine to Surgeon General's committee.] Letter to A. McCormick, July 3, 1963.

1200.13. Yeaman A. [Cable stating that it would be undesirable to release Battelle reports to Surgeon General.] Letter to A. McCormick, July 3, 1963 [same cable as {1200.12} in different form].

1200.14. McCormick A. Incoming cable. Letter to A. Yeaman, July 3, 1963.

1200.15. McCormick A. [Re: Withholding Battelle data from Surgeon General's committee.] Letter to A. Yeaman. July 4, 1963.

1200.16. Ellis C. [Transmitting *The Fate of Nicotine in the Body.*] Letter to W. Cutchins, July 31, 1963.

1200.17. Yeaman A. [Suggesting that it is time to release Project Hippo to the Scientific Advisory Board (SAB).] Letter to E. Jacob, August 5, 1963.

1200.18. Yeaman A. [Reporting that Tom Hoyt of TIRC has continued to withhold Project Hippo reports from TIRC and SAB.] Letter to C. Ellis, August 8, 1963.

1200.19. Ellis C. [Illegible.] 19??

1200.20. Geissbuhler H, Haselbach C. *The Fate of Nicotine in the Body.* Geneva, Switzerland: Battelle Institute, 1963.

1201.01. Johnson R. Comments on Nicotine. 19??

1202.01. McCormick A. Re: Ariel. Letter to A. Yeaman, July 20, 1970.

1203.01. Lisher and Company. Proposal for Low Delivery Project for Brown and Williamson. 1978?

1203.02. [Gori's efforts at NCI.] Note, June 12, 1978.

1204.01. Hughes I. Re: Relation between Nicotine and Tumorigenicity. Memo to C. McCarty, J. Edens, and D. Bryant, July 22, 1974.

1205.01. Blackhurst JD. *Further Work on "Extractable" Nicotine*. Southampton: R&DE, BAT, 1966. RD.437-R.

1205.02. Evelyn, SR. *The Transfer of Nicotine from Smoke into Blood Using a Perfused Canine Lung*. Southampton: R&DE, BAT, 1967. RD.457-R.

1205.03. Wood DJ. *Relation between "Extractable Nicotine" Content of Smoke and Panel Response*. Southampton: R&DE, BAT, 1967. L.228-R.

1205.04. Evelyn SR. *The Absorption of Nicotine via the Mouth: Studies Using Model Systems*. Southampton: R&DE, BAT, 1968. RD.560-R.

1205.05. Wood DJ. *Relation between "Extractable" Nicotine Content of Smoke and Panel Response*. Southampton: R&DE, BAT, 1968. L.228-E.

1205.06. Evelyn SR. *The Effect of Puff Volume on "Extractable Nicotine" and on the Retention of Nicotine in the Mouth*. Southampton: R&DE, BAT, 1969. L.314-R.

1205.07. Isaac PF. *The Absorption and Effects of Nicotine from Inhaled Tobacco Smoke*. Melbourne: Department of Pharmacology, University of Melbourne, 1970.

1205.08. Creighton D. *Nicotine in Smoke and Human Physiological Response*. Southampton: BAT, 1970. RD.701-R.

1205.09. Willey G, Kellett D. *Effects of Nicotine on the Central Nervous System*. Montreal: Imperial Tobacco Group, 1971.

1205.10. Creighton DE, Mcgillivray LM. *Relative Contributions of Nicotine and Carbon Monoxide to Human Physiological Response*. Southampton: R&DE, BAT, 1971. RD.839-R.

1205.11. Partial duplicate of {1220.01}.

1205.12. Creighton DE, Watts BM. *Further Studies on the Effect of Nicotine on Human Physiological Response*. Southampton: GR&DC, BAT, 1973. RD.1007-R.

1205.13. Kilburn KD, Underwood JG. *Preparation and Properties of Nicotine Analogues; Part II*. Southampton: GR&DC, BAT, 1973. RD.1048-R.

1205.14. Partial duplicate of {1221.01}.

1205.15. Comer AK, Thornton RE. *Interaction of Smoke and the Smoker. Part 3: The Effect of Cigarette Smoking on the Contingent Negative Variation*. Southampton: GR&DC, BAT, 1974. RD.1164-R.

1206.01. *Project Wheat*. 1974.

1206.02. Wood DJ, Wilkes EB. *Project Wheat—Part 1. Cluster Profiles of U.K. Male Smokers and Their General Smoking Habits*. Southampton: GR&DC, BAT, 1975. RD.1229-R.

1206.03. Wood DJ. *Project Wheat—Part 2. U.K. Male Smokers: Their Reactions to Cigarettes of Different Nicotine Delivery as Influenced by Inner Need*. Southampton: GR&DC, BAT, 1976. RD.1322.

1207.01. *Conference on Smoking Behaviour*. Southampton: GR&DC, BAT, 1976.

1208.01. Thornton RE. *Some "Benefits" of Smoking*. Southampton: GR&DC, BAT, 1977. RD.1461.

1208.02. Courtney JR, Comer AK. *The Study of Human Smoking Behaviour Using Butt Analysis*. Southampton: GR&DC, BAT, 1978. RD.1608.

1208.03. Kilburn KD. *Preparation and Properties of Nicotine Analogues: Part III*. Southampton: GR&DC, BAT, 1979. RD.1473.

1208.04. Read GA, Anderson IGM. *Method for Nicotine and Cotinine in Blood and Urine*. Southampton: GR&DC, BAT, 1980. RD.1737-C.

1208.05. Read GA, Anderson IGM, Chapman RE. *Nicotine Studies: A Second Report. Estimation of Whole Body Nicotine Dose by Urinary Nicotine and Cotinine Measurement*. Southampton: GR&DC, BAT, 1981. R&D-L023–81.

1209.01. Proceedings of the Smoking Behaviour–Marketing Conference, July 9–12, 1984, Session I, Montreal, Quebec. 1984.

1210.01. Research Conference United Kingdom 1984. BAT, 1984.

1211.01. Kersch J, Libert O, Rogg-Effront C. *Final Report on Project Hippo I*. Geneva: Battelle Institute (for BAT), 1962.

1211.02. Libert O. *Report No. 1 Regarding Project Hippo II*. Geneva: Battelle Institute (for BAT), 1962.

1211.03. Haselbach CH, Libert O. *Final Report on Project Hippo II*. Geneva: Battelle Institute, 1963.

1212.01. Libert O. *Final Report on Project Hippo I*. Geneva: Battelle Institute, 1962.

1212.02. Libert O. *Report No. 1 regarding Project Hippo II*. Geneva: Battelle Institute, 1962.

1212.03. Haselbach C, Libert O. *Final Report on Project Hippo II*. Geneva: Battelle Institute, 1963.

1213.01. Geissbuhler H, Haselbach C. *The Fate of Nicotine in the Body*. Geneva: Battelle Institute, 1963.

1214.01. Evelyn S. *The Absorption of Nicotine via The Mouth: Studies Using Model Systems*. Southampton: R&DE, BAT, 1968. RD.560-R.

1215.01. Evelyn S. *The Effect of Puff Volume on "Extractable Nicotine" and on the Retention of Nicotine in the Mouth*. Southampton: R&DE, BAT, 1969. L.314-R.

1216.01. Creighton D. *Nicotine in Smoke and Human Physiological Response*. Southampton: R&DE, BAT, 1970. RD.701-R.

1217.01. Wood D. *Quarterly Report April–June 1971*. Southampton: R&DE, BAT, 1971.

1218.01. Duplicate of {1205.09}.

1219.01. Creighton D, Mcgillivray L. *Relative Contributions of Nicotine and Carbon Monoxide to Human Physiological Response*. Southampton: R&DE, BAT, 1971. RD.839-R.

1220.01. Kilburn K, Underwood J. *Preparation and Properties of Nicotine Analogues*. Southampton: GR&DC, BAT, 1972. RD.953-R.

1221.01. Brotzge R, Kennedy J. *Human Smoking Studies: Acute Effect of Cigarette Smoke on Brain Wave Alpha Rhythm. First Report*. Louisville: Research and Development Department, B&W, 1974. 74-20.

1222.01. Kilburn K. *Preparation and Properties of Nicotine Analogues, Part III*. Southampton: GR&DC, BAT, 1979. RD.1673 Restricted.

1223.01. Thornton R. *Some "Benefits" of Smoking*. Southampton: GR&DC, BAT, 1977. RD.1461 Unclassified.

1224.01. *Proceedings of the Smoking Behaviour–Marketing Conference July 9th–12th, 1984, Session I*. 1984.

1225.01. *Proceedings of the Smoking Behaviour–Marketing Conference July 9th–12th, 1984, Session II*. 1984.

1226.01. *Proceedings of the Smoking Behaviour–Marketing Conference July 9th–12th, 1984, Session III*. 1984.

1227.01. Geissbuhler H, Haselbach C. *The Fate of Nicotine in the Body*. Geneva: Battelle Institute, 1963.

1227.02. Arwilage A. Appraisal of Report "The Fate of Nicotine in the Body" (A263). 1963.

1227.03. Fordyce W. Re: Group Research. Memo to S. Green, September 24, 1965.

1227.04. *Personality and Smoking: A Review of the Problem and Techniques*. Bristol: Imperial Tobacco Company, 1966.

1227.05. Research Services Psychology Unit. *Appendix, Note on Questionnaires from "Personality and Smoking."* Bristol: Tobacco Intelligence Department, Imperial Tobacco Company, 1966. J.4755/JGF.

1227.06. Green S. [Regarding reorienting research priorities to focus on nontobacco or reconstituted tobacco cigarettes and Project Ariel.] Memo to D. Hobson, March 2, 1967.

1227.07. Green S. *B.A.T. Group Research.* 1968.

1228.01. Partial duplicate of {1233.02}.

1228.02. Green S. [Relationship between psychological and pharmacological effects of smoking.] Memo to G. Hook, June 11, 1974.

1228.03. Frederiksen L, Martin J. Carbon monoxide and smoking behavior. *Addictive Behaviors* 1979;4:21–30.

1229.01. Constitution of the Tobacco Advisory Council. November 21, 1979.

1230.01. Lee P. Re: Note on tar reduction for Hunter to H. Bentley. July 19, 1979.

1230.02. Lee P. *Tar Reduction and Nicotine Compensation.* 1979.

1230.03. Lee P. *Reduction in Tar Yields and Trends in Male Lung Cancer Rates.* 1979.

1231.01. Mason J. [Transmitting Gallagher contribution to Tobacco Advisory Committee Ad Hoc Working Party on Tar Levels.] Letter to H. Bentley, July 25, 1979.

1231.02. Duplicate of {1230.02}.

1231.03. Duplicate of {1230.03}.

1231.04. Duplicate of {1231.01}.

1231.05. *The Lower Tar Market: Conclusion on Background Information.* 1979.

1232.01. Johnson, AH, Carreras Rothmans Limited. Market research reports relating to low tar cigarettes. Letter to H.E. Bentley, Imperial Tobacco, London, July 26, 1979.

1233.01. Roe F. Re: Nicotine Monograph. Letter to D. Beese, July 30, 1979.

1233.02. Cohen A, Roe F. *Pharmacology and Toxicology of Nicotine and Its Role in Tobacco Smoking.* Monograph, 1979.

ADDITIVES AND PESTICIDES (1300 SERIES)

1300.01. [Fragment of list of pesticides and additives, probably for coding documents.] List, 19??

1300.02. Additives Reference Guide. List, 19??

1300.03. [Illegible; appears to be a list of additives.] 19??

1301.01. Maybell H. Re: Flavor Fixatives. Memo to R. Ernst, January 28, 1953.

1302.01. Griffith R. Sucker Control Committee Discussion of Epstein Work April 27, 1967. Minutes, April 27, 1967.

1303.01. Green S. [Transmitting copy of Tobacco Research Council paper F.414 on Penar.] Letter to R. Griffith, April 16, 1968.

1303.02. [Report on the toxicity of Penar.] 1968.

1303.03. Kennedy J, Newton R. The Relative Carcinogenicity of Sucker Control Agents Maleic Hydrazide (MH) and Dimethyldodecylamine Acetate (Penar). Notes, May 31, 1968.

1303.04. Griffith R. Visit to USDA, Beltsville, September 4, 1968. Notes, September 13, 1968.

1303.05. Ayres C. Penar. Letter to W. Fordyce, I. Hughes, and R. Wade, May 18, 1970.

1303.06. Griffith R. Re: MH-30/Penar. Memo to A. Yeaman, May 1, 1968.

1304.01. Research Manager. [Regarding DDT residues in tobacco.] Letter to H. Grice, December 17, 1968.

1305.01. Harrison L, Brumleve B. Brown & Williamson Tobacco Corporation Second Wave Gross Inventory, Project Critical Document Form. January 6, 1969.

1305.02. American Mutual Insurance Alliance. *Fumigation.* Safety Information Service, January 6, 1969.

1306.01. Kennedy J. Relative Toxicity of Smoke Gas Phase Constituents/343. Notes, July 14, 1969.

1307.01. Health of Cigarette Smokers Endangered by Pesticide Residues in Tobacco. In *Congressional Record—Senate,* July 28, 1969.

1308.01. Partial duplicate of {1303.05}.

1309.01. Pepples E. [G-13 process.] Memo to I. Hughes, June 2, 1977.

1309.02. Pepples E, Ricer (?). Agreement [between B&W and Liggett Group re B&W's purchase of G-13 processed tobacco.] June 16, 1978.

1309.03. Webb J. Re: Incoming Material Inspection—Expanded Tobacco. Memo to J. Nall, D. Roth, and C. Rosene, May 1, 1978.

1309.04. Toxicological Properties of Freon 11 in Tobacco from the G13 Process. 19??

1309.05. Temko S. Memorandum to: Committee of Counsel. Memo, December 5, 1977.

1309.06. Diamond J. August 1977 Briefing Paper CPSA Petition CP-77-6 Freon-11 Refrigerants. 1977.

1309.07. Levangie, J. Petition. Letter, February 22, 1977.

1309.08. Bechtel P. Petition Guidance Memorandum; February 22, 1977 Communication from Mr. James C. Levangie. Memo to M. Freeston, March 14, 1977.

1309.09. Schmeltzer D. [Freon.] Letter to J. Levangie, March 30, 1977.

1309.10. Levangie J. Supplement to Petition CP 77-6. Letter to S. Lembery, May 27, 1977.

1309.11. Canter D. Refrigerants Used in Commercial and Residential Refrigeration and Air-Conditioning Systems (CP-77-6). Memo to F. Shacter, D. Clay, and R. Hehir, May 19, 1977.

1309.12. Bigio J. Refrigerants Used in Commercial and Residential Refrigeration and Air Conditioning Systems (CP-77-6). Memo to F. Shacter, May 6, 1977.

1309.13. Leight, W. Petition CP-77-7. Memo to D. Scott, J. Bigio, and W. West, May 3, 1977.

1309.14. Howard C. Memorandum of Jules L. Bigio, CPSC, April 26, 1977; Petition CP-77-7. Memo to W. Leight, May 2, 1977.

1309.15. CP-77–7. Letter to W. Leight, D. Scott, and J. Bigio, April 26, 1977.

1309.16. Johnson K. [Phosgene.] Letter to R. Sandler, 19??

1310.01. Boothroyd R. Additives Guidance Panel. April 9, 1965.

1310.02. Felton D. Additives Guidance Panel [meeting]. Minutes to S. Green, C. Bowra, R. Pritchard, D. Davies, D. Felton, F. Haslam, S. Liddle, T. Mcdowell, H. Morini, D. O'Brien, B. Pearson, J. Sikkel, A. Cousins, I. Hughes, S. Keshava, R. Nicholls, C. Peacock, E. Rittershaus, C. Rosene, R. Sanford, J. Sismey, and R. Wade, January 5, 1978.

1311.01. Litwin D. Real [brand of cigarette launched by R. J. Reynolds]: Claims Substantiation Meeting. Memo to E. Darrack, C. Domeck, T. Rachl, and R. Sachs, July 13, 1977.

1312.01. Pepples E. [NCI bioassay for carcinogenicity of menthol.] Memo to J. Esterle, December 26, 1978.

1313.01. Pepples E. [Compounds for NCI carcinogenicity testing.] Letter to F. Panzer, January 10, 1979.

1313.02. Esterle J. [Transmitting a list of chemicals being tested for carcinogenicity by NCI.] Memo to E. Pepples, January 8, 1979.

1313.03. [Additives currently and possibly used in cigarettes.] List, 19??

1314.01. Partial duplicate of {1315.01}.

1314.02. Esterle, J. G. Cigarette Additives: Biological Testing. Louisville: B&W, 1981.

1315.01. Esterle J. Re: Cigarette Additives. Memo to R. Sanford, September 11, 1981.

1315.02. Media Coverage of "Deer-Tongue": A Chronology. List 19??

1316.01. Wells J. Re: Additives. Memo to E. Pepples, September 25, 1981.

1317.01. Rosene C. Re: Insecticide "Fican-Plus"/490-21. Memo to K. Brotzge, June 2, 1983.

1317.02. Brotzge K. Re: Fican-Plus/Insecticide/341. Memo to C. Sawyer, June 10, 1983.

1317.03. Infestation Audit, December 7, 1987.

1317.04. Lindsay J. Pesticide Inventory. Memo to B. Alcon, June 19, 1985.

1317.05. Re: Fumigation with Phosphine Gas and Daily Application of DDVP. Memo to A. Stone, February 15, 1979.

1317.06. Tucker I. Re: Pesticide Residue Studies for Export Department. Memo to A. Up-
field, May 26, 1958.

1317.07. *Progress Report—Leaf Division.* 1971?

1317.08. Geffert G. [Analysis of DDT in tobacco.] Letter to H. Grice, December 17, 1968.

1317.09. Griffith R. Re: MH-30/Penar. Memo to A. Yeaman, May 1, 1968.

1318.01. Brotzge K. Re: Annual Pesticide Residue Meetings/367. Memo to E. Kohnhorst,
April 12, 1984.

1318.02. Sheets T. Pesticide Residues in Tobacco, Tobacco Products, and Main-Stream
Smoke. 19??

1319.01. Kohnhorst E. [Transmitting article for comment (probably regarding cocoa).]
Letter to G. Esterle and C. J. Rosene, June 4, 1984.

1319.02. Pepples E. [Handwritten note transmitting the "cocoa" article.] Notes to
T. Sandefur, May 30, 1984.

1319.03. Esterle J, Rosene C. *Cocoa.* 1984.

1320.01. Rosene C. Re: Coumarin Substitutes/490. Memo to E. Pepples, June 18, 1984.

1320.02. Kohnhorst E. Coumarin. Memo to T. Sandefur, June 6, 1984.

1321.01. Kohnhorst E. Conversation with Dr. Hughes/Ernie Pepples/Tommy Sandefur.
Notes, June 8, 1984.

1322.01. Additives Guidance Panel [meeting]. Minutes, April 9, 1965.

1322.02. Sachs R. Re: Diethylene Glycol. Memo to File, June 18, 1984.

1323.01. Esterle J. [Handwritten note: The picture remains unclear.] Notes, 19??

1323.02. Evelyn S. Re: Coumarin. Letter to E. Kohnhorst, July 19, 1984.

1323.03. Evelyn S. Brief Notes on a Visit to BAT Hamburg by Dr. S. R. Evelyn. Notes to
L. Blackman, February 15, 1982.

1323.04. Evelyn S. Re: Coumarin. Letter to F. Seehofer, August 13, 1980.

1323.05. Evelyn S. [Regarding coumarin.] Letter to J. Rouaud, August 13, 1980.

1323.06. Rouaud J. [Rat studies of coumarin.] Letter to S. Evelyn, August 4, 1980.

1323.07. Conning D. [Latest information on coumarin from the British Biological Research Association.] Letter to S. Evelyn, May 9, 1979.

1323.08. Weinberger M. [Meeting with FDA regarding coumarin.] Letter to D. Conning,
March 15, 1979.

1323.09. Ueno I, Hirono I. Non-carcinogenic response to coumarin in Syrian golden hamsters. *Food Cosmetic. Toxicol.* 1981; 19:353–355.

1324.01. Benner R, Clements E. Re: Non-Tobacco Additive or Ingredient Documents.
Memo to Brown and Williamson Smoking & Health Litigation File. November 1, 1988.

1325.01. Additives and Potentially Hazardous Additives. List, 19??

1325.02. Other Fungicides. List, 19??

1325.03. Other Herbicides. List, 19??

1325.04. Other Pesticides. List, 19??

1326.01. Additive Code Analogues. List, 19??

1327.01. Pesticides and Potentially Hazardous Additives. List, 19??

1328.01. Substances. [List of substances in smoke, with information about physical and
chemical properties.] List, 1989.

1328.02. Tinsley B. Brown and Williamson Tobacco Corp. Subjective Coding Project—
Substance Glossary. Memo to All Subjective Coders, April 25, 1989.

1329.01. Partial duplicate of {1326.01}.

1329.02. Partial duplicate of {1328.01}.

1330.01. [Partial list of organic compounds used as additives and their characteristics.]
List, 19??

1331.01. Kilburn K. *A Technological Forecast of the Future of Tobacco Processing.*
Southampton: R&DE, BAT, 1978. RD.1618 Restricted.

1332.01. S & H Item 3. Memo, March 7, 1978.

TOBACCO WORKING GROUP (1400 SERIES)

1400.01. DB. File Note [regarding Committee of Counsel meeting]. Notes, March 15, 1973.

1400.02. Hughes, IW. Letter to G. Gori, May 31, 1973.

1401.01. Panzer F. Letter from the President [of the US] to Dr. Jonathan E. Rhoads, Chairman, National Cancer Advisory Board. Letter to B. Roach, October 18, 1974.

1401.02. Tso T. Report of the Fifteenth Meeting. Tobacco Working Group, Lung Cancer Task Force, September 10 and 11, 1974, Bethesda, Maryland. Minutes, September 10, 1974.

1402.01. TWG terminated (handwritten note). Notes, August 12, 1977.

1402.02. Rauscher F. Department of Health, Education and Welfare, Charter, Tobacco Working Group, National Cancer Institute. 19??

1402.03. Functional Statement, Tobacco Working Group, National Cancer Institute. 19??

1402.04. [Note regarding Tobacco Working Group.] Notes, 19??

1402.05. Hughes I. [Clarifying role in TWG.] Letter to G. Gori, March 28, 1972.

1402.06. File Note. March 15, 1973.

1402.07. Duplicate of {1401.02}.

1403.01. Hall G. (A) NO1-CP-55666, (B) FPR 1-11.202, (C) and FPR 1-22.3(A), Purchase Order No. 39. Letter to R. Brown, September 29, 1975.

1403.02. Brown & Williamson Tobacco Co. Purchase Order. Budget to Inc. Meloy Laboratories. October 6, 1975.

1404.01. Kornegay H. [Comments on Hughes's suggestions to Gio Gori regarding draft press release.] Letter to E. Pepples, January 14, 1976.

1404.02. Pepples E. [Transmitting letter from I. W. Hughes to G. Gori arguing that NCI should not use proposed press release.] Letter to T. Ahrensfeld, J. Greer, H. Roemer, A. Stevens, D. Hardy, H. Kornegay, and F. Panzer, December 29, 1975.

1404.03. Hughes I. [Commenting on two draft press releases submitted by Gio Gori.] Letter to G. Gori, December 23, 1975.

1404.04. Copy of {1404.03}.

1404.05. Stevens A. [Transmitting Spears's comments on Gori's draft NCI press release.] Letter to T. Ahrensfeld, J. Greer, E. Pepples, H. Roemer, D. Hardy, H. Kornegay, and F. Panzer, December 22, 1975.

1404.06. Spears A. [Comments on proposed NCI press release.] Letter to G. Gori, December 18, 1975.

1404.07. Spears A. Preliminary Draft of Comments Relating to Press Release Materials. Notes to G. Gori, 1975.

1404.08. Rauscher F, Rhoads J, Levy R. Release Statement, December 10, 1975.

1404.09. Gori G. [Press release on dangers of smoking (draft).] Bethesda: National Cancer Institute, December 10, 1975.

1404.10. Pepples E. Re: Your December 8 Memo regarding Gori Releases. Letter to I. Hughes, December 16, 1975.

1404.11. Hughes I. [Transmitting proposed press release by Gio Gori.] Memo to C. McCarty, D. Bryant, and E. Pepples, December 8, 1975.

1404.12. Gori G. [Press release regarding health dangers of smoking.] To E. Pepples, 19??

1404.13. Rauscher F, Rhoads J, Levy R. [Draft press release on dangers of smoking and safe cigarette project.] 1975?

1405.01. Pepples E. [Recommending Hughes not accept voting membership on TWG.] Memo to I. Hughes, January 19, 1976.

1405.02. Tso I, Gori G. leaf Quality and Usability: Theoretical Model. 1976.

1406.01. Wells J. Re: TWG/ISC. Memo to E. Pepples, September 17, 1976.

1406.02. Public Health Service, 42 USC 286D. 19??

1414.01. Radio TV Reports Inc. *Broadcast Excerpt, 1978.*
1414.02. Radio TV Reports Inc. *The MacNeil-Lehrer Report, Broadcast Excerpt.* 1978.
1414.03. Radio TV Reports Inc. *Panorama—Interview with Dr. Gio Batta Gori.* 1978.
1414.04. Duplicate of {1413.01}.
1414.05. Smith C. Low-Tar Smoking Reports "Tolerable" Cancer Risk. August 11, 1978.
1414.06. *Congressional Record—Senate.* August 15, 1978, pp. 26040–26042.
1414.07. Congressional Record—Senate. August 16, 1978, pp. 26332–26334.
1414.08. Hughes I. Re: Phone Conversation Today with Dr. Gio Gori. Memo to C. Mc-Carty, D. Bryant, and E. Pepples, December 8, 1975.
1415.01. [Biographical information about Gio Gori.] 19??

SMOKELESS TOBACCO COUNCIL (1500 SERIES)

1500.01. Pepples E. [Transmitting press account in which employee of US Tobacco stated smokeless tobacco had the "least possible danger" of all forms of tobacco use.] Memo to J. Edens, C. McCarty, and R. Pittman, March 25, 1977.
1500.02. Kranes M. Chaws—Gripping Entertainment, Tobacco's More Than a Smoke. *New York Post,* March 16, 1977.
1500.03. Pepples E. [Transmitting $5,000 for Smokeless Tobacco Council.] Letter to Smokeless Tobacco Council and J. Chapin, February 26, 1979.
1500.04. Rossi R. Re: Smokeless Tobacco Council Scientific Research Committee. Letter to C. McCarty, February 16, 1979.
1500.05. Stevens A. [Smokeless Tobacco Council.] Letter to J. Chapin, January 17, 1978.
1500.06. Pepples E. [Justification for joining Smokeless Tobacco Council.] Memo to R. Pittman and C. McCarty, September 28, 1978.
1500.07. Bantle L. [Request to contribute $10,000 to join Smokeless Tobacco Council.] Letter to C. McCarty, September 12, 1978.
1500.08. [Handwritten note to file.] Notes, 19??
1500.09. Bantle L. [Invitation to join Smokeless Tobacco Council.] Letter to C. I. Mc-Carty, September 12, 1978. [same letter as {1500.07} with different marginalia]
1500.10. Scientific Research Committee Smokeless Tobacco Council Budget 1978. Budget, 1978?
1501.01. Stevens A. [Lorillard and Smokeless Tobacco Council.] Letter to E. Pepples, February 13, 1979.
1501.02. Mitchell G. Smokeless Tobacco Sales Reported Soaring as Munching Instead of Puffing Fad Grows. *Lexington Herald,* November 20, 1978.
1501.03. Rossi R. [Expressing gratitude that B&W joined Smokeless Tobacco Council research effort.] Letter to E. Pepples, October 16, 1978.
1501.04. Pepples E. [B&W will join Smokeless Tobacco Council and contribute $5,000.] Letter to L. Bantle, October 10, 1978.
1501.05. [Handwritten note saying "this is approved."] Notes to E. Pepples, 19??
1501.06. Duplicate of {1500.07}.
1501.07. Duplicate of {1500.01}.
1502.01. Wells J. Re: Smokeless Tobacco Council. Memo to E. Pepples, November 9, 1979.
1503.01. Kerrigan M. [Response to J. Cullen regarding request for information on smokeless tobacco.] Letter to J. Cullen, September 30, 1985.
1503.02. Kerrigan M. [Response to J. Cullen's request for information on smokeless tobacco (draft).] Letter to J. Cullen, September 5, 1985.
1503.03. Cullen J. [Requesting help for NCI's effort to evaluate the health effects of smokeless tobacco.] Letter to T. Sandefur, August 22, 1985.
1503.04. Business Card of Janet S. McClendon. 19??

1503.05. Grice H. Re: Snuff and Chewing Tobacco. Letter to Members of Tobacco Advisory Council Executive Committee and Members of Tobacco Advisory Council Research Committee, August 10, 1984.

1503.06. Firth J. Commercial—In Confidence. Letter to H. Grise, August 7, 1984.

1503.07. Harris A. [Invitation to attend Smokeless Tobacco Council.] Letter to I. Hughes, January 21, 1983.

1503.08. Sheets T. [Need for better data on pesticides.] Letter to A. Gottacho, November 4, 1982.

1503.09. Smokeless Tobacco Council—Scientific Research Committee: Status of Research Proposals and Research. November 1, 1979.

1503.10. Pepples E. [Joining Smokeless Tobacco Council.] Letter to W. Rosson, October 8, 1979.

1503.11. Rosson W. [Announcing meeting of Smokeless Tobacco Council Board.] Letter to C. McCarty, September 21, 1979.

1503.12. Cummins B. [Charges for CTR and political activity.] Memo to C. Heger, August 24, 1979.

1503.13. Pittman R. [Status of STC research projects.] Memo to E. Pepples, March 6, 1979.

1503.14. Smokeless Tobacco Council—Scientific Research Committee: Status of Research Proposals and Research. February 26, 1979.

1503.15. Smokeless Tobacco Council. Summary of Funding for Medical Research Projects (1976 through 1979 Inclusive). 1978.

1503.16. Brown & Williamson Tobacco Corporation. Voucher [to transfer $5,000 to Smokeless Tobacco Council] to the Smokeless Tobacco Council. 1979

KENTUCKY TOBACCO AND HEALTH RESEARCH INSTITUTE (1600 SERIES)

1600.01. Pepples E. [Requesting background check on Dr. David Justus prior to potential funding by UK Tobacco and Health Research Institute.] Letter to T. Finnegan, November 6, 1980.

1600.02. Justus D. [Preliminary proposal to UK Tobacco and Health Research Institute on tobacco allergies.] Letter to G. Huber, October 22, 1980.

1601.01. Pepples E. Re: Moakley Bill. Letter to J. Rupp, September 28, 1983.

1602.01. Warren P, McCuiston P. Kentucky Tobacco Research Board [meeting]. Minutes, September 10, 1984.

1602.02. Shinn W. [Kentucky Tobacco and Health Research Institute.] Letter to E. Pepples, September 20, 1984.

1602.03. McCuiston P. [Transmitting minutes of September 10 meeting of Kentucky Tobacco Research Board.] Letter to E. Pepples, September 14, 1984.

1603.01. Pepples E. [Regarding annual report of Kentucky Tobacco and Health Research Institute.] Letter to W. Shinn, September 25, 1984.

HEALTH CLAIMS (1700 SERIES)

1700.01. Burgard J. [Request to develop a campaign to bring the industry side of the smoking and health controversy to the public through product advertising.] Memo to R. Pittman, August 21, 1969.

1700.02. Objectives. List, 19??

1700.03. Come Up to Kool. Advertisement, 19??

1700.04. [List of advertising themes for various cigarette brands between the 1930s and 1960s]. List, 19??

1701.01. [Concerning refinement of Low Tar by Special Blend concept boards for advertisements.] Letter to R. Parker, February 14, 1977.

1702.01. [Minutes of strategy meeting on Barclay and epidemiology studies; may be incomplete.] Minutes, July 17, 1985.

1703.01. [Chronology of advertisements and media coverage of Viceroy cigarettes, 1950–1956.] 19??

1703.02. Historical VICEROY Positioning and Campaigns. 19??

1704.01. Viceroy [brand history, 1936–1956]. 19??

LAWYERS (1800 SERIES)

1800.01. Hill and Knowlton, Inc. Description. 19??

1800.02. Blalock JV. [Regarding concerns over upcoming Surgeon General's report, FTC, etc; page 1 missing.] Memo to J. Burgard, June 18, 1963.

1801.01. Blalock JV. Tobacco Institute, Tobacco Industry Research Committee, and Hill & Knowlton. Memo to J. Burgard, June 18, 1963.

1801.02. Finch E. Smoking and Health. Memo, October 3, 1967.

1801.03. ["Assertions" and "Facts" on smoking; partial document.] Q & A, 1967.

1801.04. Cigarette Smoking and Health—What Are the Facts? Q & A, 19??

1801.05. Those Who Expressed Doubt before United States Congress of Smoking-Disease Relationship. 1965?

1802.01. Yeaman A. [Objecting to the fact that Battelle report was sent to TIRC.] Letter to A. McCormick, June 28, 1963.

1802.02. McCormick A. Incoming cable. Letter to A. Yeaman, July 3, 1963.

1802.03. Yeaman A. [Cable regarding disclosure of nicotine research to Surgeon General's committee.] Letter to A. McCormick, July 3, 1963.

1802.04. Yeaman A. [Cable confirming that Battelle report on nicotine would be withheld from Surgeon General.] Letter to A. McCormick, July 3, 1963.

1802.05. Yeaman A. Implications of Battelle Hippo I & II and the Griffith Filter. Memo, July 17, 1963.

1802.06. Ellis C. [Transmitting *The Fate of Nicotine in the Body*.] Letter to W. Cutchins, July 31, 1963.

1802.07. Yeaman A. [Transmitting three-volume report on Project Hippo and suggesting that it may be time to give copies to the CTR Scientific Advisory Board.] Letter to E. Jacob, August 5, 1963.

1802.08. Yeaman A. [Whether to make Project Hippo results available to CTR Scientific Advisory Board.] Letter to C. Ellis, August 8, 1963.

1803.01. McCormick A. [Re: Withholding Battelle data from Surgeon General's committee.] Letter to A. Yeaman, July 4, 1963.

1804.01. Prichard? [Regarding biological testing.] Letter to E. Finch, January 2, 1964.

1804.02. Wade T. Re: Report of Sir Charles Ellis to Mr. Dobson, January 3, 1964. Memo to E. Finch, January 10, 1964.

1804.03. Ellis C. [Proposal for research program to reduce cigarette toxicity through the development of filters.] Letter to R. Dobson, January 3, 1964.

1804.04. Investigation of the Effects of Cigarette Smoke on Ciliary Activity. 19??

1804.05. Short term Carcinogenicity Test. 19??

1804.06. Development of Inhalation Techniques. 19??

1805.01. Griffith R. Report to Executive Committee. 1965.

1806.01. Griffith R. [Expressing concern about releasing results of Harrogate research on public opinion and government action.] Letter to E. Finch, J. Crume, and A. Yeaman, July 19, 1965.

1807.01. Griffith R. Re: Chemosol. Memo to A. Yeaman, July 19, 1967.

1807.02. Part Three, Summary of Tumorigenesis Experiment and Biostatistical Report and Corroboration. 1967.

1807.03. Hudson P. [Thank-you note for statistical assistance.] Letter to H. Levine, June 22, 1967.

1807.04. [Regarding Chemosol experiments.] Letter to P. Hudson, June 27, 1967.

1807.05. Schumacher J. [Sending copy of letter to Finch for his file; awaiting response.] Letter to A. Yeaman, May 2, 1967.

1807.06. Schumacher J. [Chemosol.] Letter to E. Finch, May 2, 1967.

1807.07. [Regarding Chemosol.] Letter to W. Hoyt, December 12, 1967.

1807.08. Topol A. Re: Chemosol. Memo to H.T. Austern, September 16, 1969.

1807.09. Technical Report on Chemosol: A Fuel Additive for Cigarette Tobacco. 19??

1808.01. Griffith R. Re: B&W Biological Testing. Memo to E. Finch, September 3, 1968.

1808.02. Detailed Analysis of Factors Considered Important in Assessing the Need for a Biological Testing Program. 19??

1808.03. Green S. Research Conference Held at Hilton Head Island, S.C., 24th–30th September 1966. Minutes, September 24, 1968.

1808.04. Sanford R. [Regarding conclusions of Hilton Head meeting.] Letter to S. Green, December 4, 1968.

1809.01. Yeaman A. [Information exchange through A.D. Little.] Letter to G. Hargrove, November 27, 1968.

1809.02. Hargrove G. [Transmitting documents F.1193 and F.1224.] Letter to A. Yeaman, December 4, 1968.

1809.03. Finch E. [Exchange of information between B&W and BAT.] Letter to R. Dobson, December 11, 1968.

1810.01. BAT/B&W R&D Cost and Risk Pooling Agreement. July 9, 1969.

1811.01. B.A.T. Research, Canada, Australia, Germany, R. & D. Cost-Sharing Agreement with B. & W. July 18, 1969.

1811.02. B.A.T./B.&W. R.&D. Cost Sharing Agreement, Actual Expenses 1/10/70–30/9/71. 19??

1812.01. [Summary of public policy issues confronting the tobacco industry; partial document.] 1973?

1813.01. Green S. [Transmitting an unspecified list.] Letter to J. Ravlin, July 18, 1969.

1814.01. Pepples E. [Request for articles in popular press on topics of interest to tobacco industry.] Memo to J. Blalock, February 14, 1973.

1815.01. [Regarding cost- and risk-pooling agreement between BAT and B&W.] Letter to I. Hughes, February 7, 1977.

1815.02. [Handwritten notes regarding B&W/BAT cost- and risk-pooling agreement.] Notes, 1969?

1815.03. R&D Cost and Risk Pooling Agreement [including handwritten notes]. Notes, 1969.

1815.04. BAT/B&W R&D Cost and Risk Pooling Agreement [incomplete copy]. 19??

1816.01. Pepples E. [Gardner's request to study smoke fractions.] Memo to A. Yeaman, March 10, 1977.

1816.02. Partial duplicate of {1817.03}.

1816.03. Hockett R. Re: Press Reports on Paper by Drs. C. G. Becker and T. Dubin of Cornell University College of Medicine. Memo to A. Yeaman, October 31, 1977.

1816.04. Hoel D. Re: Dr. Carl C. Seltzer. Letter to T. Ahrensfeld, J. Greer, A. Henson, E. Pepples, H. Roemer, and A. Stevens, April 28, 1978.

1816.05. Pepples E. [Re: Memo by Bill Shinn on public relations and political value of CTR.] Memo to C. McCarty, September 29, 1978.

1817.01. Pepples E. [Transmitting Gardner's research proposal, with Pepples's comments.] Letter to A. Yeaman, March 10, 1977.

1817.02. Pepples E. [Gardner's request to study short-term effects of smoke fractions.] Memo to A. Yeaman, March 10, 1977.

1817.03. Pepples E. [Does not agree with Dr. Gardner's idea to study short-term effects of smoke fractions.] Memo to I. Hughes and C. McCarty, February 28, 1977.

1817.04. Finnegan T. [Funding Dr. Salvaggio to confirm Dr. Becker's work on tobacco glycoproteins.] Letter to W. Shinn, April 19, 1977.

1817.05. Yeaman A. [Dr. Rasmussen's work and grant application.] Letter to E. Pepples, July 6, 1978.

1817.06. Duplicate of {1816.03}.

1818.01. Pepples E. CTR Budget. Letter to J. Edens, B&W Industries, C. McCarty, I. Hughes, and D. Bryant, April 4, 1978.

1818.02. Pepples E. [Value of CTR in shielding tobacco industry from "unfavorable" research results funded with industry money.] Memo to C. McCarty, September 29, 1978.

1819.01. M.S. (?). Information Retrieval System. Memo to (?) Kw, June 28, 1978.

1819.02. Yeaman A. [Budget for 1978 literature retrieval, divided among tobacco companies based on cigarettes sales.] Letter to T. Ahrensfeld, J. Greer, A. Henson, E. Pepples, and H. Roemer, December 6, 1977.

1819.03. Hoyt W, Bryant D. [Assessing contributions from industry to CTR.] Letter to American Brands, B&W, Liggett & Myers, Philip Morris, and R. J. Reynolds, December 28, 1970.

1819.04. Duplicate of {1818.01}.

1820.01. Partial duplicate of {1817.05}.

1820.02. Pepples E. [Transmittal of report on CTR Microbiological Associates project.] Letter to T. Ahrensfeld, A. Holtzman, M. Crohn, J. Greer, A. Henson, H. Roemer, W. Shinn, and A. Stevens, June 30, 1978.

1820.03. Jacob E. [Status report on CTR funding of Microbiological Associates.] Letter to E. Pepples, June 22, 1978.

1820.04. Jacob and Medinger. Current Status of CTR's Consideration of Microbiological Associates Contract Proposals. 1978.

1821.01. Duplicate of {1818.02}.

1822.01. Pepples E. [NCI bioassay for carcinogenicity of menthol.] Memo to J. Esterle, December 26, 1978.

1822.02. Pepples E. [Chemicals included in NCI program.] Letter to F. Panzer, January 10, 1979.

1822.03. Esterle J. [Transmitting a list of chemicals being tested for carcinogenicity by NCI.] Memo to E. Pepples, January 8, 1979.

1822.04. Chemicals Which Are Currently Used/Chemicals Which May Be Present in Current Additives. List, 19??

1823.01. Pepples E. Re: Estimates of the Fraction of Cancer in the United States Related to Occupational Factors, Dated 1/15/78. Memo to J. Keehan and I. Hughes, January 22, 1979.

1824.01. Wells J. Re: Procedure for Handling BAT Scientific Documents. Memo to E. Pepples, November 9, 1979.

1824.02. Wells J. Re: Southampton Smoking and Health Material. Memo to E. Pepples, June 15, 1979.

1824.03. Wells J. BAT Science. Memo to E. Pepples, February 17, 1986.

1825.01. Wells J. Re: Smoking and Health—Tim Finnegan. Memo to E. Pepples, July 24, 1981.

1826.01. Witt S. Re: CTR—Tax Credit for Contributions. 1983.

1827.01. Pepples E. [Tax aspects of CTR contributions.] Letter to A. Stevens, February 25, 1983.

1827.02. Witt S. Re: CTR—Tax Credit for Contributions. 1983.

1827.03. Duplicate of {1826.01}.

1828.01. *Legal Considerations on Smoking and Health Policy.* 19??

1828.02. Johnson A. *Smoking and Health Issues.* BAT, 1985.

1829.01. Baker R. [Letter transmitting legal memo on attribution of statements by BAT subsidiaries.] Letter to D. Schechter, February 4, 1985.

1829.02. Baker R. [Legal analysis of the attribution problem.] Notes, 1985.

1829.03. Board of B.A.T. Industries P.L.C. List, 19??

1829.04. Tobacco Companies, B.A.T. Industries. Organizational chart, 19??

1829.05. Non Tobacco Companies, B.A.T. Industries. Organizational chart, 19??

1829.06. Ricketts P. Legal Considerations in Smoking and Health Issues to Operating Group Chairmen and Liaison Directors. 19??

1829.07. Scientific Information. [Legal approaches to evidence that smoking causes disease.] 19??

1830.01. Wells J. Re: Conference with BAT Legal on U.S. Products Liability Litigation. Notes to File, June 12, 1984.

1831.01. Pepples E. [Addiction vs. changes in functional behavior.] Memo to E. Kohnhorst, August 16, 1984.

1832.01. Hoel D. [Scheduling meeting of Public Smoking Advisory Group.] Letter to E. Pepples, September 24, 1984.

1832.02. Hoel D. [Reactivating the Public Smoking Advisory Group.] Letter to J. Chapin, A. Henson, A. Holtzman, J. Murray, E. Pepples, A. Stevens, and S. Witt, September 13, 1984.

1833.01. Wells J. [Suggested changes to Blackman paper.] Letter to H. Morini, October 25, 1984.

1833.02. Blackman, LCF. *The Controversy on Smoking and Health—Some Facts and Anomalies.* Draft paper, BAT, 1984.

1834.01. Wells J. Re: Document Retention. Notes to File, January 17, 1985.

1834.02. Griffith R. Report to Executive Committee. 1965.

1835.01. Wells J. Re: Document Retention. Memo to File, January 17, 1985.

1836.01. Schechter D. [BATUS and litigation.] Letter to R. Baker, August 30, 1985.

1836.02. Rosdeitcher S. [Concerns that BAT research could be discovered in a US lawsuit.] Memo to D. Schechter, July 8, 1985.

1837.01. Wells J. Re: BAT Science. Memo to E. Pepples, February 17, 1986.

1837.02. [Abstracts of various BAT research projects on smoke mutagenicity, nicotine and sidestream smoke.] 19??

1837.03. Excluded Projects, Summary. List, 19??

1838.01. [Handwritten notes on history of B&W/BAT cost- and risk-pooling agreement from 1958 through 1980.] Notes, 19??

1838.02. [Handwritten notes mentioning risk- and cost-sharing agreement between B&W and Canada.] Notes, 19??

1838.03. R&D Cost and Risk Pooling Agreement [including handwritten notes.] Notes, 1969.

1839.01. [Handwritten note saying that parts of attached document should be changed or deleted.] Notes to P. Tighe, June 3, 1978.

1840.01. Hardy D. [Warning to B&W about problems created by "careless" statements by B&W and BAT scientists at research conferences and problems created by the B&W/BAT cost- and risk-pooling agreement.] Letter to D. Bryant, August 20, 1970.

1840.02. Hardy D. [Status report on B&W's pending health litigation.] Letter to D. Bryant, October 27, 1970.

1840.03. Bryant D. [Concern that BAT might become involved in products liability litigation in the US through B&W.] Letter to E. Langford, November 5, 1970.

1840.04. Langford E. [Reaction to David Hardy's opinion (1840.01) regarding problems created by "careless" statements by B&W and BAT scientists.] Letter to D. Bryant, November 11, 1970.

1840.05. [A number of cigarette advertisements which appear to have been published in British newspapers and magazines.] 19??

TIRC AND CTR (1900 SERIES)

1900.01. Tobacco Industry Research Committee. A Frank Statement to the Public by the Makers of Cigarettes. December 28, 1960.

1901.01. Tobacco Industry Research Committee. A Frank Statement to Cigarette Smokers. *The Tobacco Leaf,* January 1954.

1902.01. Blalock J. Re: Tobacco Institute, Tobacco Industry Research Committee, and Hill & Knowlton. Memo to J. Burgard, June 18, 1963.

1902.02. Tobacco Industry Research Committee, Executive Committee [membership]. List, 19??

1902.03. Tobacco Industry Research Committee, Industry Technical Committee [membership]. List, 19??

1902.04. Hill and Knowlton, Inc. Staff (Relative to T.I. and T.I.R.C.). List, 19??

1902.05. Hill and Knowlton, Inc. 19??

1903.01. Pepples E. 10 Assertions about Smoking and Health vs. the True Facts. October 3, 1967.

1903.02. Cigarette Smoking and Health: What Are the Facts? October 3, 1967.

1903.03. Tobacco Industry Research Committee Organization and Policy. 1967?

1903.04. Tobacco Industry Research Committee Members. List, 19??

1903.05. Tobacco Industry Research Committee, Scientific Advisory Board. List, 19??

1903.06. Tobacco Industry Research Committee Staff. List, 19??

1903.07. Those Who Expressed Doubt before United States Congress of Smoking-Disease Relationship. [Excerpts of testimony before House and Senate committees.] 1965?

1903.08. Tobaccotalk Concerns. 19??

1904.01. Hockett R. Smoking-Disease Links Continue to Lack Scientific Proof. *American Automatic Merchandiser,* October 1, 1970.

1905.01. Hoyt W, Bryant D. [Confirming financial commitments from individual companies to CTR.] Letter to American Brands, B&W, Liggett & Myers, Philip Morris, and R. J. Reynolds, December 28, 1970.

1906.01. Review of the Liaison Meeting at St. Thomas. 1972.

1907.01. Kornegay H. Re: Shubik Blasts Tobacco Industry Scientists. Memo to Committee of Counsel, October 10, 1974.

1907.02. Tobacco Industry Scientists Are Prostitutes, Shubik Charges. *Cancer Newsletter* 1974;1:35.

1907.03. [Description of TIRC.] 19??

1907.04. Partial duplicate of {1903.01}.

1907.05. Duplicate of {1903.04}.

1907.06. Duplicate of {1903.05}.

1907.07. Duplicate of {1903.06}.

1907.08. Duplicate of {1902.02}.

1907.09. Duplicate of {1902.03}.

1907.10. Hill & Knowlton, Inc., Staff (Relative to T.I. and T.I.R.C.). List, 19??

1907.11. Duplicate of {1902.05}.

1908.01. Report to CTR Annual Meeting, January 31, 1975.

1908.02. *Use of the Nitromethane Fraction Index (NMFI) as an Indicator of Biological Activity of Smoke: Summary.* 19??

1909.01. Pepples E. [Hypnosis to help people quit smoking.] Memo to I. Hughes, April 18, 1977.

1909.02. Shinn W. [Hypnosis to treat nicotine addiction.] Letter to T. Ahrensfeld, J. Greer, C. Hetsko, E. Pepples, H. Roemer, and A. Stevens, April 14, 1977.

1910.01. Duplicate of {1816.03}.

1910.02. Partial duplicate of {1816.01}.

1910.03. Yeaman A. [Work by Dr. Rasmussen on DNA repair.] Letter to E. Pepples, July 6, 1978.

1910.04. Partial duplicate of {1817.03}.

1910.05. Shinn W. [Encouraging attendance at scientific meetings.] Letter, February 9, 1978.

1910.06. Finnegan T. [Providing funds for Dr. Salvaggio to confirm Dr. Becker's work on tobacco glycoproteins; partial document.] Letter to W. Shinn, April 19, 1977.

1910.07. Hockett R. [Cancellation of Dr. Becker's grant after he found undesirable results about tobacco glycoproteins; partial document.] Letter to A. Yeaman, October 31, 1977.

1911.01. Jacob E. [Recommending funding for Prof. Eysenck.] Letter to W. Shinn, January 18, 1978.

1911.02. Finnegan T. Re: Dr. Henry Rothschild. Letter to W. Shinn, February 17, 1978.

1911.03. Hughes I. [Re: Salvaggio abstract and manuscript.] Letter to D. Hoel, February 6, 1978.

1911.04. Pepples E. Re: Dr. John Salvaggio. Letter to W. Shinn, May 18, 1977.

1911.05. Shinn W. [Regarding funding Dr. Salvaggio.] Letter to T. Ahrensfeld, J. Greer, C. Hetsko, E. Pepples, H. Roemer, and A. Stevens, April 28, 1977.

1911.06. Finnegan T. Re: Dr. John Salvaggio. Letter to W. Shinn, April 19, 1977.

1911.07. Jacob and Medinger. Current Status of CTR's Consideration of Microbiological Associates Contract Proposals. 1978.

1911.08. Duplicate of {1820.02}.

1911.09. Jacob E. [Current status of CTR's project with Microbiological Associates.] Letter to E. Pepples, June 22, 1978.

1912.01. Nobile P. Researcher Doubts Safety of Low-Tar Smoking. *Journal-News,* August 11, 1978.

1913.01. Waite C. Re: The Addiction Research Foundation, A) Mr. Pepples's Letter of 11 September 1978, B) Mr. Cornell's Letter to Wm. Shinn of 9 August 1978. Memo to H. Kornegay, September 19, 1978.

1913.02. Shinn W. Re: Addiction Research Foundation. Letter to T. Ahrensfeld, M. Crohn, J. Greer, A. Henson, E. Pepples, and A. Stevens, August 24, 1978.

1913.03. Shinn W. [Request for funding from Addiction Research Foundation.] Letter to T. Ahrensfeld, M. Crohn, J. Greer, A. Henson, E. Pepples, and A. Stevens, August 15, 1978.

1913.04. Cornell L. [Requesting financial support for the Addiction Research Foundation.] Letter to W. Shinn, August 9, 1978.

1913.05. Cornell L. [Soliciting financial support from Lorillard Tobacco for the Addiction Research Foundation.] Letter to A. Stevens, September 6, 1978.

1913.06. Stevens A. [Lorillard will not support Dr. Goldstein's request to construct a nicotine laboratory.] Letter to L. Cornell, August 22, 1978.

1913.07. Stevens A. [Lorillard will not be supporting Dr. Goldstein.] Letter to L. Cornell, November 30, 1977.

1913.08. Yeaman A. [Addiction Research Foundation.] Letter to C. McCarty, May 19, 1977.

1913.09. Shinn W. [Dr. Goldstein's application for CTR special funding.] Letter to E. Pepples, April 14, 1977.

1913.10. Fields S. [Transmitting material from the Addiction Research Foundation to Shook, Hardy, and Bacon.] Letter to W. Shinn, April 1, 1977.

1913.11. Goldstein A. The Council for Tobacco Research U.S.A. Inc. Application for Research Grant. December 15, 1976.

1914.01. Pepples E. [Handwritten note to E. Clements, saying B&W has no more money for research grants.] 19??

1915.01. Pepples E. [Information on nicotine for discussion with Dr. Bourne.] Letter to J. Edens, December 15, 1977.

1915.02. Waite C. Re: The Addiction Research Foundation. Memo to H. Kornegay, September 19, 1978.

1916.01. [Memo to staff regarding how to respond to CTR-funded project by Gary Friedman implicating smoking as a cause of heart disease.] Memo, February 1, 1979.

1917.01. Pepples E. [Draft press release regarding UCLA project.] Letter to L. Stanford, May 29, 1979.

1917.02. Pepples E. Re: UCLA Medical School Research. Memo to C. McCarty, I. Hughes, R. Pittman, and R. Roach, May 29, 1979.

1917.03. Stanford L. Re: UCLA Three-Year Extension. Letter to E. Pepples, T. Ahrensfeld, M. Crohn, and J. Chapin, May 22, 1979.

1917.04. Shinn W. [Re: Gloria Powell, Director of Child Psychology at UCLA.] Letter to E. Pepples, May 15, 1979.

1917.05. Stanford L. [Extension of UCLA agreement.] Letter to I. Hughes, C. Goldsmith, W. Hobbs, and J. Chapin, May 9, 1979.

1917.06. Extension Agreement for Research by and between the Regents of the University of California and Brown & Williamson Tobacco Corporation; Philip Morris. April 20, 1979.

1917.07. Cline Fined. 19??

1917.08. M.S. Re: Research Contracts [at UCLA, Washington University, and Franklin Institute.] Memo to Mr. P., October 1, 1981.

1918.01. Charitable Contributions Grants Payable before March 15, 1981. List, December 23, 1981.

1919.01. Sirridge P. [Information on Drs. Craig Daniels and Charles Erwin.] Letter to E. Pepples, June 17, 1981.

1919.02. Stone W. [Providing requested background information on Charles Erwin and Craig Daniels.] Memo, 19??

1919.03. Pepples E. [Requesting background information on Daniels and Erwin.] Letter to P. Sirridge, May 19, 1981.

1919.04. Pepples E. [Acknowledging receipt of background information on Daniels and Erwin.] Letter to P. Sirridge, June 23, 1981.

1919.05. [Note to Ernie regarding Dr. Daniels and Erwin.] 19??

1920.01. [Detailed description of CTR.] 19??

SPECIAL PROJECTS (2000 SERIES)

2000.01. Parmele H. [Sending a sample of tobacco tar dissolved in acetone.] Letter to R. Roberts, February 4, 1955.

2000.02. Proposed study by Alvan R. Feinstein, M.D., of the Natural Course and Post-Therapeutic Outcome of Cancers of the Lung, Larynx, and Rectum [partial document]. Proposal, 19??

2000.03. Fudenberg H. [Request for research funding.] Letter to E. Jacob, July 20, 1972.

2000.04. Yeaman A. Meeting of General Counsel on December 17, 1965. Memo, December 17, 1965.

2001.01. Hardy D. [Theodor Sterling, progress report and continued funding.] Letter to A. Yeaman, December 26, 1968.

2001.02. Hardy D. [Theodor Sterling.] Letter to P. Grant, F. Haas, C. Hetsko, H. Ramm, P. Smith, and A. Yeaman, December 26, 1968.

2002.01. Sterling T, Pollack S. The incidence of lung cancer in the U.S. since 1955 in relation to the etiology of the disease. *Am J Pub Health*, February 1972.

2002.02. Sterling T. [Requesting $5,000 for panel on effects of environmental pollution on human health.] Letter to W. Shinn, February 29, 1972.

2002.03. Rodin E. [ALEPH Foundation's role as intermediary for Sterling's symposium in Israel.] Letter to T. Sterling, February 24, 1972.

2002.04. Society of Engineering Science in Tel Aviv, Israel. Pollution: Engineering and Scientific Solutions. June 12, 1972.

2002.05. Shinn W. [Value of Sterling's work to tobacco industry.] Letter to T. Ahrensfeld, D. Bryant, F. Haas, C. Hetsko, H. Roemer, A. Stevens, and A. Yeaman, March 1, 1972.

2002.06. Bryant D. [Regarding recommendation to grant $5,000 to ALEPH Foundation for a panel on "Effects of Pollutants on Human Health."] Letter to W. Shinn, March 7, 1972.

2003.01. Washington University Special Project. 19??

2003.02. UCLA Special Project [budget and grantees]. Budget, 19??

2003.03. Harvard Special Project [budget and donors]. List, 19??

2004.01. Hoel D. Re: Dr. Carl C. Seltzer. Letter to T. Ahrensfeld, D. Bryant, J. Greer, C. Hetsko, H. Roemer, and A. Stevens, April 16, 1976.

2004.02. Shinn W. [Recommend continuing Seltzer's funding as CTR special project.] Letter to T. Ahrensfeld, D. Bryant, J. Greer, C. Hetsko, H. Roemer, and A. Stevens, March 23, 1977.

2004.03. Pepples E. Re: Dr. Carl Seltzer. Letter to W. Shinn, April 5, 1977.

2004.04. Pepples E. Re: Dr. Carl Seltzer. Letter to W. Shinn, August 9, 1978.

2004.05. Shinn W. [Recommend supporting Dr. Seltzer through a CTR special project.] Letter to T. Ahrensfeld, J. Greer, A. Henson, E. Pepples, H. Roemer, and A. Stevens, August 7, 1978.

2004.06. Pepples E. Re: Dr. Carl C. Seltzer. Letter to D. Hoel, May 3, 1978.

2004.07. Hoel D. Re: Dr. Carl C. Seltzer. Letter to T. Ahrensfeld, J. Greer, A. Henson, E. Pepples, H. Roemer, and A. Stevens, April 28, 1978.

2004.08. Hoel D. Re: Dr. Carl Seltzer. 1979.

2004.09. Hoel D. Re: Dr. Carl Seltzer. Letter to T. Ahrensfeld, M. Crohn, J. Greer, A. Henson, E. Pepples, and A. Stevens, April 4, 1979.

2004.10. Pepples E. Re: Carl C. Seltzer. Letter to D. Hoel, April 6, 1979.

2004.11. Hoel D. [Renewal of Seltzer's funding.] Letter to T. Ahrensfeld, M. Crohn, J. Greer, A. Henson, E. Pepples, and A. Stevens, April 16, 1979.

2004.12. Hoel D. [Transmitting media coverage of Carl Seltzer's trip to Australia and New Zealand.] Letter to T. Ahrensfeld, M. Crohn, J. Greer, A. Henson, E. Pepples, and A. Stevens, May 17, 1979.

2004.13. Wilson P. Smokers—Take Heart! [Victoria, Australia] *Sun*, May 5, 1979.

2004.14. Former-Smoker Studies Challenged. *Canberra Times*, May 2, 1979.

2004.15. Whong L. Doctor Slams Link between Smoking and Heart Disease. *The Australian*, May 2, 1979.

2004.16. Channel 10, 6:00 P.M. News, January 5, 1979.

2004.17. Convinced Stopping Smoking Does Not Reduce Heart Disease. 1979.

2004.18. Channel 7, 11:00 A.M., July 5, 1979.

2004.19. Theory Up in Smoke [regarding Carl Seltzer]. [Victoria, Australia] *Herald*, 19??

2004.20. Hoel D. Re: Dr. Carl C. Seltzer. Letter to J. Greer, A. Henson, A. Holtzman, E. Pepples, A. Stevens, and S. Witt, July 1, 1982.

2004.21. Sirridge P. Re: Dr. Carl C. Seltzer. Letter to J. Greer, A. Henson, A. Holtzman, E. Pepples, A. Stevens, and S. Witt, April 4, 1983.

2004.22. Pepples E. Re: Dr. Carl C. Seltzer. Letter to P. Sirridge, April 7, 1983.

2004.23. Pepples E. Re: Carl Seltzer's Letter to Robin MacNeil. Memo to I. Hughes, J. Alar, and T. Humber, February 20, 1984.

2004.24. Kornegay H. [Regarding Seltzer's challenge to Castelli's appearance on Mac-Neil/Lehrer.] Letter to E. Pepples, February 17, 1984.

2004.25. Seltzer C. [Re: Interview with Dr. Castelli on MacNeil/Lehrer.] Letter to R. Mac-Neil, January 31, 1984.

2004.26. Sirridge P. Re: Dr. Carl C. Seltzer. Letter to A. Henson, A. Holtzman, J. Murray, E. Pepples, A. Stevens, and S. Witt, April 9, 1984.

2004.27. Pepples E. [Agrees to renew Seltzer's project.] Letter to P. Sirridge, April 13, 1984.

2004.28. Pepples E. Re: Dr. Carl Seltzer. Letter to T. Finnegan, July 9, 1985.

2004.29. Finnegan T. Re: Dr. Carl Seltzer. Letter to A. Holtzman, (?) Murray, A. Henson, E. Pepples, A. Stevens, and S. Witt, July 2, 1985.

2004.30. Seltzer C. The effect of cigarette smoking on coronary heart disease: Where do we stand now? *Arch Environ Health* March 1970; 29:418–423.

2004.31. Seltzer C. Proposal. July 29, 1978.

2004.32. Oechsli F, Seltzer C. Teenage smoking and antecedent parental characteristics: A prospective study. *Publ Hlth* (Lond.) 1983;98:103–108.

2004.33. *Smoking Does Not Cause Heart Disease and Drinking in Moderation Actually Reduces It.* 1979.

2005.01. CTR Special Projects. List, 19??

2006.01. Heimstra N, Fallesen J, Kinsley S, Warner N. The effects of deprivation of cigarette smoking on psychomotor performance. *Ergonomics* 1980;23:1047–1055.

2006.02. Dille J, Linder M. The effects of tobacco on aviation safety. *Aviation, Space and Environ Med* 1981;52:112–115.

2006.03. Hoel D. Re: Response Analysis Corporation Project. Letter to T. Ahrensfeld, D. Bryant, C. Hetsko, H. Roemer, and A. Stevens, November 10, 1976.

2006.04. Pepples E. [Funding of Response Analysis Corp.] Letter to D. Hoel, July 6, 1977.

2006.05. Hoel D. Re: Response Analysis Corporation Project. Letter to T. Ahrensfeld, C. Hetsko, E. Pepples, H. Roemer, and A. Stevens, June 17, 1977.

2006.06. Pepples E. [Acknowledging receipt of letter regarding Response Analysis Corp. project.] Letter to D. Hoel, November 12, 1976.

2006.07. Duplicate of {2006.05}.

2007.01. Pepples E. [Agrees to fund Dr. Domingo Aviado.] Letter to W. Shinn, May 13, 1977.

2007.02. Shinn W. [Regarding Dr. Aviado's request for funding.] Letter to T. Ahrensfeld, J. Greer, C. Hetsko, E. Pepples, H. Roemer, and A. Stevens, May 9, 1977.

2007.03. Hoel D. [Transmitting program for International Symposium on Mechanisms of Airways Obstruction to be held in South Africa.] Letter to E. Pepples, January 19, 1978.

2007.04. Mechanisms of Airways Obstruction. March 28, 1978.

2007.05. Shinn W. [Dr. Aviado's request for funding.] Letter to T. Ahrensfeld, M. Crohn, J. Greer, A. Henson, E. Pepples, and A. Stevens, October 24, 1979.

2007.06. Aviado D. Curriculum Vitae. 19??

2007.07. Pepples E. Re: Dr. Domingo Aviado. Letter to W. Shinn, October 31, 1979.

2007.08. Sirridge P. [Regarding financial support for Dr. Aviado.] Letter to T. Ahrensfeld, J. Greer, E. Pepples, A. Stevens, M. Crohn, and A. Henson, February 6, 1981.

2007.09. Pepples E. [Agrees to continuing to support Dr. Aviado.] Letter to P. Sirridge, February 12, 1981.

2007.10. Sirridge P. [Recommending financial support for Aviado.] Letter to J. Greer, A. Henson, A. Holtzman, E. Pepples, A. Stevens, and S. Witt. February 8, 1982.

2007.11. Copy of {2007.08}, without letterhead.

2007.12. Pepples E. [Agrees to fund Dr. Aviado.] Letter to P. Sirridge, February 17, 1982.

2007.13. Sirridge P. [Re: Funding Dr. Aviado.] Letter to J. Greer, A. Henson, A. Holtzman, E. Pepples, A. Stevens, and S. Witt, January 26, 1983.

2007.14. [Re: granting Domingo Aviado $102,000 for 1983.] Letter to P. Sirridge, January 31, 1983.

2007.15. Pepples E. Re: Dr. Domingo Aviado. Letter to P. Sirridge, February 6, 1984.

2007.16. Sirridge P. [Recommends further support of Aviado.] Letter to A. Henson, A. Holtzman, J. Murray, E. Pepples, A. Stevens, and S. Witt, February 1, 1984.

2007.17. Pepples E. Re: Dr. Domingo Aviado. Letter to P. Sirridge, February 12, 1985.

2007.18. Sirridge P. [Recommends further support for Dr. Aviado.] Letter to A. Henson, A. Holtzman, J. Murray, E. Pepples, A. Stevens, and S. Witt, February 8, 1985.

2008.01. Wells J. [*Medical World News* article about Dr. Alan Blum.] Letter to W. Kloepfer, December 6, 1977.

2008.02. Kloepfer W. [Transmitting *Medical World News* article regarding Dr. Alan Blum.] Letter to J. Wells, December 1, 1977.

2008.03. Rothschild H. [Progress report, budget, and future plans.] Letter to T. Finnegan, February 8, 1978.

2008.04. Rothschild H. Respiratory System Cancer In Louisiana [grant proposal]. 1977?

2008.05. Proposed Budget for 1978–1979. January 1, 1978.

2009.01. [Summary of research plan by H. Rothschild to investigate causes of lung cancer other than smoking.] 1979?

2009.02. Proposed Budget for 1979–1980. April 10, 1979.

2009.03. Rothschild H. Abstract of Application—Research. Memo to J. Finerty, April 10, 1979.

2009.04. Duplicate of {1911.02}.

2009.05. Finnegan T. [Transmitting a copy of Henry Rothschild's "The Bandwagons of Medicine."] Letter to T. Ahrensfeld, A. Henson, E. Pepples, H. Roemer, and A. Stevens, October 31, 1978.

2009.06. Cohen L, Rothschild H. The Bandwagons of Medicine. Department of Medicine, Louisiana State University Medical Center, 19??

2009.07. Landau R. [Tentative acceptance letter regarding "The Bandwagons of Medicine" from *Perspectives in Biology and Medicine*.] Letter to H. Rothschild, September 19, 1978.

2009.08. Finnegan T. [Circulating Dr. Rothschild's recent report.] Letter to T. Ahrensfeld, A. Hensen, E. Pepples, H. Roemer, and A. Stevens, June 13, 1978.

2009.09. Finnegan T. [Transmitting report from Henry Rothschild.] Letter to T. Ahrensfeld, A. Hensen, E. Pepples, H. Roemer, and A. Stevens, June 1, 1978.

2009.10. Pepples E. Re: Dr. Rothschild. Letter to W. Shinn, April 6, 1978.

2009.11. Finnegan T. Re: Dr. Henry Rothschild. Letter to W. Shinn, February 17, 1978.

2009.12. Rothschild H. [Progress report, budget, and future plans.] Letter to T. Finnegan, February 8, 1978.

2009.13. Rothschild H. Respiratory System Cancer in Louisiana. 19??

2009.14. Proposed Budget for 1978–1979. January 1, 1978.

2009.15. Finnegan T. [Regarding funding Henry Rothschild.] Letter to W. Shinn, February 26, 1977.

2009.16. Pepples E. [Agrees with recommendation to fund Rothschild.] Letter to W. Shinn, March 16, 1977.

2009.17. Rothschild H. Proposal for a Pilot Study of the Disproportionately High Mortality Due to Respiratory Tract Cancer in Southern Louisiana. 19??

2009.18. [Phone message to MP from Dr. Hughes.] March 1, 19??

2009.19. Rothschild H. [Preliminary results regarding genetics and cancer causation.] Letter to Brown & Williamson Tobacco Corp., February 24, 1976.

2010.01. Shinn W. [Importance of encouraging attendance at scientific meetings.] Letter to T. Ahrensfeld, M. Crohn, J. Greer, A. Henson, E. Pepples, and A. Stevens, February 9, 1978.

2010.02. Pepples E. Re: CTR Budget. Letter to J. Edens, B&W Industries, C. McCarty, I. Hughes, and D. Bryant, April 4, 1978.

2010.03. Pepples E. [Value of having CTR fund work that may "go sour."] Memo to C. McCarty, September 29, 1978.

2011.01. Pepples E. Re: Dr. La Via. Letter to W. Shinn, March 29, 1978.

2011.02. Shinn W. [Re: Dr. La Via.] Letter to T. Ahrensfeld, J. Greer, A. Henson, E. Pepples, H. Roemer, and A. Stevens, March 24, 1978.

2011.03. Finnegan T. Re: Dr. Mariano La Via. Letter to W. Shinn, February 17, 1978.

2011.04. Curriculum Vitae, Mariano F. La Via, M.D. 19??

2012.01. Duplicate of {2011.04}.

2012.02. Shinn W. [Payment of Dr. Gibbons at University of Alabama.] Letter to T. Ahrensfeld, J. Greer, A. Henson, E. Pepples, H. Roemer, and A. Stevens, March 24, 1978.

2012.03. Hoel D. [Proposal for funding from A. Szent-Gyorgyi.] Letter to E. Pepples, November 30, 1977.

2012.04. Szent-Gyorgyi A. [Seeking common interest in cancer research (handwritten note).] Letter to D. Hoel, November 1, 1977.

2012.05. Hoel D. [Expressing interest in providing funding.] Letter to A. Szent-Gyorgyi, November 9, 1977.

2013.01. Sterling T. Blue-Collar Work May Be Hazardous to Your Health. *Courier-Journal* [Louisville], September 24, 1978.

2013.02. Pepples E. [Agrees to extend funding for Eysenck.] Letter to E. Jacob, May 31, 1978.

2013.03. Jacob E. [Report on Prof. Eysenck's work.] Letter to M. Crohn, A. Henson, A. Holtzman, E. Pepples, and A. Stevens, May 25, 1987.

2013.04. Pepples E. [Summary of Dr. Gardner's proposals.] Letter to A. Yeaman, March 10, 1977.

2014.01. Wells J. Re: Harvard Air Quality/Lung Health Study. Memo to E. Pepples, April 28, 1978.

2014.02. Harvard University Air Quality/Lung Health Study. School of Public Health. Brochure, 19??

2015.01. Shinn W. [Projects from Eysenck and Franklin Institute.] Letter to T. Ahrensfeld, J. Greer, A. Henson, E. Pepples, H. Roemer, and A. Stevens, March 9, 1978.

2015.02. Finnegan T. Re: Dr. Henry Rothschild. Letter to J. Greer, A. Henson, A. Holtzman, E. Pepples, A. Stevens, and S. Witt, February 15, 1982.

2015.03. Pepples E. Re: Perry/Sterling Project. Letter to W. Shinn, October 29, 1980.

2015.04. Sirridge P. Re: Dr. Theodor Sterling. Letter to J. Murray, A. Henson, A. Holtzman, E. Pepples, A. Stevens, and S. Witt, January 23, 1984.

2015.05. Budget for a Continuing Critical Review of Major Factors in the Area of Smoking and Health, May 1, 1984 to April 30, 1985, T. D. Sterling Limited. Budget, May 1, 1984.

2016.01. Pepples E. [Conversation with Cooper and Gori regarding letter of intent.] Memo to J. Edens, C. McCarty, R. Kirk, I. Hughes, and R. Pittman, May 23, 1979.

2016.02. Pepples E. [Agreement to fund Cornell University for five years.] Letter to T. Cooper, May 24, 1979.

2016.03. Pepples E. Re: Letter to Dr. Cooper. Memo to J. Edens, C. McCarty, R. Kirk, I. Hughes, and R. Pittman, May 24, 1979.

2016.04. Pepples E. [Possibility of B&W's supporting epidemiological research at Cornell University.] Letter to T. Cooper, May 24, 1979.

2017.01. Blass J. [Description of research on brain function at Cornell University, in an effort to secure funding.] Letter to T. Finnegan, February 5, 1980.

2017.02. McDowell F. [Seeking financial support for Burke Rehabilitation Center.] Letter to B. Myerson, October 1, 1980.

2017.03. No document at this number.

2017.04. Stevens A. [Nicotine research at Burke Rehabilitation Center.] Letter to T. Finnegan, October 13, 1980.

2017.05. No document at this number.

2017.06. Duplicate of {1825.01}.

2017.07. Blass J. [Reporting preliminary data that nicotine has beneficial effects on brain diseases in animals.] Letter to T. Finnegan, June 16, 1981.

2017.08. Sturchio P. Report of Expenditures Brown and Williamson Tobacco Company for Period 10/1/80–3/31/81. Budget, March 31, 1981.

2017.09. Finnegan T. [Re: John Blass.] Letter to E. Pepples, August 10, 1981.

2017.10. Finnegan T. Re: Dr. John P. Blass. Letter to E. Pepples, September 30, 1981.

2017.11. Blass JP. [Transmitting two preprints "heavily stamped with our new 'Priviledged Communication' stamp."] Letter to T. Finnegan, September 16, 1981.

2017.12. Blass J, Gibson G, Duffy T, Plum F. Cholinergic Deficiency in Metabolic Encephalopathies. Ithaca, NY: Cornell University Medical College and Burke Rehabilitation Center, 1980?

2018.01. Shinn W. [Consulting agreement with Dr. Aviado.] Letter to T. Ahrensfeld, M. Crohn, A. Henson, E. Pepples, and A. Stevens, January 30, 1980.

2019.01. Shinn W. [Site visit to Washington University. Letter to P. Lacy, February 21, 1980.

2019.02. Stevens A. Re: Washington University. Letter to T. Ahrensfeld, A. Holtzman, M. Crohn, J. Greer, E. Pepples, H. Kornegay, and W. Shinn, February 14, 1980.

2019.03. Pepples E. [Transmitting press accounts on Dr. Paul Lacy's research.] Memo to J. Edens, C. McCarty, R. Kirk, I. Hughes, R. Pittman, B. Cummins, F. Kiernan, and W. Dewitt, April 18, 1979.

2019.04. Research on Insulin-Producing Cells May Lead to New Diabetes Treatment/ Diabetes Research Advances. *Courier-Journal* [Louisville], April 13, 1979.

2019.05. Shinn W. [Re: Funding Dr. Lacy.] Letter to T. Ahrensfeld, J. Chapin, M. Crohn, E. Pepples, and C. Wayne, January 22, 1980.

2019.06. Pepples E. Washington University Project—For June 5 Trip. Memo to I. Hughes, June 2, 1980.

2019.07. Hoel D. [Arranging site visit to Washington University.] Letter to E. Pepples, April 29, 1980.

2019.08. Washington University Site Visit Participants, June 5–6, 1980. List, 1980.

2019.09. Speake M. Washington University Project. 1980.

2019.10. Pepples E. [Site visit to Washington University.] Letter to W. Shinn, March 6, 1980.

2020.01. Shinn W. Re: Perry/Sterling Project. Letter to T. Ahrensfeld, M. Crohn, J. Greer, A. Henson, E. Pepples, and A. Stevens, October 22, 1980.

2020.02. Pepples E. Re: T. D. Sterling: Feasibility Study on Office Environments. Letter to R. Northrip, August 13, 1980.

2020.03. Northrip R. Re: T. D. Sterling: Feasibility Study on Office Environments. Letter to T. Ahrensfeld, M. Crohn, J. Greer, A. Henson, E. Pepples, and A. Stevens, July 17, 1980.

2025.03. Finnegan T. Re: Dr. John P. Blass. Letter to E. Pepples, September 30, 1981.

2025.04. Pepples E. [Possible research grant to Cornell University.] Letter to T. Cooper, May 24, 1979.

2025.05. Blass J. [Discussion of nicotine and Alzheimer's or Parkinson's disease.] Letter to E. Pepples, February 21, 1984.

2026.01. Sirridge P. Re: T. D. Sterling: Office Building Syndrome Investigation. Letter to T. Ahrensfeld, J. Greer, A. Henson, E. Pepples, A. Stevens, and S. Witt, November 20, 1981.

2027.01. Comprehensive Smoking Prevention Education Act, Appendix to Hearings before the Subcommittee on Health and the Environment of the Committee on Energy. 1982.

2028.01. Pepples E. [List of projects for review.] Memo to J. Esterle, March 11, 1982.

2028.02. Pepples E. [Proposals for funding of research by B&W.] Memo to M. Reynolds, March 10, 1982.

2028.03. Esterle J. Re: Proposals for Industry Funding. Memo to E. Pepples, March 23, 1982.

2029.01. Duplicate of {2028.03}.

2029.02. Pepples E. [Recent proposals for industry funding of scientific proposals.] Memo to J. Esterle, March 11, 1982.

2029.03. Pepples E. [Proposals for B&W funding.] Memo to M. Reynolds, March 10, 1982.

2029.04. Pepples E. [Proposal to continue funding V. Riley's work.] Memo to R. Sanford, March 10, 1982.

2030.01. Sirridge P. [Updated list of CTR special projects.] Letter to J. Greer, A. Henson, A. Holtzman, E. Pepples, A. Stevens, and S. Witt, April 2, 1982.

2031.01. CTR Special Projects. 1982.

2032.01. Lederberg J. [Inviting attendance at symposium at Rockefeller University.] Letter to E. Pepples, September 17, 1982.

2032.02. Nichols R. [Personal note regarding visit to Rockefeller University.] 1982.

2032.03. Pepples E. [Meeting for lunch; also telling him that Dr. Gori is still "studying the matter for us."] Letter to J. Lederberg, September 27, 1982.

2032.04. Table of Contents. *Br J Addiction* 1982;77(2):35.

2032.05. Pepples E. [Grant to Rockefeller University.] Letter to J. Lederberg, December 31, 1981.

2032.06. Pepples E. [Effects of depriving smokers of cigarettes.] Letter to J. Lederberg, November 30, 1981.

2032.07. Lederberg J. [Soliciting contributions.] Letter to E. Pepples, September 6, 1984.

2033.01. Pepples E. Re: Dr. Irving Zeidman. Letter to W. Shinn, May 31, 1983.

2033.02. Shinn W. [Recommends funding Zeidman's project.] Letter to J. Greer, A. Henson, A. Holtzman, E. Pepples, A. Stevens, and S. Witt, May 6, 1983.

2033.03. Zeidman I. Curriculum Vitae—Irving Zeidman, M.D. 19??

2034.01. Pepples E. Re: Dr. Henry Rothschild. Letter to T. Finnegan, May 20, 1983.

2034.02. Finnegan T. Re: Dr. Henry Rothschild. Letter to J. Greer, A. Henson, A. Holtzman, E. Pepples, A. Stevens, and S. Witt, May 16, 1983.

2034.03. Rothschild H. Statement of Henry Rothschild, M.D., Ph.D. in Response to S.772, The Smoking Prevention Health and Education Act of 1983. 1983?

2034.04. Rothschild H. *Genetic Aspects of Lung Cancer—Progress Report (1982–1983).* 1982.

2034.05. Rothschild H. Request for Funding 1983–1984. Proposal, January 1, 1983.

2034.06. Pepples E. Re: Dr. Henry Rothschild. Letter to T. Finnegan, March 10, 1982.

2034.07. Budget [for Henry Rothschild research project]. 1982.

2034.08. Pepples E. Re: Dr. Henry Rothschild. Letter to T. Finnegan, August 11, 1980.

2034.09. Finnegan T. Re: Dr. Henry Rothschild. Letter to T. Ahrensfeld, M. Crohn, J. Greer, A. Henson, E. Pepples, and A. Stevens, August 4, 1980.

2034.10. Rothschild H. *Progress Report (1979–1980)*. 1979.

2034.11. Rothschild H. Request for Funding 1980–1981. Proposal, January 1, 1980.

2034.12. Finnegan T. Re: Dr. Henry Rothschild. Letter to T. Ahrensfeld, M. Crohn, J. Greer, A. Henson, E. Pepples, and A. Stevens, July 15, 1980.

2034.13. Rothschild H, Mulvey J. *An Association between Respiratory System Cancer Mortality and Sugarcane-Related Occupation.* 19??

2034.14. Pepples E. [Considering continued funding of Dr. Rothschild's research.] Memo to R. Sanford and J. Esterle, June 12, 1979.

2034.15. Pepples E. [Approves funding Dr. Rothschild's research.] Letter to P. Sirridge, June 11, 1979.

2034.16. Sirridge P. [Recommending third year of support for Dr. Rothschild.] Letter to T. Ahrensfeld, M. Crohn, J. Greer, A. Henson, E. Pepples, and A. Stevens, June 8, 1979.

2034.17. McClendon J. Re: Dr. Henry Rothschild. Letter to W. Shinn, May 21, 1979.

2034.18. Rothschild H. [Past accomplishments and proposal for next year.] Letter to T. Finnegan, April 17, 1979.

2034.19. Rothschild H. Request for Funding 1979–1980. Proposal, April 17, 1979.

2035.01. CTR Special Projects. 1983.

2036.01. Pepples E. [Relationship between smoking and various forms of dementia.] Letter to J. Lederberg, December 12, 1983.

2037.01. Pepples E. Dr. Theodor D. Sterling. Letter to P. Sirridge, January 24, 1984.

2037.02. Sterling T. Are Regulations Needed to Hold Experts Accountable for Contributing "Biased" Briefs of Reports That Effect [*sic*] Public Policies? 1983.

2037.03. Pepples E. [Agrees to continue funding Sterling.] Letter to P. Sirridge, March 8, 1982.

2037.04. Sirridge P. [Extension of Sterling's funding; value in responding to congressional investigations.] Letter to J. Greer, A. Henson, A. Holtzman, E. Pepples, A. Stevens, and S. Witt, March 1, 1982.

2037.05. Sterling T. Budget for: A Continuing Critical Review of Major Factors in the Area of Smoking and Health, May 1, 1984 to April 30, 1985, T. D. Sterling Limited. Budget, May 1, 1984.

2037.06. Question and/or Comment Sheet for Technical and Symposia Papers Only. 1982.

2037.07. Sterling T. Non-smoking wives of heavy smokers have a higher risk of lung cancer [letter to editor]. *Br Med J* 1981;282:1156.

2037.08. Pepples E. Re: Dr. Arvin S. Glicksman Perry/Sterling Project on Occupational Exposures. Letter to B. O'Neill, December 1, 1981.

2037.09. O'Neill B. Re: Dr. Arvin S. Glicksman Perry/Sterling Project on Occupational Exposures. Letter to T. Ahrensfeld, J. Greer, A. Henson, E. Pepples, A. Stevens, and S. Witt, November 18, 1981.

2037.10. Pepples E. Re: T. D. Sterling—Office Building Syndrome Investigation. Letter to P. Sirridge, December 1, 1981.

2038.01. Sirridge P. [Updated chart of CTR special projects.] Letter to A. Henson, A. Holtzman, J. Murray, E. Pepples, A. Stevens, and S. Witt, September 4, 1984.

2038.02. CTR Special Projects. 1989.

2039.01. Pepples E. Re: Dr. John C. Gruhn. Letter to M. Davidson, March 12, 1985.

2039.02. Davidson M. Re: Dr. John C. Gruhn. Letter to T. Ahrensfeld, J. Murray, A. Henson, E. Pepples, A. Stevens, and S. Witt, March 5, 1985.

2040.01. Finnegan T. Re: Dr. Carl Seltzer. Letter to A. Holtzman, J. Murray, A. Henson, E. Pepples, A. Stevens, and S. Witt, July 2, 1985.

2040.02. Pepples E. Re: Dr. Carl Seltzer. Letter to T. Finnegan, July 9, 1985.

2040.03. Seltzer C. The effect of cigarette smoking on coronary heart disease: Where do we stand now? *Arch Environ Health* March 1970;20:418–422.

2040.04. Seltzer C. Proposal. July 29, 1978.

2040.05. Duplicate of {2004.32}.

2041.01. Pepples E. Re: ACVA Atlantic, Inc. Letter to D. Hoel, July 8, 1985.

2041.02. Hoel D. Re: ACVA Atlantic, Inc. Proposal. Letter to J. Chapin, A. Henson, A. Holtzman, J. Murray, E. Pepples, A. Stevens, and S. Witt, June 27, 1985.

2041.03. ACVA Atlantic Inc. and G. Robertson. Residential Inspection—Indoor Air Pollution. Proposal, May 2, 1985.

2041.04. Robertson G. Quotation: Residential Inspection—Indoor Air Pollution. Quotation, ACVA Atlantic, Inc., May 2, 1985.

2042.01. Special Account Number 4 Recipients. List, June 20, 1986.

2043.01. Special Projects and Special Accounts. List, February 23, 1989.

2044.01. Sirridge P. [Enclosing chart of CTR special projects.] Letter to A. Henson, A. Holtzman, J. Murray, E. Pepples, A. Stevens, and S. Witt, September 4, 1984.

2044.02. CTR Special Projects. 1989.

2045.01. Shook, Hardy, and Bacon Special Account: Consultancies. List, 1989.

2046.01. Shook, Hardy, and Bacon. [Regarding CTR budget.] Letter to J. E. Edens, C. I. McCarty, I. W. Hughes, and DeBaun Bryant, 19??

2047.01. [Handwritten note mentioning Dr. Domingo Aviado.] 19??

2048.01. Harvard University Special Project. List, 19??

2048.02. UCLA Special Project. 19??

2048.03. Washington University Special Project. 19??

2048.04. [Handwritten note on special projects.] 19??

2048.05. Special Account #4: Consultancies. List, 19??

2048.06. CTR Special Projects. List, 19??

2048.07. Special Account #4: Consultancies. List, 19??

2048.08. Special Account #4: Consultancies. List, 19??

2048.09. Special Account #5: List, 19??

2048.10. [Fragment of University Special Project budget.] List, 19??

2048.11. CTR Special Projects under Consideration. List, 1977.

2048.12. Non-CTR Special Projects. List, 1977.

2048.13. CTR Special Projects. List, 1978.

2048.14. CTR Special Projects. List, 1979.

2048.15. CTR Special Projects. List, 1979.

2048.16. CTR Special Projects. List, 1979.

2048.17. CTR Special Projects. List, 1979.

2048.18. CTR Special Projects. List, 1980.

2048.19. CTR Special Projects. List, 1980.

2048.20. CTR Special Projects. List, 1983.

2048.21. CTR Special Projects. List, 1983.

2048.22. CTR Special Projects. List, 1984.

2048.23. CTR Special Projects. List, 1984.

2048.24. Sirridge P. [List of CTR Special Accounts 4 and 5 projects and consultancies and other special projects.] Letter to A. Henson, A. Holtzman, J. Murray, E. Pepples, A. Stevens, and S. Witt, September 4, 1984.

2048.25. Sirridge P. [CTR Special Accounts 4 and 5 and consultancies.] Letter to A. Henson, A. Holtzman, J. Murray, E. Pepples, A. Stevens, and S. Witt, October 8, 1985.

2048.26. Sirridge P. [List of CTR Special Accounts 4 and 5 and consultancies.] Letter to W. Juchatz, A. Holtzman, J. Murray, E. Pepples, P. Randour, and A. Stevens, October 24, 1986.

PUBLIC RELATIONS (2100 SERIES)

2131.02. Kornegay H. [Plans to lobby editors to oppose Hatch-Packwood bill.] Letter to E. Pepples, February 8, 1983.

2131.03. Judge C. [Presentation to editor of *Time* magazine to rebut Surgeon General's report.] Letter to S. Chilcote, February 8, 1983.

2131.04. Humber T. [Preventing anti-smoking ads and editorial content in magazines.] Memo to I. Hughes, February 8, 1983.

2131.05. Pepples E. Re: Industry Contacts with Editors. Memo, February 14, 1983.

2131.06. Covington and Burling. Memorandum to the Committee of Counsel Re: Proposed Compromise Legislation Concerning Cigarette Labeling and Advertising. 1983.

2132.01. Wells J. [Transmitting "B&W's Public Issues Environment."] Memo to T. Olges, July 22, 1985.

2132.02. B&W's Public Issues Environment. 19??

2133.01. Tobaccotalk Concerns. 19??

2134.01. Hope for Cigarettes. 19??

2135.01. ICOSI Background Briefing Paper: International tobacco companies are using double standards in the selling of high 'tar' and nicotine cigarettes in developing countries. 1979.

2135.02. ICOSI Background Briefing Paper: Tobacco growing in Third World countries inhibits the production of food crops. 1979.

2135.03. ICOSI Background Briefing Paper: International tobacco companies use in developing countries advertising methods not considered acceptable in the Western World. 1979.

2135.04. ICOSI Background Briefing Paper: The tobacco companies encourage farmers in Third World countries to use wood for the flue-curing of tobacco[,] thus depriving the poor man of his national fuel resources. 1979.

2135.05. ICOSI Background Briefing Paper: Smoking and pregnancy. 1979.

2135.06. ICOSI Background Briefing Paper: Smoking and youth. 1979.

2135.07. ICOSI Background Briefing Paper: The use of the terms "evidence" and "proof" in papers relating to smoking and health. 1979.

2135.08. ICOSI Background Briefing Paper: Advertising restrictions do not have the intended effects. 1979.

2135.09. ICOSI Background Briefing Paper: Effect of warning labels on cigarette use is questionable. 1979.

2135.10. ICOSI Background Briefing Paper: Taxation and cigarette use. 1979.

2135.11. ICOSI Background Briefing Paper [regarding WHO report "Controlling the Smoking Epidemic"]. 1979.

2135.12. ICOSI Background Briefing Paper: International cigarette companies do not include warning clauses on cigarette packs or in cigarette advertising in developing countries. 1979.

2135.13. ICOSI Background Briefing Paper: In most developing countries international tobacco companies are opposed to the publication of "tar" and nicotine tables and decline to reveal the "tar" and nicotine deliveries of their brands. 1979.

2135.14. ICOSI Background Briefing Paper: Smoking and health—A perspective. 1979.

2135.15. ICOSI Background Briefing Paper: Smoking and lung cancer. 1979.

2135.16. ICOSI Background Briefing Paper: Smoking and cardiovascular disease. 1979.

2135.17. ICOSI Background Briefing Paper: Chronic obstructive pulmonary disease. 1979.

2136.01. World-Wide Political and Social Aspects of Smoking and Health, 19??

2136.02. Scientific Developments in Smoking and Health and the Role of Group Research and Development. Minutes, 19??

2136.03. Direction and Future Activities of Group R. & D. Minutes, 19??

POLITICS (2200 SERIES)

2200.01. Federal Government Involvement in the Smoking Controversy. 19??

2201.01. Clements E. [Forwarding third Hudson report.] Letter to A. Yeaman, July 13, 1967.

2202.01. Burgard J. Suggested Reply to Senator Kennedy's Letter. (Second draft), October 20, 1967.

2203.01. Cigarette Advertising and Labeling. In Hearing before the Consumer Subcommittee of the Committee on Commerce, United States Senate, July 22, 1969.

2203.02. Duplicate of {2120.07}.

2203.03. Duplicate of {2120.05}.

2203.04. Duplicate of {2120.06}.

2203.05. Duplicate of {2102.01}.

2203.06. Duplicate of {2120.08}.

2203.07. Duplicate of {2120.01}.

2203.08. Duplicate of {2120.02}.

2204.01. Cigarette Labeling, 15 U.S.C.A. Section 1336. 19??

2205.01. Pepples E. *Industry Response to Cigarette/Health Controversy.* 1976.

2206.01. Duplicate of {2120.04}.

2207.01. Waite C. Re: Hearings on the National Cancer Program, NCI and the ACS, 14–16 June 1977: Overview and Comments Concerning. Memo to H. Kornegay, June 17, 1977.

2207.02. Renewal of U.S. Cancer Grant Held Up Pending Federal Audit. *Washington Post,* July 5, 1977.

2207.03. Mintz M. "Startling" Cancer Rise among Nonwhite Adult Males Cited. *Washington Post,* June 15, 1977.

2207.04. Experts Say Cancer War Is Mismanaged, Worthless. *Wall Street Journal,* June 15, 1977.

2207.05. Russell C. Possible Conflict Cited in Travel by Cancer Official. *Washington Star,* June 6, 1977.

2207.06. Mintz M. House Probers Question Cancer Expert's Expenses. *Washington Post,* June 16, 1977.

2208.01. Duplicate of {2207.02 through 2207.06}.

2209.01. Edwards T. [Releasing letter to President Carter from Albert Clay, chairman of board of Burley Auction Warehouse Association.] Press Release, November 28, 1977.

2209.02. Clay A. [Praise for Peter Bourne's position on tobacco.] Letter to President Jimmy Carter, November 23, 1977.

2210.01. Pepples E. Re: Morgan's Paper [see 2211.01]. Memo to J. Edens, C. McCarty, R. Kirk, R. Pittman, and D. Bryant, August 14, 1978.

2210.02. FTC Is Seeking Ways to Decide If Pictures in Advertising Convey False Impressions. *Wall Street Journal,* August 11, 1978.

2211.01. *Up from the Bombshelter* [incomplete copy]. [Position paper by Charles Morgan, a civil rights attorney.] 1978.

2212.01. *Cigarette Smuggling.* 1978.

2213.01. Panzer F. Letter from the President [of the US] to Dr. Jonathan E. Rhoads, Chairman, National Cancer Advisory Board. To W. Roach, October 18, 1974.

2213.02. Duplicate of {2126.01}.

2213.03. Duplicate of {2126.06}.

2213.04. Duplicate of {2126.03}.

2214.01. Duplicate of {2117.01}.

2215.01. Pepples E. [Preparation of congressional testimony regarding passive smoking.] Memo to R. Roach, September 6, 1978.

2216.01. Duplicate of {2215.01}.

2217.01. Tobacco Institute. *New Cigarette Warnings, The Legislative Situation: Executive Summary.* 1982.

2218.01. Pepples E. [Young "Starters."] Letter to W. Ford, August 26, 1982.

2219.01. No document at this number.

2220.01. Sachs R. Re: Committee of Counsel Meeting—12/8/83. Memo to H. Frigon, I. Hughes, J. Alar, R. Pittman, E. Kohnhorst, and J. Wells, December 9, 1983.

2221.01. Covington and Burling. Memorandum to the Committee of Counsel Re: Proposed Compromise Legislation Concerning Cigarette Labeling and Advertising. January 19, 1983.

2222.01. Duplicate of {2220.01}.

2223.01. Duplicate of {2220.01}.

2224.01. Wells J. Pending Cigarette Sampling Legislation. Memo to D. Sharp, August 23, 1984.

2224.02. Wells J. [Boston ordinance prohibiting free sampling of cigarettes.] Memo to I. Hughes, J. Alar, T. Sandefur, R. Blott, E. Pepples, R. Sharp, J. Hendricks, T. Olges, B. Freedman, and L. Amos, September 7, 1984.

2225.01. Duplicate of {2218.01}.

2225.02. Pepples E. [B&W position on comprehensive tobacco control legislation in Congress.] Letter to W. Ford, September 13, 1984.

2226.01. Duplicate of {2225.02}.

2227.01. Business Card of Ernest Pepples. 19??

2227.02. Pepples E. Re: Cigarette Labeling and Advertising Legislation. Memo to I. Hughes, October 24, 1984.

2228.01. Wells J. [Transmitting "B&W's Public Issues Environment."] Memo to T. Olges, July 22, 1985.

2228.02. B&W's Public Issues Environment. 1985.

2229.01. Wells J. State Activities Division 1987 Proposed Budget. Tobacco Institute. 1986.

2230.01. Closing Statement by Senator Cook. Congressional Hearing, US Congress. 19??

2231.01. Haddon R. Smoking and Health: U.K. Strategy Report, July 1977.

2231.02. B.A.T. Board Strategies, Smoking and Health, Questions and Answers. 1977.

2231.03. Blackman L. Ten Key Facts on Smoking and Health Controversy. November 20, 1981.

2231.04. Sir John Partridge K.B.E., Chairman of Imperial Group Ltd. Answers Questions Put at the Annual General Meeting on "Action on Smoking and Health." Imperial Group Ltd., 19??

2231.05. No document at this number.

2231.06. Green S. *Basis for Research in Smoking.* 1975.

2231.07. Green S. *Safety Evaluation of Cigarettes.* 1976.

2231.08. Green S. *Cigarette Smoking and Causal Relationships.* 1976.

2231.09. Green S. Suggested Questions for CAC.III. Memo, August 26, 1977.

2231.10. I.T.L./B.A.T. Notes of a Joint Meeting Held in Bristol on Tuesday 9th January, 1979. Minutes, January 30, 1978.

2232.01. Leach M. Re: Westminister and Whitehall. Memo to P. Sheehy, C. Lockhart, I. Bluett, D. Dunbar, B. Garraway, N. Goddard, S. Green, M. Marjoram, R. Pritchard, P. Wright, R. Crichton, R. Gilderdale, M. Noakes, T. Tice, H. Verkerk, J. Drummond, E. Knight, D. Lobb, D. Price, P. Richardson, and P. Short, August 3, 1979.

CALIFORNIA PROPOSITIONS 5 AND 10 AND OTHER STATE
ACTIVITIES (2300 SERIES)

2300.01. Wells J. Re: New Jersey Sanitary Code—Proposed No Smoking Amendment. Memo to R. Pittman, E. Pepples, W. Wyatt, J. Broughton, W. Ogburn, G. Nolan, and R. Roach, October 11, 1977.

2301.01. Pepples E. Re: California Initiative. Memo to Brand Group, February 15, 1978.

2302.01. Pepples E. [California Proposition 5.] Letter to J. Swaab, January 23, 1979.

2302.02. California Proposition 5. Payback Calculations Based on Assumed Unit Cigarette Declines (per Day per Smoke). 1978?

2302.03. Swaab J. [Requesting information on California Proposition 5.] Letter to P. Cacciatore, December 1, 1978.

2302.04. Swaab J. [Requesting information on California Proposition 5.] Letter to E. Pepples, January 15, 1979.

2302.05. Pepples E. Campaign Report—Proposition 5, California 1978. January 11, 1979.

2302.06. Pepples E. "Everyone Must Help": Article for Use in *Farm News* (Dr. Ira Massie). 1980?

2303.01. Johnson J. [Editorial letter challenging evidence that passive smoking is dangerous.] Letter to Editors, No on Prop. 10, October 7, 1980.

2303.02. Californians Against Regulatory Excess. The Public Smoking Question (No on Prop 10). News release, 1980.

MOVIES (2400 SERIES)

2400.01. Scott D. [Procedures for documenting that product placement in movies actually occurs.] Memo to N. Domantay, October 26, 1983.

2400.02. Pepples E. [Recommendation that B&W end cinema advertising.] Memo to J. Coleman, November 8, 1983.

2400.03. Domantay N. [Regarding AFP's involvement with Plitt Theaters.] Letter to R. Kovoloff, January 12, 1984.

2400.04. Freedman B. Re: Termination of Cinema Relationships. Memo to N. Domantay, T. McAlevey, and J. Coleman, January 26, 1984.

2400.05. McAlevey T. Re: Cinema Concepts. Memo to N. Domantay, January 25, 1984.

2400.06. Cinema Concepts. Theatre Chains for "Kool-Jazz" Advertisement. List, January 24, 1984.

2400.07. Coleman J. [Summary of phone call from R. Kovoloff at AFP regarding payment.] Memo to T. McAlevey, February 8, 1984.

2400.08. Neville T. [Re: Plitt Theater in cinema advertising program.] Letter to R. Kovoloff, November 10, 1982.

2400.09. Coleman J. [Request to arrange audit of AFP.] Letter to J. Ripslinger, August 8, 1983.

2400.10. Broderson J. Re: Associated Film Productions Inc. Memo to J. Coleman, August 8, 1983.

2400.11. Ripslinger J. [Need to reschedule audit appointment.] Letter to J. Coleman, August 4, 1983.

2400.12. Pepples E. [Decision to end cinema advertising.] Letter to R. Ellis, February 21, 1984.

2400.13. Coleman J. Re: Apocalypse Now—Marlboro. Memo to N. Domantay, December 5, 1983.

2400.14. Coleman J. Re: AFP. Memo to N. Domantay, February 2, 1984.

2400.15. Domantay N. Re: Cinema Advertising. Memo to I. Hughes, August 4, 1983.

2403.04. Kovoloff R. [Response to query about bill.] Letter to T. Neville, October 12, 1981.

2404.01. Ripslinger J. [Summarizing agreement between Sylvester Stallone and AFP on behalf of B&W.] Letter to S. Stallone, June 14, 1983.

2404.02. Stallone S. [Agrees to use B&W products in five films for $500,000.] Letter to R. Kovoloff, April 28, 1983.

2404.03. Neville T. [Re: Providing Barclay billboards for placement in film.] Letter to Robert Kovoloff (American Film Productions), August 13, 1981.

2404.04. Exhibits I and II, AFP Payments. List, 1983.

2405.01. [Notes on agreement with Cinema Concepts for B&W product placement in films.] 19??

2405.02. Freedman B. Re: Cinema Concepts, Inc. Memo to N. Domantay and C. Heger, February 3, 1984.

2405.03. Leach C. Re: Cinema Concepts, Inc. Letter to B. Freedman, February 1, 1984.

2405.04. McAlevey T. Re: Cinema Concepts Settlement. Memo to D. Johnston, April 2, 1984.

2405.05. Freedman B. Re: Cinema Letters. Memo to File, March 12, 1984.

2405.06. Freedman B. Re: Cinema Concepts Settlement. Memo to E. Pepples, March 8, 1984.

2405.07. Duplicate of {2405.06}, without Pepples's response.

2405.08. Reed J. Re: Cinema Concepts, Inc. Letter to B. Freedman, March 7, 1984.

2405.09. Conorqui K. [Notification of Cinema Concepts that B&W cinema advertising is being terminated.] Letter to S. Harnell, March 5, 1984.

2405.10. Freedman B. [Transmitting copy of B&W letter to Cinema Concepts.] Letter to J. Reed, February 22, 1984.

2405.11. Pepples E. Re: Cinema Concepts. Memo to B. Freedman, February 16, 1984.

2405.12. Duplicate of {2405.11}, with different marginalia.

2405.13. Duplicate of {2405.11}, with different marginalia.

2405.14. Freedman B. Re: Cinema Concepts—Terminated January 30, 1984. Memo, February 13, 1984.

2406.01. Tobacco Issues (Part 1), Hearings before the Subcommittee on Transportation and Hazardous Materials of the Committee on Energy and Commerce, House of Representatives, H.R. 1250. July 25, 1989.

2406.02. Exhibit I, AFP Payments [made in connection with product placement in movies]. List, 19??

2406.03. Duplicate of {2404.02}.

2406.04. Tye J. [Congressional testimony.] July 16, 1989.

2406.05. Statement of Charles O. Whitley. July 16, 1989.

2406.06. Wilson MG. [Regarding product placement of Lark cigarettes in *License to Kill*.] Letter to Congressman Thomas A. Luken, July 19, 1989.

2406.07. Tobacco Issues (Part 2), Hearings before the Subcommittee on Transportation and Hazardous Materials of the Committee on Energy and Commerce, House of Representatives. November 6, 1989.

MISCELLANEOUS (2500 SERIES)

2500.01. Williams M. Tobacco's Hold on Women's Groups, Anti-Smokers Charge Leaders Have Sold Out to Industry Money. *Washington Post,* November 14, 1991.

2500.02. Williams M. Feminism's Unaddressed Issue: Health Risks to Women Who Smoke. 19??

2500.03. Williams M. The Funding Habit Women's Groups Can't Resist. 19??

2500.04. [Fragment of congressional testimony regarding smoking on television.] February 1, 1982.

2501.01. [Description of Gary Huber's career.] Notes, 19??

2502.01. What Kentucky Spends on Health Care. *Courier-Journal,* August 2, 1992.

2502.02. Why Wait to Ban Tobacco? *Courier-Journal,* 19??

2502.03. Readin', Writin' and Smokin'? 19??

2502.04. Daniel J. Dangers of Smoking [letter to editor]. 19??

2502.05. Cross A, Jennings M. Clinton Ends Silence, Backs Tobacco Supports. 19??

2502.06. Tobacco Talk. 19??

2503.01. Levin M. Secret Cigarette Additives, What Goes Up in Smoke? *The Nation,* December 23, 1991.

2504.01. Blanton J. "Trivial" Animal Research Protested at UK Center. 19??

2504.02. Duplicate of {2120.06}.

2504.03. Duplicate of {2120.03}.

2505.01. National Health Goals. Hearing before the Committee on Labor and Human Resources, United States Senate. January 12, 1987.

2506.01. *The Dark Side of the Marketplace.* 19??

2506.02. Mintz M. Liggett Officer Said Opposed to Sale of "Safe" Cigarette. *Washington Post,* February 19, 1988.

2506.03. Mintz M. "Safe" Cigarette Lobby Effort Detailed. *Washington Post,* 19??

2506.04. Miller G. The "Less Hazardous" Cigarette: A Deadly Delusion. *New York State Journal of Medicine,* 1985.

2507.01. Porter J. The Last Cigarette Advertisement. *New York State Journal of Medicine,* 1985.

2507.02. Mintz M. Toxic Residue Said Found on Firm's Cigarettes. *Washington Post,* January 6, 1988.

2507.03. Egerton J. Burley Growers Cautioned about Chemical Usage. 19??

2508.01. [Re: Report to Executive Committee 7/1/65.] Notes, 19??

About the Authors

Stanton A. Glantz, Ph.D., is professor of medicine and member of the Institute for Health Policy Studies and the Cardiovascular Research Institute at the University of California, San Francisco. In 1983 he helped to defend the San Francisco Workplace Smoking Ordinance against a tobacco industry attempt to repeal it by referendum. The San Francisco victory represented the tobacco industry's first electoral defeat and is now viewed as a major turning point in the battle for nonsmokers' rights. He is one of the founders (with Peter Hanauer and others) of Americans for Nonsmokers' Rights. In 1982 he resurrected the film *Death in the West*, suppressed by Philip Morris, and developed a curriculum that has been used by an estimated one million students. In addition, he helped write and produce the films *Secondhand Smoke*, which concerns the health effects of involuntary smoking, and *On the Air*, which describes how to create a smoke-free workplace. An associate editor of the *Journal of the American College of Cardiology* and a member of the California State Scientific Review Panel on Toxic Air Contaminants, Dr. Glantz has served as a consultant to the National Institutes of Health, Environmental Protection Agency, Occupational Safety and Health Administration, National Science Foundation, and numerous scientific publications. He conducts research on cardiovascular function, passive smoking, applied biostatistics, and tobacco policy and politics, and is the author of six books, including *Primer of Biostatistics* and *Primer of Applied Regression and Analysis of Variance* (published by McGraw-Hill), two software packages, including SigmaStat (published by Jandel Scientific), and over ninety scientific papers, including the first major review that identified involuntary smoking as a cause of heart disease.

John Slade, M.D., is associate professor of clinical medicine at the Robert Wood Johnson Medical School of the University of Medicine and Dentistry of New Jersey. He practices at St. Peter's Medical Center in New Brunswick. Frustrated by the difficulty in helping his patients stop smoking and by the lack of attention this problem received in medical education, he began studying the clinical and public health aspects of tobacco in the early 1980s. This work has led Dr. Slade to make substantial contributions to both clinical and public health practice. He coedited the first comprehensive clinical textbook on nicotine addiction, *Nicotine Addiction: Principles and Management* (published by Oxford University Press), and has helped produce seven annual, national conferences on nicotine dependence for the American Society of Addiction Medicine. He has worked on tobacco control problems at the local, state, and national levels, including matters related to tobacco product regulation. He is an associate editor of *Tobacco Control: An International Journal,* a journal published by the British Medical Association, and he served as president of STAT, Stop Teenage Addiction to Tobacco, from 1994 through 1995.

Lisa A. Bero, Ph.D., is assistant professor of clinical pharmacy and health policy at the University of California, San Francisco. Prior to joining the faculty at UCSF, she received her Ph.D. in pharmacology from Duke University and completed a Pew Fellowship in Health Policy at the Institute for Health Policy Studies. Her current studies focus on assessing the quality of published medical research and examining how research is translated into effective clinical practice and health policy, including tobacco control policy.

Peter Hanauer, LL.B., has been involved in the nonsmokers' rights movement for more than twenty years and is a founder and past president of Americans for Nonsmokers' Rights, which is based in Berkeley, California. In 1977 he coauthored a clean indoor air ordinance that was adopted by the city council in Berkeley by a vote of 9–0. The ordinance was one of the first comprehensive local laws in the nation that regulated smoking in public places. In 1978, and again in 1980, he coauthored initiative measures on the California ballot that would have regulated smoking in public places and workplaces throughout the state. He was also the statewide treasurer of both campaigns. In 1983 he helped to write the

San Francisco Workplace Smoking Ordinance, which was approved by the San Francisco Board of Supervisors, and then played a key role in helping to defend the ordinance against an attempt by the tobacco industry to repeal it by referendum. Two years later, his analysis of that referendum battle was published in the *New York State Journal of Medicine*. In 1986 he was the lead author of *Legislative Approaches to a Smoke Free Society* (published by the American Nonsmokers' Rights Foundation), a primer on how to enact local ordinances regulating smoking. In 1988 he was one of fourteen people presented with the Dr. Luther L. Terry Award, by the United States Public Health Service Professional Association, for "A Unique Contribution Toward a Smoke-Free Society." He received a B.A. from Dartmouth College and an LL.B. from Columbia Law School. For more that thirty years, he has been a law book editor at Bancroft-Whitney Company in San Francisco, where he has specialized in jurisprudence writing. He lives in Berkeley with his wife and two children.

Deborah E. Barnes, B.A., is a research associate at the Institute for Health Policy Studies, University of California, San Francisco, where she works in public health and health policy research, including work with Dr. Bero analyzing the quality and use of research sponsored by the tobacco industry. Ms. Barnes received a bachelor's degree in human biology from Stanford University in 1987 and a graduate certificate in science writing from the University of California, Santa Cruz, in 1990.

Document Index

Name Index

Subject Index

Compositor:	BookMasters, Inc.
Text:	10/13 Sabon
Display:	Sabon
Printer:	Haddon Craftsmen, Inc.
Binder:	Haddon Craftsmen, Inc.